What's this?

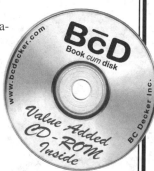

Residents Manual of Medicine

For House Staff, by House Staff

Balamurali K. Ambati, MD
Harvard Medical School
Boston, Massachusetts

W. Tyler Smith, MD
Marie T. Azer-Bentsianov, MD
Albert Einstein College of Medicine
Bronx, New York

2001
BC Decker Inc
Hamilton • London

BC Decker Inc
20 Hughson Steet South
P. O. Box 620, L.C.D. 1
Hamilton, Ontario L8N 3K7
Tel: 905-522-7017; Fax: 905-522-7839
E-mail: info@bcdecker.com
Website: www.bcdecker.com

BC Decker

01 02 03 / PC / 9 8 7 6 5 4 3 2 1
ISBN 1-55009-153-0
Printed in Canada

Sales and Distribution

United States
BC Decker Inc
P.O. Box 785
Lewiston, NY 14092-0785
Tel: 905-522-7017 / 1-800-568-7281
Fax: 905-522-7839
E-mail: info@bcdecker.com
Website: www.bcdecker.com

Canada
BC Decker Inc
20 Hughson Street South
P.O. Box 620, L.C.D. 1
Hamilton, Ontario L8N 3K7
Tel: 905-522-7017 / 1-800-568-7281
Fax: 905-522-7839
E-mail: info@bcdecker.com
Website: www.bcdecker.com

Foreign Rights
John Scott & Company
International Publishers' Agency
P.O. Box 878
Kimberton, PA 19442
Tel: 610-827-1640
Fax: 610-827-1671

*U.K., Europe, Scandinavia,
Middle East*
Harcourt Publishers Limited
Customer Service Department
Foots Cray High Street
Sidcup, Kent
DA14 5HP, UK
Tel: 44 (0) 208 308 5760
Fax: 44 (0) 181 308 5702
E-mail: cservice@harcourt_brace.com

Australia, New Zealand
Harcourt Australia Pty. Limited
Customer Service Department
STM Division
Locked Bag 16
St. Peters, New South Wales, 2044
Australia
Tel: (02) 9517-8999
Fax: (02) 9517-2249
E-mail: stmp@harcourt.com.au
Website: www.harcourt.com.au

Japan
Igaku-Shoin Ltd.
Foreign Publications Department
3-24-17 Hongo
Bunkyo-ku,Tokyo,
Japan 113-8719
Tel: 3 3817 5680
Fax: 3 3815 6776
E-mail: fd@igaku.shoin.co.jp

*Singapore, Malaysia, Thailand,
Philippines, Indonesia, Vietnam,
Pacific Rim, Korea*
Harcourt Asia Pte Limited
#09/01, Forum
583 Orchard Road
Singapore 238884
Tel: 65-737-3593
Fax: 65-753-2145

Contents

Preface

One man cannot summon the future. — Spock
But one man can change the present. — Kirk, in "Mirror, Mirror,"
Star Trek

This book was designed with the hope of breaching the barriers between the black-board and the bedside. A deep and vast divide runs like a fault line between the academic and clinical practice of medicine, all too often breeding mutual disdain and contempt. It is a sad commentary on our medical education that many emerge from this crucible with their intellectual prowess warped and unable to appreciate or practice one or the other. Those just commencing their careers in our noble profession are caught in the crossfire and must also cope with the powerful centrifugal demands on their time and energy, having to accumulate a vast fund of knowledge while tending to large ward services.

In the fond hope of bridging the yawning gulf between theory and practice, we have aimed for three objectives that are essential to the physician-in-training:

- Develop a reservoir of knowledge that is rapidly accessible for practical application
- Lay a firm foundation of facts for the clinical evaluation and management of patients and develop a flexible framework of concepts for the ongoing assimilation of new knowledge
- Synthesize a crystallized distillate of clinical experience, pathophysiology, and esoterica with enough breadth and depth to look good on rounds and help prepare for tests

During the course of our training, we were disappointed in the available guides and manuals, which presented too much, too little, or impertinent information; were too expensive; and all too often did not fit in our lab coat's pockets! We hope we have struck the right balance here. We have heeded the old saying that brevity is the soul of wit but have tried to keep the concise nature of this endeavor from sacrificing essential knowledge. A companion guide for the trials and tribulations of medical school, internship, and residency must be brief yet provide much more than the bare bones of the subject. Certain topics (eg, parasitology) may seem far afield from the daily life of the average house officer, but we felt that several uncommonly encountered problems nonetheless merited inclusion for the sake of completeness and, more importantly, a well-rounded introduction to medicine. In keeping with the spirit of user friendliness, we have divided the book into three parts: first, a review of general topics, then the core section of individual wards that form the bulk of training, and, finally, a concise overview of primary care areas. Chapter references have been organized into groups of important guidelines, reviews, and clinical trials that the house officer should have a working knowledge of in this age of evidence-based medicine. Appendices have been included in areas of special interest: key formulas, common phrases in medical Spanish, a grouping of signs and syndromes, and our personal opinions on roundsmanship, books and supplies, and reading.

This book differs from others in its genre in several important ways. First, it was written by three residents, which should help provide the freshness of perspective so vital to insight. That this book was written entirely by three individuals should also preserve a clarifying unity of purpose while tapping into the vitality of diverse voices. We organized commonly encountered problems and entities along a format of quick points, initial management, and further discussion. But many areas do not lend themselves to a "one-size-fits-all approach," and as we considered it Procrustean to use the same format for all topics, we have taken the liberty of using different writing styles and formats best suited for different issues. The informal style of writing will likely be considered unorthodox: we make no apology for our frankness or levity, which we hope will not be misconstrued for irreverence or frivolity.

We realize that certain chapters may overlap. With the use of cross-referencing and selectively strategic streamlining, we trust that we have navigated the waters between redundancy and disconnected writing, keeping each chapter whole but the book brief. A small measure of redundancy can confer a great amount of resilience. It is inevitable that errors of omission and commission have occurred; we trust that the reader will bring these to our attention, and we look forward to hearing your comments, compliments, and criticisms in the months and years to come.

It is no mean task to try to weave myriad concepts and disparate factoids into a tapestry of wisdom and wit. Each of us had our misgivings when we embarked on this ambitious venture, but once we put our hands to the plough, we could not turn back. With equal parts of knowledge and experience, humor and candor, this book, we hope, achieves a measure of success in the daring but important task of constructing a sound scaffold for both the academic and clinical growth of students, interns, and residents. It is our sincere wish that this book is found helpful by the next generation of physicians. If it assists their care of patients and their growth as physicians, then we will have succeeded.

BKA
WTS
MTAB
April 2001

Inspired by our patients

In honor of our families

Dedicated to our teachers, colleagues, and students

Advisors

Special Advisors
Jayakrishna Ambati, MD
Ambati M. Rao, DHEd

Section Advisors
Jayakrishna Ambati, MD
Stephen Baum, MD
Peter Bluestone, MD
Adrienne Fleckman, MD
Donald Kaminsky, MD
Paul Mayo, MD
Patricia Villamena, MD
Emanuel Wurm, MD
Ian Yudelman, MD

Acknowledgments

If I have seen farther, it is because I have stood on the shoulders of giants.
—Sir Isaac Newton

Such a work cannot be produced in a vacuum. Through our lives and training, we have incurred many debts of gratitude that we can never repay; through this work, we hope merely to pass this on to others. This passing of the torch is the nature of things and is as it should be.

Quite a few individuals deserve special mention. Jayakrishna Ambati, Bala's brother, has been a font of imagination and a wellspring of encouragement throughout this project. Ambati M. Rao, Bala's father, has been the bedrock of support required for any such endeavor, especially when undertaken during a training program. Both have provided a sage lens of analytic objectivity needed to pare and polish this book. No tribute can do them justice.

Many others have devoted substantial amounts of time and effort to this book. Jennifer Sun, Nadia Waheed, and Ann-Marie Huang all made critical suggestions in their exhaustive reviews of the manuscript.

All of the authors have completed or are training in internal medicine at Beth Israel Medical Center in New York. We would like to thank all of the faculty, staff, patients, and residents of Beth Israel for their contribution to our development and maturation in residency. Drs. Baum and Fleckman, especially, have always been available and able to guide and teach us during our training.

Finally, we would like to thank Brian Decker, Jack Farrell, Paula Presutti, Susan Ball, Joanne Islip, David LeGallais, and the production team at BC Decker Inc for their efforts and counsel in sheperding this book to fruition.

GENERAL TOPICS

1

Floor Operations

Though we are not now that which in old days moved earth and Heaven, that which we are, we are—one equal temper of heroic hearts, made weak by time and fate, but strong in will, to strive, to seek, to find, and not to yield.—Alfred Lord Tennyson

It is not important that ideal things should exist in fact; it is only important that they should be kept in mind so that men may take their bearings by them and not get lost amid the confusions and pretense of the actual world.—Prof. G. Whicker, Harvard University

WORK-UPS AND INITIAL MANAGEMENT

Remember when you were told as a second-year medical student, "The history is 90% of the diagnosis"? Well, it's true. Unfortunately, that gets forgotten sometime in the second month of internship. As a second-year student, you used to take 2 hours to do a full history and physical examination (H&P). As a third-year student, you would take an hour. Subinterns take 30 minutes. Then, in the middle of internship, you will finish an H&P in under 15 minutes! Of course, it will not be complete, which is why you have a resident who will take a bit longer (~30 minutes). With time, luck, good role models, and a lot of experience, you will learn to ask just the relevant probing questions in rapid succession. It is harder to bite your tongue and listen; the nuances and details of the patient's words will give clues easily overlooked but that are treasures both for your learning and academic care.

As for physical examination, in many residencies, it is becoming a lost art, especially the cardiac and neurologic examinations. That is a sad but not irresistible force. Take your time, listen to and observe your patient carefully, watch the (good) attending physicians and your good residents closely, and always try to correlate the results of further tests (ie, echocardiography and magnetic resonance imaging [MRI]) with your findings.

Your ample rewards will include personal satisfaction, prestige, faster pick-ups of diagnoses, and a reliable fallback when technology is not available (none of which should be discounted).

What tests should you order? Certain residency programs inculcate an attitude of admission labs (complete blood count [CBC]; chemistry 7 [sodium, potassium, chloride, bicarbonate, blood urea nitrogen, creatinine, glucose] [SMA-7]; prothrombin time/partial thromboplastin time [PT/PTT]; urinalysis [U/A]), which really is not indicated. True, you probably will and should get a CBC and SMA-7 on most of your patients, but try to think before you blindly order a whole panel of tests. First, try to discern the diagnosis or at least narrow the differential on clinical grounds. Second, ask the Cochrane-Wright question, "What will you do if the test is positive and what will you do if it is negative?" If the answer is the same, then *don't get the test.* Of course, CBCs and SMAs aren't positive or negative, but the concept remains: how will the test's different possible results affect your management? The only exceptions to this are the academic setting, where there is a certain pleasure in confirming your diagnosis, and the medicolegal situation, when every last corner must be covered.

Initial orders will, of course, vary with the patient. You should know the ADCVANDALISM mnemonic for admission orders (*A*dmit, *D*iagnosis, *C*ondition, *V*ital Signs, *A*llergies, *N*ursing, *D*iet, *A*ctivity, *L*abs, *I*ntravenous [IV] fluids, *S*pecial orders, *M*edications). IV fluids and antibiotics will be discussed subsequently. Always think about the *prns* ("as-needed" orders that can be given at the nurses' discretion): common problems include pain/fever, indigestion, constipation, and trouble with sleep. You should form your own personal *prn* cocktail lest you or the overnight person be bothered unnecessarily for simple constipation. Our personal favorites are acetaminophen (Tylenol), magnesium hydroxide/aluminum hydroxide (Maalox), temazepam (Restoril), and senna (Senokot) (Table 1–1).

Also remember the orders that are easily forgotten: activity (get the patient mobilized as soon as possible), allergies, input and output, and deep vein thrombosis (DVT) prophylaxis in the immobile (Ted stockings or subcutaneous heparin).

Do not resuscitate (DNR) orders should be pursued vigorously, with alacrity, and not in an à la carte fashion. Approach the patient during periods of stability if at all possible. When approaching the patient, couch

Table 1–1. Commonly Used As-Needed Medications

Indication	Medication and Dose	Key Contraindication(s)
Pain	Acetaminophen (Tylenol) 650 mg PO q6h prn	Hepatic failure
Indigestion	Magnesium hydroxide/ aluminum hydroxide (Maalox) 15–30 cc PO q6h prn	Renal failure
Insomnia	Temazepam (Restoril) 15 mg PO qhs prn	Altered mental status
Constipation	Senna (Senokot) 2 tabs PO qhs prn	Diarrhea

the DNR status in routine terms; don't send the message that you think something bad is going to happen. Even if the patient is unstable or crashing, as long as they are conscious and competent, try to convey that the patient still has choices and control over those choices. Do not ask about individual components of the code: don't ask separately about shock, compressions, intubation, and pressors. Since the code is supposed to be a concert of interventions, offering choices on each component vitiates the point of the code. Present the question tactfully but firmly; for example, does the patient want violent and uncomfortable measures that will most likely not work (you may or may not choose to state "burning the skin, breaking ribs, puncturing lungs, and putting a tube down your throat" as possible complications)?

COMMON ENTITIES

Many of the issues dealt with below will also be discussed in Chapter 16. What follows is a rapid-fire playbook of problems, thoughts you should have, things you should do, and small arsenals of available treatments. Gastrointestinal (GI) bleed, altered mental status, shortness of breath (SOB), hypotention/hypertension (HTN), tachycardia/bradycardia, back pain, abdominal pain, and chest pain will be covered in Chapter 2 and the subsequent appropriate chapters.

Agitation

Do no harm.

Quick Points
- Find out if there are any medications or medical conditions that are causing this.
- Try to keep delirious patients in quiet, stable rooms with lots of reminders about time.

Initial Management
- Treat the underlying cause and discontinue any offending medications.
- Restrain the patient only if he or she is a danger to himself/herself or others (be very good about documenting restraints and renewing them according to protocol).
- Four-point restraints should be used in only the most extreme cases.
- Haloperidol (Haldol) and lorazepam (Ativan) (each 0.5–2.0 mg PO/IM/IV q2h–q6h prn) are the workhorses for agitation; remember that lorazepam is sedating, whereas haloperidol can be associated with neuroleptic malignant syndrome.

Clogged Nasogastric Tube or Percutaneous Endoscopic Gastrostomy Tube

Quick Point
- Try to prevent this by frequent flushes.

Initial Management
- Pancreatin (Viokase) usually comes in tablet form for those with pancreatic insufficiency. You can crush one tablet, mix the powder with 5 to 10 cc normal saline (NS), and flush the clogged tube. Wait 5 minutes and, usually, presto! The tube is open.
- If the tube is irreversibly clogged, you can replace it (percutaneous endoscopic gastrostomy [PEG] replacements need to be done by Gastroenterology).

Constipation

This is the bane of every intern's existence. Management of constipation revolves around one simple truth: disimpaction equals your total, supreme, and abject failure.

Quick Points
- Prevent constipation by making stool softeners/gentle laxatives available before problems start.
- Determine if constipation implies increased hardness (where softening is helpful) or decreased frequency.
- As always with any patient issue, look at the patient's medications; iron, calcium blockers, and a host of other drugs can cause constipation.
- Rule out intestinal obstruction (signs and symptoms of which would be pain, vomiting, absence of flatus, decreased bowel sounds after the obstruction, and loss of distal air on x-ray along with intestinal dilation or air-fluid levels).

Initial Management
Table 1–2 shows the common treatments in increasing power.

Table 1–2. Constipation Treatments (in Increasing Power)

Docusate (Colace) 100 mg PO tid (stool softener)
Senna (Senekot) 2 tabs PO qhs (softener/gentle laxative)
Bisacodyl (Dulcolax) suppository
Milk of magnesia 30 cc PO q4–q6h prn (laxative)
Cascara 5 cc PO q4–q6h prn (laxative)
Sorbitol 15–30 cc PO q4–q6h prn (osmotic)
Magnesium citrate ½ bottle PO q12h prn (osmotic)
Fleet enema
Tap water enema
High-colonic enema

Don't be afraid to use combinations (black and white of milk of magnesia + cascara or cascara + sorbitol are popular, even with the patients). You can often use both oral and rectal cathartics; however, don't give oral cathartics if there is an obstruction. *If there is an obstruction, all of this flies out the window. Call Gastroenterology or Surgery if there is an obstruction and place a nasogastric (NG) tube to prevent aspiration and for comfort.*

Diarrhea

This will be discussed in detail in Chapter 13.

Quick Points
- Assess for blood in the stool (history, guaiac) if it is watery or smells foul.
- If a patient has been in the hospital for more than 3 days, there is no point in getting a stool ova and parasites or even culture (except in patients with human immunodeficiency virus [HIV]).
- If the patient is on antibiotics, make sure to get a *Clostridium difficile* toxin.
- Always do a guaiac.
- Fecal fat and white blood cell count (WBC) may or may not be helpful.

Initial Management
- Keep close track of the patient's fluid status and replace it as necessary.
- As long as the diarrhea is not infectious, it is okay to give antidiarrheals (Table 1–3).

Table 1–3. Commonly Used Antidiarrheals and Doses

Diphenoxylate + atropine (Lomotil)	1–2 tabs or 10 cc PO q4–q6h prn
Attapulgite (Kaopectate)	15–30 cc PO q4–q6h prn
Loperamide (Immodium)	2 mg PO as needed up to a maximum dose of 8 mg per day

Gastroparesis

Quick Points
- This is common in patients recovering from acute illness, chronic patients, and diabetics.
- Signs are high residual volumes in PEG or NG feeding tubes.
- Again, make sure there is no obstruction.

Initial Management
- Cisapride and erythromycin, promotility agents, have lots of drug interactions (Table 1–4).
- Another option if these don't work is to place a long tube (Cantor) or percutaneous endoscopic jejunostomy (PEJ) tube into the jejunum (done by Surgery or Gastroenterology).

Table 1–4. Agents to Promote Gastrointestinal Motility and Doses

Cisapride (Propulsid)	10–20 mg PO/G-tube qid
Metoclopramide (Reglan)	10 mg PO/G-tube q6h
Erythromycin	250 mg PO/G-tube q6h (not IV)

Hematuria

Quick Points
- Check for infection, bleeding disorder, medications, traumatic Foley insertion, or maintenance.
- Make sure the patient is hemodynamically stable.

Initial Management
- A standard work-up for unexplained gross hematuria in a male or nonmenstruating female is urine cytology, intravenous pyelography (IVP), and cystoscopy (to rule out bladder cancer, renal cancer, and kidney stones).
- Start blood transfusion or IV fluid as necessary.

Hemoptysis

Quick Points
- Make sure the patient is hemodynamically stable.
- The most common cause is nonspecific bronchitis.
- Get a history to rule out chronic lung disease, tuberculosis (TB), and pneumonia.

Initial Management
- Treat the cause.
- If the patient is at risk and hemoptysis is unexplained, evaluate for cancer (chest x-ray [CXR], consider computed tomography [CT]/bronchoscopy).
- If unstable, start blood transfusion and IV fluids, and call Pulmonary and/or Interventional Radiology for emergent bronchoscopy and/or angiography.

Insomnia

This is a very common problem and understandably so: how would you sleep when there's always activity outside the door, lights go on and off without your control, your vital signs are checked every few hours, and people come and go from your room as they please?

Quick Points
- When prescribing sleeping medications, follow the Hippocratic oath: *primum, non nocere* (first, do no harm).
- A lot of sleeping medications are long-lasting, causing needless work-ups for altered mental status in the morning (diphenhydramine [Benadryl] especially throws elderly patients for a loop).
- Try also to avoid medications that cause dependence (medium- and long-acting benzodiazepines are a big culprit in this regard).
- Be aware that sleeping medications often accumulate in patients with liver dysfunction.

Initial Management
Agents used for insomnia are listed in Table 1–5.
- Chloral hydrate (found in Mickey Finn drinks) is cheaper but should be avoided in cirrhotics.

Table 1–5. Commonly Used Sleeping Medications and Doses

Temazepam (Restoril)	15 mg PO qhs prn
Zolpidem (Ambien)	5–10 mg PO qhs prn
Chloral hydrate	500 mg PO qhs prn

Itching/Rash

Quick Point
- Look at the medications (we know, it's starting to sound like a broken record).

Look for any systemic diseases that could be responsible (liver/kidney failure, Hodgkin's disease, and jaundice for itch; any number of infectious, endocrine, or rheumatologic diseases for rash).

Initial Management
Don't be afraid to call Dermatology (they are generally very nice and helpful). See Chapter 17.
Antipruritic agents are listed in Table 1–6.

Table 1–6. Commonly Used Antipruritic Agents

Topical Creams/Lotions	Oral Agents
Calomine lotion	Diphenhydramine (Benadryl) 25–50 mg PO q4–q6h prn (watch out for sedation)
Aqua-phor (especially for dryness)	Hydroxyzine (Atarax) 10 mg PO tid
Lac-Hydrin cream	
Eucerin cream	

Mouth Pain

Sore throat will be discussed in Chapter 16. Mucosal ulcers occur for many reasons (see Chapters 5, 10, and 11).

Initial Management
- Magic mouthwash (attapulgite, diphenhydramine, and lidocaine mixture in 1:1:1 ratio) 15 to 30 cc PO q4 to q6h prn
- Viscous lidocaine
- Hurricaine or Cetacaine (aerosolized lidocaine) spray

Nausea/Vomiting

Quick Points
- Make sure nothing bad is happening (eg, cardiac infarct, acute abdomen, central nervous system [CNS] disease).
- Examine the abdomen carefully.
- Look at medications (chemotherapy and narcotics are major causes of nausea).

Initial Management

Antiemetic agents are listed in Table 1–7.
- Prochlorperazine works on the dopaminergic system, so watch out for dystonic reactions.
- Metoclopramide works on both the dopaminergic and serotonergic (5-hydroxytryptamine [(5-HT]) systems.
- Ondansetron and granisetron work just on the 5-HT pathway and thus have few side effects. As these antiemetics are very expensive, most hospitals restrict their use to chemotherapy patients.

Table 1–7. Commonly Used Antiemetics

Prochlorperazine (Compazine)	10 mg PO/IM/IV q4–q6h prn
Metoclopramide (Reglan)	10 mg PO/IM/IV q4–q6h prn
Ondansetron (Zofran)	8 mg PO bid
Granisetron (Kytril)	1 mg PO bid
Trimethobenzamide (Tigan)	250 mg PO tid prn
Lorazepam (Ativan) (yes, Ativan)	1–2 mg PO/IM/IV q4h–q6h prn

Pain

This is a problem that cuts to the core of most problems and cuts across several fields, especially cancer and chemical dependency. Know the World Health Organization (WHO) stepladder of pain medications (discussed in Chapter 10).

Quick Points
- As a general rule, try to go along with what the nurses want to do, especially in substance abuse patients.
- However, patients who have chronic, terminal illnesses (cancer, substance abuse) realize that there's little to lose, and the primary objective should be palliation, even at the expense of just about everything else. Sometimes stupor and, not uncommonly, death are preferred by many to continued suffering.
- Ethically, the entity of double effect is accepted: if the primary aim of treatment is relief of suffering, then it is acceptable if a consequence of that treatment is death.

Initial Management

Analgesic agents are listed in Table 1–8.

- All nonsteroidal anti-inflammatory drugs (NSAIDs) have essentially the same maximum efficacy, although some patients may respond better to certain drugs. The only exception is ketorolac, which has the analgesic efficacy of some narcotics. Watch for stomach ulcers and renal toxicity when giving NSAIDs.
- Be careful with acetaminophen use in patients with liver or renal failure.
- Percocet = acetaminophen + oxycodone; Percodan = aspirin + oxycodone.
- Narcotics can be given at a frequency of your discretion. Don't oversedate the patient (when you write the order for narcotics, write "hold for respiratory rate < 14").
- The common stepladder of many house staff is acetaminophen (Tylenol), NSAIDs (ibuprofen, ketoprofen), ketorolac (Toradol), weak narcotics (codeine, hydrocodone, Percocet/Percodan), and strong narcotics (morphine, meperidine, hydromorphone) (Figure 1–1).
- Conversion to long-acting agents. After 1 to 2 days of as-needed narcotics in a patient with a need for long-term pain control, calculate the total daily dose he or she is on, and then switch to long-acting forms (morphine [MS Contin] [a bid drug equivalent to total morphine dosing] or fentanyl patch [25–100 µg/hr patch] one patch every 3 days). Methadone is another alternative.
- For real pain (acute or chronic), use an around-the-clock (ATC) regimen with as-needed rescue doses at half the ATC rate (eg, Percocet 1 tab q6h ATC + Percocet 1 tab q3h prn).
- Avoid meperidine (Demerol) in general due to toxicity (seizures, problems in liver/renal failure patients, interactions) and limited efficacy (short duration). The only exceptions are pancreatitis (it doesn't cause sphincter contraction, unlike morphine) and sometimes sicklers (who traditionally like the drug and for whom comfort takes precedence).
- In terms of what to do in difficult-to-manage cases, pain consult services are usually very helpful and receptive; don't hesitate to call them in.
- If someone has a good prognosis, try to minimize chronic narcotic use.
- But for patients with an acute, self-limited problem (eg, kidney stones), narcotics can be great. For the substance abuse patient, there is rarely one

correct answer. Quite often, you just want the patient to leave you alone, but the nurse doesn't want to keep giving narcotics. Diplomacy is the one thing that might help you cross this tightrope; never lose your cool.
- Adjunctive pain medications can sometimes be quite helpful (sleeping medications, hydroxyzine [Vistaril 10–25 mg PO qid prn]) without giving in to the demand for narcotics. In the outpatient setting, where acetaminophen and NSAIDs just don't cut it, but you don't want to start chronic narcotics for, let's say, nonspecific back pain, you can use tramadol (Ultram 100 mg PO qid)—of uncertain efficacy but still with the power of placebo.

Table 1–8. Commonly Used Analgesics

Acetaminophen (Tylenol)	650 mg–1 g PO/PR q6h prn
Ibuprofen (Motrin)	200–800 mg PO q6h prn
Ketorolac tromethamine (Toradol)	15–30 mg PO/IM/IV q6h prn (up to 5 days)
Acetaminophen + oxycodone/aspirin + oxycodone (Percocet/Percodan)	1–2 tabs PO q4–q6h prn
Morphine	2–30 mg PO/SQ/IM/IV prn
Hydromorphone (Dilaudid)	1–3 mg PO/SQ/IM/IV
Meperidine (Demerol)	25–150 mg SQ/IM

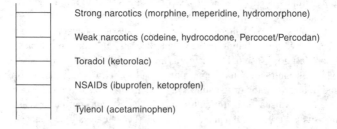

Strong narcotics (morphine, meperidine, hydromorphone)

Weak narcotics (codeine, hydrocodone, Percocet/Percodan)

Toradol (ketorolac)

NSAIDs (ibuprofen, ketoprofen)

Tylenol (acetaminophen)

Figure 1–1. Commonly used stepladder for analgesia.

Urinary Problems

Initial Management

- *Incontinence:* Differentiate stress, urge, functional, and overflow incontinence (see Chapter 13). For stress incontinence, the patient may need pelvic muscle exercises or procedures to correct anatomic abnormalities (such as cystoceles). For urge incontinence (detrusor dyssynergia), you can use oxybutynin (Ditropan). For overflow incontinence, the patient may need a chronic indwelling catheter or intermittent catheterization; sometimes bethanechol can help. If there is benign prostatic hyperplasia (BPH), stricture, or other obstruction, you can do surgery/transurethral prostatic resection (TURP). For functional incontinence (as with Alzheimer's disease), the patient may need prompted voiding.
- *Low urine output:* Check if the patient was sleeping overnight (an eternal staple of night shift anuria), was going to the bathroom without recording volume, and if the Foley catheter is kinked. Check medication and look for a distended bladder, dehydration/volume status, pulmonary edema, and evidence of renal failure. If everything checks out, observe. If not, do what you have to do (fluid challenge for dehydration, furosemide [Lasix] for congestive heart failure [CHF]).
- *Pain on urination:* Check urinalysis and culture and sensitivity. Consider antibiotics; pyridium is also a good palliative for cystitis pain (just tell the patient that the urine will be red). If the patient has renal colic, hydrate and give plenty of analgesia (don't hesitate to give ketorolac and narcotics).

READING X-RAYS

The sooner you learn how to read an x-ray, the better able you are to treat your patient and the wiser you will seem to the powers that be. It is vital that you learn how to read a CXR, abdominal films, head CTs, and cervical spines (C-spines). When first learning, you should master the formal method of reading, which may seem tedious but confers the twin benefits of a shield against omission and an aura of authority. Just remember that most of the reading revolves around silhouettes and symmetry.

Chest X-Ray

Assess the quality of the film, based on the following:

- Technique. posteroanterior (PA) films are better than anteroposterior (AP) films because the heart shadow is smaller relative to the thorax as the heart is closer to the film. You can tell technique by looking for the marking on the x-ray (it's okay to cheat on this kind of stuff) or, more academically, noting the relative size of anterior and posterior rib shadows: in a PA film, the posterior rib shadow is larger as it is closer to the x-ray source relative to the anterior rib shadow.

- Penetration (you should lose the vertebral bodies about halfway down; seeing them below indicates overpenetration).

- Inspiration (you should see the lung down to the 9th to 10th rib; too little indicates poor inspiratory effort or volume loss, whereas too much goes for hyperinflation consistent with emphysema). Rib counting is a rapidly acquired skill, once you recognize that you will miss the first rib in the beginning as it practically dives down from the neck.

- Rotation (assess symmetry of sternoclavicular angles).

Start from the outside in. Note the condition of soft-tissue and bony structures (look for fractures, foreign bodies, subcutaneous emphysema). Look at pleura by tracing the contour of pleura bilaterally down to the costophrenic angles; if there are any irregularities or blurring, consider effusion and pleural masses and correlate clinically. Look at lung volumes (are they appropriate or is there asymmetric volume loss?). Then look at lung fields and compare both sides, looking for opacities and characterizing them as consolidation, infiltrates, and edema and by pattern (reticulonodular, granular, interstitial, fluffy). Localize infiltrates: lower lobes and upper lobes are easy. Right middle lobe (RML) infiltrates obscure the right heart border, whereas lingular ones obscure the left. Retrocardiac opacities are given away when the heart shadow is as white left of the spine as it is when overlying the spine. Look for hilar nodes and obliteration of the aorticopulmonary window. When looking for the carina, an old surgeon's trick is to look at the film end-on against the light source; an angle > 90 degrees indicates splaying of the carina and is consistent with subcarinal nodes. Assess cardiomegaly: if, in a good PA film, the heart shadow is larger than one hemithorax, then there is cardiomegaly (usually left ventricle [LV] enlargement). AP films and those with poor inspiratory effort (wherein the heart is pushed up, yielding a widening of the shadow) are notoriously difficult to interpret.

The lateral is very important and should be obtained whenever possible. Loss of the retrosternal air space filling indicates either right ventricle (RV) enlargement or an anterior mediastinal mass (thymoma). Left atrium (LA) enlargement in the old days could be diagnosed with a lateral film post barium swallow: the LA would impinge on the esophagus, and that area would be highlighted. Loss of the retrocardiac black triangular air space indicates abnormal opacification. RML infiltrates give a wedge-shaped whiteout over the middle of the heart in the lateral film.

Look at air space volume and character to see if they are symmetric in the size and density of bronchovascular markings, which should be evident two-thirds of the way out. If they are more so, either there is CHF with pulmonary congestion or the film is underpenetrated. If less so, the patient may have interstitial loss (emphysema, bullae), overpenetrated film, or pneumothorax (think of this if there is asymmetry and if there is an abnormal area of pitch-black lung fields.)

Other Films

The main use of abdominal films is for obstruction (dilated loops, air-fluid levels seen on upright). Free air is seen better on CXR. For roundsmanship and occasional clinical use, sentinel loops and mid-abdominal calcification go for pancreatitis. Pneumobilia occurs when a gallstone has made a chole-enteric fistula, which can subsequently lead to gallstone ileus (the stone gets trapped in the ileocecal valve). Thumbprinting indicates mucosal edema seen in mesenteric or colonic ischemia. Psoas abscesses and retroperitoneal hemorrhage obliterate psoas shadow. Treat accordingly. For further discussion, refer to Chapter 13.

Head CT reading is an art that takes years to master. The house officer needs to be able to recognize blood, gross masses, edema, and cerebrovascular accidents (CVAs) to some extent (stuff that can kill a patient before you can get a radiology report). On CT without contrast, blood appears white. If there is intracerebral hemorrhage, call your resident and Radiology immediately. Epidural hematomas have a biconvex shape, causing impingement on brain tissue, whereas subdurals have a concave configuration against the brain. Look for mass effect, midline shift, loss of sulci, and ventricular compression to assess the degree of edema.

Acute CVAs in general will not be seen on CT until 24 to 72 hours later (often appearing as darkening of brain tissue). Remember that head CT is not good for posterior fossa disease due to bony artifact.

C-spine films are important simply because you will need to have some familiarity with them in any emergency room (ER) experience as you will have to make decisions prior to orthopedic evaluation. Look at three bony lines (anterior and posterior vertebral body lines and vertebral spine line). Look for obvious dislocation/subluxation and fractures. Look at the soft-tissue shadow anterior to the vertebra; you should see a bulge at about C3, representing the start of the esophagus; if there is none, then there might be retropharyngeal hemorrhage obscuring the shadows. Use the Waters view (shot through the mouth) to look at the odontoid process (C1–C2); again, you're looking for all lines and spaces to be symmetric and obvious fractures.

PROCEDURES

All procedures require practice and patience, confidence and competence. Also, positioning is of the utmost importance (both for success and your back).

Phlebotomy

Practice first on fellow medical students. This will be good practice for getting everything together before you enter the patient's room (remember a needle [preferably 23 gauge], vacutainer/syringe, tubes, gauze, tourniquet, gloves, band-aid, specimen bags, forms, and stamped labels). You don't want to play with bloody tubes and gloves at the nurses' station, lest the clerk bite your head off. As for the actual procedure, you should know how to do it (at least in theory) by now.

Intravenous Lines

Learning this is vital to looking like a star to your residents. Don't give up until you've tried the antecubitals. This procedure involves identifying a vein that is juicy and won't roll, making it big by tourniquet, hand squeeze, alcohol, and patting. Insert the angiocath at a 30-degree angle; once you get a flash, advance the catheter over the stylet. Make sure to have gauze under the catheter (both to stabilize the insertion point and to keep the sheets from getting bloodied). Also remember to take the tourniquet off once the stylet is out. Have the IV start-up kit with flush ready to go before insertion. Have tape at the bedside as well.

Arterial Blood Gases

This is perhaps the easiest procedure to do because you know exactly where to go. Go at a 30- to 45-degree angle, pointing toward one of your fingers, which is on the pulse. Traditionally, students were taught to put two fingers on the pulse and go in between; although this is effective, it risks twice as many fingers to being stuck and forces you to go at 90 degrees, which is harder than 30 degrees. Don't give up until you try the brachial and femoral arteries.

Paracentesis

This is also a relatively easy procedure. Tap out where the fluid is; generally, the left lower quadrant (LLQ) is the site you go in. Make sure the PT/PTT and platelets are okay (which is key because many patients you want to tap have liver problems). Use an angiocath and Z-track (puncture skin, move laterally, then puncture peritoneum) to minimize fistula formation. If you're taking off a lot of fluid (> 2–3 L), consider replacing it with saline and/or albumin. Get out of there if you see blood or air.

Thoracentesis

Have the patient lean forward with arms on a pillow over a table. Make sure he or she takes slow breaths (also with paracentesis). Aim above the ribs (avoid the neurovascular bundle, which is below). Make sure the PT/PTT and platelets are okay. Consider ultrasonography localization. Insert the needle as low on the back as possible. If you take off more than 1 L, the risk for post–re-expansion pulmonary edema goes up.

Lumbar Puncture

Take all of the time in the world for proper positioning. Make a mark at the midpoint between the iliac crests. You can have patients lean forward on a table or lie in the fetal position. Either way, you want maximum exposure, so have the patient bend the head and knees into the chest as much as possible. You will feel a pop when you get to the subarachnoid space, which is where the cerebrospinal fluid (CSF) is. Numb the periosteum as much as you can (that's the most sensitive area you're going through). If the L4 interspace doesn't work, just work your way up the spine.

2

Selected Emergencies

In the physician or surgeon no quality takes rank with imperturbability.
— Sir William Osler

There are three kinds of people in life — people who make things happen, people who watch things happen, and people who don't know what happened. — Anonymous

Emergencies demand a playbook in your head for rapid evaluation and management. The general rules are
- Get as much information as quickly as possible (emergencies are the only situation when and "H&P" is not "what you should do first." The patient's medex is critical information.
- Rule out life-threatening things.
- Treat treatable things.
- Call for back-up.

ABDOMINAL PAIN

Quick Points
- Check the medex (narcotics, anticholinergics, and others can cause vomiting or obstruction).
- Rule out surgical abdomen (appendicitis, cholecystitis).
- Look also for pancreatitis, bowel obstruction, constipation, enteritis, peptic ulcer disease/gastritis, and GI bleeding. Tables 2–1 and 2–2 display diagnostics for abdominal conditions and differential diagnosis of obstruction.
- Intussusception is usually in the pediatric population; it can present with currant jelly stool, which is also seen in Meckel's diverticulum (another pediatric entity) and in enteric or colonic ischemia. In adults, intussusception usually occurs when a leading edge of mass pulls one segment of GI tract into another.

Table 2–1. Diagnostics of Choice for Abdominal Conditions

Condition	Diagnostic
Appendicitis	CT (classically, laparotomy was taught as right approach for high suspicion, but a 1997 *N Engl J Med* article showed that CT with contrast was cost effective)
Cholecystitis	HIDA (nuclear medicine) scan
Pancreatitis	CT with contrast; ultrasound has role later in course to look for pseudocyst
Cholelithiasis	Ultrasound
Diverticulitis	Enema (use meglumine diatrizoate [Gastrografin] if any question of perforation); colonoscopy
Obstruction	History and physical; upright radiography
Peptic ulcer disease	Esophagogastroduodenoscopy

Table 2–2. Differential for Obstruction

Adhesions (usually after prior surgery)

Inflammatory bowel disease

Colon carcinoma

Hernia

Intussusception (see text)

Management depends on the cause; get Gastroenterology and/or Surgery involved earlier rather than later.

ALTERED MENTAL STATUS

Look for medication effects, other causes of delirium, a history of dementia, acute medical conditions (especially toxic-metabolic encephalopathies), and sundowning (common in alert elderly patients with a new change in environment [eg, intensive care unit (ICU) psychosis]). Do a proper neurologic examination. Consider head CT. Consider a neurologic evaluation. Haloperidol (Haldol) and lorazepam (Ativan) (0.5–2 mg PO/IM/IV prn) are effective for severe agitation.

BACK PAIN

Quick Points
- Rule out epidural abscess, cord compression, and aortic dissection (a lot of this can be done just by H&P).
- Perform a thorough neurologic examination looking for sensory levels and Babinski reflexes; muscle strength is essential. Symptoms of bowel/bladder dysfunction, radiation of pain, dermatomal numbness, and weakness are also vital.
- If the patient is an injection drug user (IDU), has endocarditis, or has had recent spine surgery, epidural abscess is high up in the differential.
- For those with cancer, new-onset back pain is metastatic until proven otherwise. MRI is essential to rule out cord compression and epidural abscess (consider emergent radiation therapy for cord compression and neurosurgery evaluation for cord compression and epidural abscess).
- Dissection often occurs in smokers and those with a history of vascular problems and presents with excruciating pain.
- Look for asymmetric pulses and HTN.
- Transesophageal echocardiography (TEE) and MRI are procedures of choice for dissection.
- For dissection, use labetalol and/or nitroprusside to control blood pressure (BP).
- Surgical dissections are those involving the aortic arch, not the descending aortic dissections (unless other vessels are being compromised [eg, subclavian, renal]).
- For nonspecific and chronic pain, see Chapter 16.

BRADYCARDIA

Quick Points
- Look at the electrocardiogram (EKG) carefully for blocks.
- Look at the medex (beta-blockers, alpha-2 agonists, and calcium blockers can cause bradycardia).
- Consider cardiac and cerebral disease.

Initial Management

If the patient is hemodynamically unstable or symptomatic, consider the interventions in Table 2–3.

See Chapter 6 for more information.

Table 2–3. Interventions for Bradycardia

Atropine 1 mg IV

Epinephrine 1 mg IV

Isoproterenol drip

Pacemaker (transcutaneous or transvenous)

TACHYCARDIA

Quick Points
- Rule 1: If it is sinus tachycardia, then the patient has a separate problem that needs to be treated (myocardial infarction [MI], fever/sepsis, hypotension, hypovolemia, pulmonary embolus [PE], etc).
- If it is not sinus tachycardia, determine the heart's rhythm.

Initial Management

The following are the usual options to slow heart rate:
- Beta-blockers (eg, metoprolol [Lopressor]) 5 mg IV or esmolol drip (load 500 µg/kg, then 50–200 µg/kg/min)
- Diltiazem (Cardizem) 25 mg IV followed by drip (5–15 mg/hr)
- Adenosine 6 mg, then 12 mg, and then another 12 mg IV

Try to avoid verapamil. Use procainamide for Wolff-Parkinson-White syndrome. Use lidocaine and procainamide for ventricular tachycardia. Use ibutilide (Corvert) for atrial flutter. Shock is always a consideration; shock immediately if the patient is hemodynamically unstable. See Chapter 6 for an in-depth review of bradycardia and tachycardia.

CHEST PAIN

Quick Points
- As soon as you are called for this by the floor or ER, tell the person calling over the phone to get an EKG so that by the time you arrive, it is waiting for you.
- A description of the pain and the number of risk factors (see Chapter 6 for a full discussion) are essential to how aggressive you will be in your work-up.
- Basic differential:
  - Acute coronary syndrome (unstable angina/MI)
  - Stable angina
  - Costochondritis (pain to palpation at costochrondral junction; can be pleuritic in nature)
  - Aortic dissection
  - Pericarditis (pleuritic and positional pain; friction rub; sinus tachycardia elevation all over EKG; young patient after recent viral illness); treat with indomethacin
  - Gastroesophageal reflux
  - Pneumonia or other causes of pleuritic pain

Initial Management
The vital measures to perform in patients with acute MI are listed in Table 2–4.

Table 2–4. Critical Interventions in Acute Myocardial Infarction

Aspirin 325 mg PO × 1

Nitroglycerin 0.4 mg sublingual q5 min × 3

Oxygen

Beta-blockers (metoprolol [Lopressor] 5 mg IV q10 min × 3; hold for pulse < 60)

Heparinization (as for pulmonary embolus)

Consider enalapril (Vasotec) 1.25 mg IV × 1

Call Cardiology for consideration of thrombolytics or angioplasty

For more information, see Chapter 6.

LOWER GASTROINTESTINAL BLEED

Quick Points
- Differential:
  - Arteriovenous malformations (AVMs)/angiodysplasia
  - Colon cancer (the right colon causes more anemia, whereas the left colon causes more obstruction)
  - Diverticulosis (not diverticulitis)
  - Mesenteric/colonic ischemia (look for postprandial pain, clinical set-up [a history of atrial fibrillation, vascular disease, and HTN/diabetes])

Initial Management
- Support with fluids and blood.
- Surgery and Gastroenterology need to be involved early.
- Consider colonoscopy, angiography, and tagged-cell scan. Angiography can be used as a therapeutic measure with options for embolization. Red blood cell (RBC) scans are very sensitive but not specific.
- If the source is unclear but the patient is bleeding out, hemicolectomy is the option of last resort. See Chapter 13 for further discussion.

UPPER GASTROINTESTINAL BLEEDING

Quick Points
- Differential:
  - Peptic ulcer disease (PUD)
  - Esophageal varices
  - Esophagitis
  - In Mallory-Weiss and Boerhaave's syndromes a history of retching and vomiting is important; Boerhaave's syndrome causes pleural effusion and can be diagnosed with barium swallow; do not use meglumine diatrizoate [Gastrografin] if Boerhaave's is a concern [vice versa for colonic perforation]).
  - Dieulafoy's lesions (rare)
- Diagnostics revolve around esophagogastroduodenoscopy (EGD), and management should be as per Gastroenterology.

Initial Management
- Aggressively resuscitate with fluids and blood.
- Table 2–5 lists commonly used agents to reduce acid production.
- In renal failure patients, halve the dose given (eg, use qd dosing).
- Cimetidine (Tagamet; older H_2-blocker) is falling out of favor due to drug interactions.
- Beta-blockers (eg, propranolol [Inderal] 40 mg PO bid) are indicated for varices.
- Antibiotics should be used for infectious esophagitis.

Table 2–5. Acid Reduction Agents

H_2-Blockers	Proton-Pump Inhibitors
Famotidine (Pepcid) 20 mg PO bid	Omeprazole (Prilosec) 20–40 mg PO qd
Nizatidine (Axid) 150 mg PO bid	Lansoprazole (Prevacid) 15–30 mg PO qd
Ranitidine (Zantac) 150 mg PO bid	

HYPOTENSION

Quick Points
- Get a clinical picture of events leading to hypotension and general medical condition.
- Check to see how BP has been running. Get a good handle on volume status and lung status.
- The basic differential is shown in Table 2–6.
- Differential diagnosis of addisonian crisis: rapid steroid taper in a dependent patient, TB/cytomegalovirus (CMV) adrenalitis, classic Addison's, adrenal infiltration, Waterhouse-Friderichsen syndrome (see Chapter 5).

Initial Management
- Treat the cause.
- Fluids (nomal saline [titrate to patient's weight, BP, and cardiorespiratory status])
- Hespan (hetastarch; artificial colloid) 250 to 500 cc IV bolus

- Blood (for bleeding patients)
- Pressors: norepinephrine (Levophed) (16 mg/250 cc 5% dextrose in water [D_5W] titrated to BP) is a mainstay. Many use dopamine (400 mg/250 cc D_5W) initially.
- For anaphylaxis, see Table 2–7.

Table 2–6. Differential of Acute Hypotension

Cardiac (congestive heart failure, myocardial infarction)

Sepsis

Hypovolemia/severe blood loss

Anaphylaxis

Neurogenic (spinal cord trauma)

Addisonian crisis

Table 2–7. Acute Pharmacologic Interventions in Anaphylaxis

Epinephrine 0.1 mg SQ × 1

Diphenhydramine (Benadryl) 50 mg IV × 1

Hydrocortisone 100 mg IV × 1

Further Discussion

Crystalloids (NS, Ringer's lactate) are the standard fluid resuscitation measure employed. However, significant amounts of crystalloids leave the vasculature within hours. Colloids (eg, albumin, hetastarch) stay in the vasculature much longer. Another advantage of hetastarch and albumin is that they provide equivalent amounts of hemodynamic support as crystalloids with far less volume, which can be a great plus in patients with cardiac, hepatic, or renal failure. For reasons of expense, hetastarch is generally preferred to albumin, except in patients with cirrhosis. In the actively bleeding patient, blood is, of course, the preferred fluid replacement. For management of shock, see Chapter 15.

HYPERTENSION

Quick Points
- Check the medex (see if the patient is due to get BP medications in an hour; if so, give them now).
- Check trends on vital signs (200 mm Hg may not be a big deal acutely in someone who lives at 180 but 160 can be a problem in a patient whose baseline is 90).
- Look for end-organ damage, which indicates a hypertensive emergency (ie, altered mental status, headache, visual changes, retinal hemorrhages, cardiac ischemia, renal dysfunction).

Initial Management
- If no end-organ signs of dysfunction are present and BP is less than 200/100 and not that much higher than baseline, it can be okay to tell the nurse "Okay, let's watch it."
- Find out if there is a reason for an acute rise in BP, especially following serious causes (Table 2–8).
- If you feel that you have to intervene or just need to fix the number, bear in mind the following:
  - Rule 1: *Nifedipine (Procardia) is bad.* In the 1980s and early 1990s (and still in other industrialized countries), nifedipine is often used just to fix the numbers. It's very effective, but its induction of reflex tachycardia can be very detrimental as it can cause MI. By the way, *sublingual nifedipine is really bad.*
  - Rule 2: If the patient is having or recently had a CVA, don't lower the BP to normal. Systolic BP of ~160 to 180 is necessary in these patients to maintain cerebral perfusion.

Table 2–8. Differential of Serious Causes of Acute Hypertension

Stroke

Myocardial infarction

Renal stenosis

Pheochromocytoma

Aortic dissection

- When the nurse calls you with a high BP, determine if it is malignant or not.
  - If not malignant, you may want to use extra doses of what the patient is already on or use the patient's current drugs sooner than the schedule frequency. Other options are listed in Table 2–9.
- Remember that exact drip formulations vary from hospital to hospital and that over 48 hours of nitroprusside can lead to cyanide toxicity.

Table 2–9. Commonly Used Drugs for Acute Rise in Blood Pressure

Nonmalignant Hypertension	Malignant Hypertension
Clonidine 0.1 mg PO × 1	Nitroprusside drip
Nitro-paste 1 inch to chest wall	Labetalol drip
Enalapril (Vasotec) 10 mg PO	Esmolol drip

HYPERTHERMIA

Quick Points
- Look for infection, stroke/intracranial hemorrhage, and malignant hyperthermia.
- Causes of malignant hyperthermia include anesthetics, phenothiazines, haloperidol, and tricyclic antidepressants.
- Signs and symptoms include hyperthermia, muscle rigidity, rigors, dry skin, increased creatine phosphokinase (CPK), renal failure, and pupillary dilation.

Initial Management
- Treat the cause.
- Replete IV fluids generously.
- Give an ice/cooling blanket.
- Use acetaminophen and NSAIDs to break fever.
- If the hyperthermia is malignant, use dantrolene 100 mg PO bid-qid and/or bromocriptine.
- Procainamide (2–6 mg/min) can prevent ventricular fibrillation in a patient with malignant hyperthermia; stop if QRS widens > 50%, hypotension occurs, or after 1 g is given.

- As this group of patients frequently develops rhabdomyolysis, acidosis, and renal failure, consider alkalinizing urine with sodium bicarbonate IV.
- Meperidine (Demerol) 25 mg IV as needed is useful for rigors due to amphotericin B.

HYPOTHERMIA

Look for sepsis and cold exposure. Use a warming blanket and warm all IV fluids and blood.

SHORTNESS OF BREATH

Quick Point
Think of the etiologies of dyspnea listed in Table 2–10.

Table 2–10. Differential of Common Causes of Dyspnea

Cardiac	Pulmonary
Congestive heart failure	Pneumonia
Myocardial infarction	Chronic obstructive pulmonary disease/asthma
	Pneumothorax
	Interstitial disease (cancer, pneumonoconiosis)
	Pulmonary embolus

Initial Management (Table 2–11)
- Do a quick physical (vitals, rales, wheezes, breath sounds should help you focus your diagnosis).
- In general, always get an arterial blood gas (ABG), CXR, and an EKG. Know the alveolar-arterial gradient (Appendix D).
- Knowing whether the blood gas is venous or arterial is important: skill and technique are critical, depending on drawing only when you see pulsation and arterial-color blood.
- Pulse oximetry is handy too, but it can be fooled: carboxyhemoglobin (smokers, carbon monoxide) and methemoglobinemia (which occurs after exposure to many agents, including dapsone, nitrite,

nitrates, primaquine, and sulfonamides) give falsely elevated levels, and patients with poor extremity perfusion have falsely low levels.

- Intubation. The decision to intubate is primarily clinical (how the patient is doing and what his or her reserve is), not based on ABG or x-ray.
- Not uncommonly, at 2 AM, you will be called on an elderly smoker with chronic obstructive pulmonary disease (COPD) and heart disease with features of pneumonia, CHF, COPD, cancer, and PE. You may not get the diagnostic of choice (CT/ventilation-perfusion [V/Q] scan/bronchoscopy) at that hour, in which case, it is often all right to use all of the interventions in Table 2–11 as long as there are no major contraindications.
- For PE, the index of suspicion is critical and is based on a history of cancer/DVT/immobilization and symptoms (acuteness and severity) (Figure 2–1).
- If spiral CT is inconclusive, go to the angiogram. The V/Q scan is out of favor because studies showed that 30% of people with low-probability V/Q and a high index of suspicion had a PE. In our experience, too many V/Qs are indeterminate, intermediate, or low probability for them to be of use.
- For roundsmanship, know that the most common sign of PE on EKG is sinus tachycardia; the most classic sign is the S wave in I, Q in III, and inverted T in III. The most common sign of PE on CXR is a normal x-ray; the most classic sign is Westermark's hump/sign (a wedge-shaped opacity in the area of infarction). You can also get pleural effusion.

THE CODE

It is vital to keep in your pocket an Advanced Cardiac Life Support (ACLS) card (the CodeRunner from the Committee of Interns and Residents is great), with the management algorithms (which will not be included here, as this is meant more as a general and philosophical discussion). Also, don't take bad results to heart. As someone once said, "If you can't save them when they're alive, how can you save them when they're dead?" Critical initial steps are to

- Ensure IV access (and rapid central line placement),
- Manage airway and rapidly intubate,
- Perform chest compressions, and
- Make sure someone is running the code.

Table 2–11. Basic Management Options for Dyspnea

Intervention	Dose	Indication	Comment
Oxygen	Discretionary	Hypoxemia	Use carefully in chronic obstructive pulmonary disease
Antibiotics	Discretionary	Pneumonia	
Furosemide (Lasix)	40–100 mg PO/IV	Congestive heart failure	Use aggressively if patient is wet
Nebulized albuterol (Proventil) Nebulized ipratropium (Atrovent)	1 unit dose at discretionary frequency	Asthma, chronic obstructive pulmonary disease	Be cautious with nebulized albuterol in patients with heart disease
Steroids	Prednisone 40–100 g PO bid Methylprednisolone 40–125 IV q6h	Asthma, chronic obstructive pulmonary disease	Doses depend on weight and severity of disease
Heparin	5,000 U IV bolus, then 25,000 U/250 cc D_5W at 10 cc/hr	Pulmonary embolus, myocardial infarction	Screen patients for hemorrhage elsewhere (especially gastrointestinal or central nervous system)
Needle aspiration		Pneumothorax	

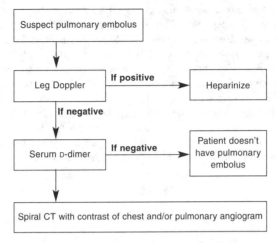

Figure 2–1. Diagnostic approach for pulmonary embolism.

You only need four or five doctors in the room. The only laboratories you need are those that can make a difference: potassium, magnesium, and calcium. ABG will not be of use until the patient is stable on a ventilator. In general, one of the medical residents should try intubation before Anesthesia. Let the juniors and interns do as much as possible.

The ethics of coding are important, from a personal and professional perspective. "Slow" and "Hollywood" codes (going through the motions of the code) should be avoided if at all possible; it does the patient no service but does cause considerable indignity. Proper communication with the patient, family, and attending physician prior to a crisis is essential. However, sometimes you have little choice, especially if you are the covering house staff in the middle of the night. If you feel you are running a futile code, keep the code brief and simple.

In terms of technical aspects, bear in mind the following rules of thumb:
- Shock is good for almost everything except aystole.
- You can never go wrong with epinephrine or atropine.
- Atropine, lidocaine, and epinephrine can be given by endotracheal (ET) tube.

- Don't give bicarbonate unless the patient has a history of metabolic acidosis (the addition of bicarbonate in a setting of poor ventilation causes paradoxical intracellular acidosis; see Chapter 15).
- If there is no response after 20 to 30 minutes, call the code; in a patient whom you are coding futilely for whatever reason (unreasonable/ adamant patient or family), call it after three epinephrines/atropines if there is no response.

As background, the code is not really meant for medically ill patients; it works in acute trauma and cardiac settings, but for the elderly patient with multiple medical problems, 99% of patients do not live to 1 year after the code, and probably more than 90% don't leave the hospital alive.

3

Fluids, Electrolytes, Nutrition, and Acid-Base Status

It takes all the running you can do to stay in the same place. — The Red Queen (*Alice in Wonderland*)

Don't learn the tricks of the trade. Learn the trade. — Anonymous

An important piece of medical care, this area is often managed ad hoc in a haphazard way, with numbers seemingly being picked out of thin air. But there is a formal process that should be invoked here as well (see also Appendix D).

MAINTENANCE FLUIDS

Quick Points
- Maintenance hydration is indicated when the patient is euvolemic but can have nothing by mouth (NPO) (eg, awaiting surgery, run-of-the-mill shortness of breath [SOB], uncomplicated pancreatitis, etc).
- Always assess electrolyte status, cardiac state, and renal function prior to starting fluids.

Initial Management
- The standard fluid is ½NS.
- Rate is given by the 4, 2, 1 rule: 4 cc/kg for the first 10 kg, 2 cc/kg for the next 10 kg, and then 1 cc/kg for each kg above. This equals $x + 40$ (where x is weight in kg) for adults.
- Generally, the patient who is NPO could use a few calories as well, so the fluids used would include 5% dextrose (D_5) and some potassium supplement (20 mEq KCl/L is usually sufficient). For example, an order for a 70-kg adult would be D_5½NS + 20 mEq KCl/L @ 110 cc/hr.

- In surgery, never use NS or ½NS. Always use Ringer's lactate (RL) (the clinical significance is purely your not getting yelled at by the surgeons; surgeons like to believe that since lactated Ringer's solution has some bicarbonate and potassium, it more closely resembles plasma than what medicine people use).
- In pediatrics, the standard maintenance fluid is ¼NS.
- Adjust the rate downward if someone is liable to develop pulmonary edema or fluid overload.

ELECTROLYTES

Hypernatremia/Repletion of Free Water

Quick Points
- Free water deficit is given by the formula
$$0.6 \times wt\ (kg) \times ([Na - 140]/140).$$
- The ensuing discussion assumes that the patient's hypernatremia is due to fluid loss; occasionally, patients can be hypernatremic and hypervolemic, which occurs in settings of hyperaldosteronism (Conn's syndrome, congenital adrenal hyperplasia/enzyme deficiencies). In these instances, urine sodium is usually > 20 mEq/L.

Initial Management (Figure 3–1)
- You should first give NS in a dehydrated patient until the patient's hemodynamic status is okay.
- Then give D_5W (sterile water will alone cause hemolysis) at a rate replacing half of the water deficit in the first 24 hours, and then replace the rest over the next 48 hours.
- For a 70-kg patient with a sodium of 160 mEq/L, the water deficit is $0.6 \times 70 \times 20/140 = 6$ L; for the first day, you would give 3 L/24 hr = 125 cc/hr D_5W. *Too fast repletion leads to cerebral edema.*
- Check urine sodium (if > 20 mEq/L, this indicates renal losses from renal failure or diuretics).

Hyponatremia

The dangers of hyponatremia include lethargy and seizures. Also, this disorder illustrates the danger of the "euboxic" approach to medicine (ie,

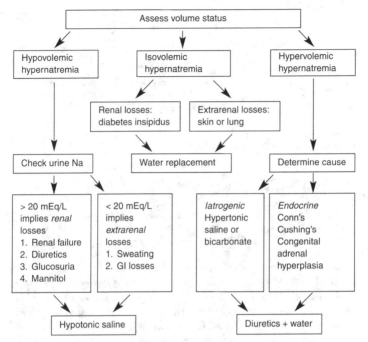

Figure 3–1. Evaluation and management of hypernatremia.

viewing the patient as a box and trying to fix all of the numbers in the box). Classically, if you don't have enough of something, the doctor should give that something, so in hyponatremics, simple logic would lead to you giving salt. *Wrong!* In general, hyponatremia is not due to a sodium deficit but to too much water in the body. (Hypovolemic hyponatremia indicates a sodium deficit and occurs in adrenal or renal failure.)

Quick Points
• Most inpatients with hyponatremia will be euvolemic or hypervolemic, and much of this will be due to iatrogenic administration of too much fluid.

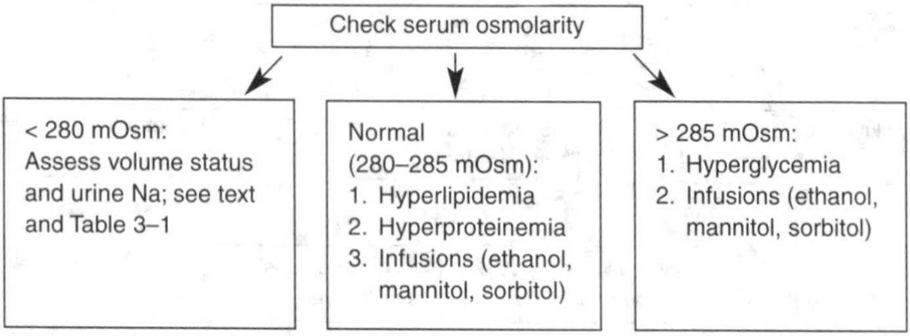

Figure 3–2. Initial evaluation of hyponatremia.

- Hypervolemic hyponatremia often occurs in CHF, liver failure, and renal failure.
- Urine sodium < 10 mEq/L indicates that the kidney is holding onto sodium, whereas urine sodium > 20 mEq/L indicates inappropriate concentration of the urine (see Figure 3–2 for differential).

Initial Management (Table 3–1)

- Treatment should first focus on treating the cause; *treat the patient, not the labs.*
- If fixing the number is needed, first start with fluid restriction to less than 1 L. This includes all fluids entering the patient; so calculate how much IV fluid, Solu-sets, PEG feedings, and voluntary drinking

Table 3–1. Causes and Management of Hypo-osmotic Hyponatremia

	Urine Sodium < 10 mEq/L	Urine Sodium > 20 mEq/L	Treatment
Hypovolemic	Extrarenal losses (vomiting, diarrhea, pancreatitis, sweating)	Renal losses (diuretics, renal failure, nephritis, urinary obstruction, renal tubular acidosis)	Isotonic saline
Isovolemic	Water intoxication	SIADH, renal failure	Water restriction
Hypervolemic	Nephrosis, congestive heart failure, cirrhosis	Renal failure	Water restriction

SIADH = syndrome of inappropriate antidiuretic hormone.

is occurring. Fluid restriction is difficult to force, requiring compliance by the patient and enforcement by the nurses.

- If the sodium is still going down, you can sometimes give NS + furosemide.
- Demeclocycline (a tetracycline with the side effect of blocking the antidiuretic hormone [ADH] receptor) 300 mg PO bid can also be tried.
- If the patient is having seizures or severe mental status changes from hyponatremia, then you can go to hypertonic saline (3% or 5% based on the hospital; NS is 0.9%). Don't give this unless it is absolutely necessary. Don't raise the sodium more than 1 point every 2 hours. If the sodium dropped acutely (eg, from sorbitol administration), you can raise it 2 points every 2 hours. This means that you have to check SMA-7 q2h; such frequent blood drawing can only be maintained in the ICU, where the patient should be placed for hypertonic saline anyway because a toxicity of its use if correction is too rapid is central pontine myelinolysis, which manifests as quadriplegia (may or may not be reversible). Now you should see the double entendre of euboxia: not just treating the patient as a box but also causing the patient to "box" (ie, die).

Potassium

Many people panic whenever the patient has a potassium problem. There is rarely a need to panic.

Hyperkalemia

Quick Points
- See if the blood is hemolyzed, if the patient is in tumor lysis, or if the patient is in adrenal or renal failure or is acidotic.
- The most fear-inducing symptom of hyperkalemia is cardiac: first high T waves, then sine wave, and then ventricular arrhythmias. Table 3–2 lists the causes of hyperkalemia.

Initial Management
- Furosemide 40 to 100 mg IV depending on potassium (will work only if there is significant urine output).

Table 3–2. Differential of Hyperkalemia

Normal total body K	Pseudohyperkalemia	Test tube hemolysis, high WBC or platelet
	Redistribution	Acidosis, GI bleeding, tissue necrosis, drugs (digitalis, beta-blockers, succinylcholine)
Elevated total body K	Excess ingestion	Penicillin K, salt substitute in diets
	Impaired excretion	Renal or adrenal failure

- Sodium polystyrene sulfonate (Kayexalate) enema or 15 g orally as often as needed.
- Insulin + D_{50} (insulin promotes cellular uptake of potassium; this is only a temporizing measure).
- Calcium gluconate 1 ampule intravenously (should be used only if cardiac effects are occurring from hyperkalemia; this is only a temporizing measure).
- Sodium bicarbonate 1 ampule intravenously (alkalosis promotes kaliuresis).
- Dialysis (indications for dialysis are reviewed in Chapters 9 and 15)

Hypokalemia

Quick Points
- Alkalosis, vitamin B_{12} therapy, and insulin overdose can cause hypokalemia.
- You can see the U wave and flattening of T waves and sometimes prolongation of QT as well.
- Muscle cramps may also be a symptom.
- See Figure 3–3 for evaluation of hypokalemia.

Initial Management
- KCl 20 mEq PO tid or KCl 10 mEq × 4.
- Replacing potassium can be done orally (remember that KCl pills can cause esophagitis and are difficult to swallow, so elixir might be a consideration) or intravenously (most hospitals don't let you give

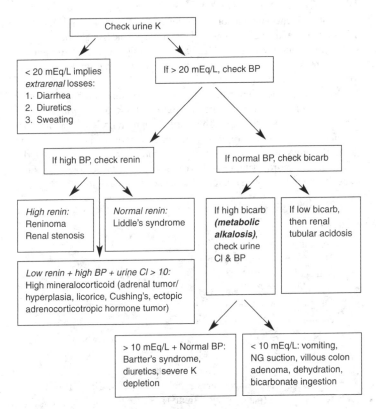

Figure 3–3. Evaluation of hypokalemia and metabolic alkalosis.

more than 10 mEq × 4 or 20 mEq × 3 without a repeat check). KCl burns when given peripherally (can be alleviated somewhat by adding bicarbonate to the mixture or you can give it centrally).
• If you continually replace potassium but it doesn't budge, check for low calcium and magnesium, as both ions are needed for the body to retain potassium.

Some residents and attending physicians "like a potassium level of 4." You should treat the patient, not the labs; some people live at home just fine with a potassium level of 3.2. Mildly low potassium is only detrimental if the patient is on digoxin or has a cardiomyopathy or history of arrhythmia. You don't need to chase a low potassium all day in most patients.

Why is high potassium worse than low potassium? Intracellular potassium is over 100 mEq/L, whereas extracellular potassium is about 4 mEq/L, so the polarization of the cardiac membrane is kept in place by a transmembrane concentration gradient in a ratio of about 25. If the potassium goes up to 6, 7, or 8, that ratio drops precipitously, making the left ventricle more irritable and arrhythmogenic, but a low potassium doesn't affect matters that much with respect to polarization.

Hypercalcemia

Quick Points
- Differential:
  - Hyperparathyroidism (Table 3–3)
  - Milk-alkali syndrome
  - Sarcoidosis
  - Drugs (vitamin A, lithium, androgens, estrogens, thiazides)
- High calcium can also cause sinus bradycardia and shortening of QT.

Initial Management
1. NS (key) (start at at least 100 cc/hr if the cardiac status is okay)
2. Furosemide (increases calciuresis, unlike thiazides, which decrease it)
3. Bisphosphonates (pamidronate [Aredia] has become standard now for IV use and reduces rates of pathologic fractures in breast cancer and multiple myeloma and may even decrease skeletal metastases in breast cancer)

Table 3–3. Mnemonic for Symptoms of Hyperparathyroidism

Stones	Renal calculi (due to high calcium)
Bones	Bone resorption/pain (due to parathyroid hormone)
Moans	Pancreatitis; peptic ulcers (due to high calcium)
Psychic overtones	Lethargy (due to high calcium)

4. Calcitonin (comes in Miacalcin nasal spray and has the added benefit of being an adjuvant analgesic in cancer patients)
5. Mithramycin (rarely used)

Hypocalcemia

Quick Points
- Symptoms include cardiac irritability, longer QT interval, and neuromuscular irritability (Chvostek's and Trousseau's signs).
- Differential:
  - Osteoblastic metastases (breast/prostate)
  - Vitamin D deficiency
  - Overtransfusion (citrate in blood chelates calcium)
  - Renal failure

Initial Management
- Replete with oral calcium (calcium carbonate 500 mg PO tid) or IV (1 ampule calcium gluconate as often as indicated).
- If calcium repletion isn't working, check for low magnesium, which is needed for calcium retention.

Calcium at the cell membrane is about 6 mEq/L intracellularly and 8 mEq/L extracellularly. This very close ratio explains why any change in calcium is so much more important than a similar change for other ions. The mnemonic is "Just as milk helps you sleep, high calcium calms the cell membranes, and just as monkeys eating bananas always jump around, high potassium makes cell membranes more excitable."

Magnesium

This shadow ion underlies potassium and calcium. If you are having trouble repleting potassium, calcium or magnesium might be low. Magnesium is essential for the body to hold onto both potassium and calcium, and calcium is needed to hold onto potassium.

The differential diagnosis of low magnesium equals GI losses, hungry bone syndrome (after parathyroidectomy), osteoblastic metastases, insulin overdose, renal failure, and cisplatin/amphotericin/diuretics. The symptoms are similar to hypocalcemia. Hypermagnesemia occurs in renal failure and leads to coma and heart blocks. Treatment for hypermagnesemia is IV calcium, along with fluids, furosemide, and dialysis.

Phosphorus

High phosphorus occurs in renal failure, tumor lysis, hypoparathyroidism, and rhabdomyolysis and leads to ossification (calcium phosphate deposits in muscles). You can give calcium carbonate or Ampho-Jel. Low phosphorus is generally not a thing to worry about; however, very low phosphorus can lead to adenosine triphosphate (ATP) depletion and rhabdomyolysis. Further, low phosphorus can reduce muscle strength, which is of importance in weaning off the ventilator.

METABOLIC ACID-BASE DISTURBANCES

Metabolic Acidosis

Quick Points
- Anion gap versus non-anion gap. Serum anion gap = $Na - (Cl + HCO_3)$; > 15 is high. The anion gap may be artificially lowered by hypoalbuminemia or hyperparaproteinemia (eg, multiple myeloma [MM]).
- The mnemonic for anion-gap acidosis is MUDPILES (Table 3–4).
- For non–anion-gap acidosis, check
  - Urine anion gap (urine Na + K – Cl). If negative, it may be from diarrhea. If positive, that means there is renal tubular acidosis (RTA).
  - Serum K: If low, think diarrhea, acetazolamide use, or type 1 RTA. If potassium is normal or high, think renal failure, hypoaldosteronism, or ingestion of acids.

Table 3–4. Mnemonic for Anion-Gap Acidosis

M	Methanol
U	Uremia
D	Diabetic ketoacidosis
P	Paraldehyde
I	Infection
L	Lactic acidosis
E	Ethanol
S	Salicylates

Initial Management

- Treat the cause (eg, renal failure, sepsis).
- Bicarbonate. Give only if the pH is < 7.1 (diabetic ketoacidosis [DKA] patients can usually tolerate even lower pH without bicarbonate). The danger of bicarbonate is paradoxical intracellular acidosis (converted to CO_2 in serum and enters cells, where CO_2 is an acid). Thus, if there is no good way of blowing off CO_2 generated by the body (ie, if there is defective ventilation, beware of bicarbonate), then you are causing more harm than good.
- Bicarbonate drips. The main indications are severe acidosis, excretion of toxins (aspirin, tricyclics), and rhabdomyolysis. Know that NS + 1 ampule $NaHCO_3$ is wrong, as it is a hypertonic solution. You can give ½NS + 1 ampule, ⅓NS + 2 ampules, D_5W + 3 ampules, or ½RL + 2 ampules.

SPECIAL SITUATIONS

Alcoholic Ketoacidosis

Serum ketones may be undetected due to assay (treat with D_5NS).

Table 3–5 presents the characteristics of different alcohol-induced acidoses.

D-Lactic Acidosis

Unexplained anion gap due to D-isomer may not be detected on routine assay for lactate. It is produced in patients after bowel surgery and diarrhea.

Table 3–5. Acidosis in Different Alcohol Ingestions

Type	Breath	Ketones	Osmolar Gap	Degree of Acidosis	Affected Organ
Ethanol	+++	Possible	High	Minimal	Liver
Alcoholic ketoacidosis	+	Possible	Normal	Mild	
Methanol	No change	None	High	Severe	Eyes
Ethylene glycol	No change	None	High	Severe	Kidney (oxalate crystals in urine)

Metabolic Alkalosis

Quick Points
See Figure 3–3 for an evaluation of metabolic alkalosis.

- Check urine chloride. If it is < 15 mEq/L, this indicates chloride conservation (eg, NG tube suction, volume contraction) or diuretics (especially furosemide or thiazides). If it is >15 mEq/L, check BP.
- If BP is high, consider renal artery stenosis or Conn's and Cushing's syndromes. If BP is normal, look for potassium or magnesium depletion.
- Remember that volume contraction and steroids often cause metabolic alkalosis.

Initial Management
- If urine chloride is low, you can give NS.
- If potassium is low, give KCl.
- You can give acetazolamide (Diamox) 500 mg PO bid to cause bicarbonate wasting to fix the number (you still need to find and treat the cause).
- You can also give 1% HCl to fix the number (you need to give this via the central line).
- If there is too much mineralocorticoid, you can give spironolactone (Aldactone).

NUTRITION

Diet Order

Bear in mind the patient's diseases and dental and mental states.

- Cardiac patients and hypertensives should receive 2 g sodium and a low-cholesterol diet.
- Diabetics should, in general, get an order for an 1,800- or 2,000-calorie American Diabetic Association (ADA) diet (adjust calories for weight).
- Renal failure patients should have restrictions on sodium, potassium, and protein (based on renal function; a safe bet is 2 g sodium, 80 g protein, and 40 mEq potassium).
- Cirrhotics should have protein restriction and sometimes sodium restriction.

- Edentulous patients probably need puree; stroke patients should also start on puree.
- Get Speech and Swallow involved early in situations of CNS injury.
- Try to accommodate the native foods of patients from different cultures.

Remember that caloric requirements increase with fever, burns, trauma, and hyperthyroidism. Protein requirements in the catabolic patient can rise from 0.8 g/kg/d (normal) to 1.5 g/kg/d. Protein losses can be approximated by the following equation: (24-hr urine urea nitrogen + 4) × 6.25; you can supplement protein intake if the patient is losing lots of protein.

Supplements

Different hospitals have different formulations for supplements. Examples include Ensure and Jevity for the routine patient, Suplena and Nepro for the renal failure patient, Glucerna or Diabetic Resource (for, you guessed it, diabetics), and Peptamen (elemental amino acids for the patient with difficulty absorbing) (Table 3–6). Remember that enteral is preferable to IV for reasons of expense and efficacy. Try to get total parenteral nutrition (TPN) orders in early (generally before 1 PM) so that the pharmacy can prepare it and the patient will get it the same day.

Nutritional Support

The decision to start feeding tubes or parenteral nutrition is often agonizing to physicians, patients, and families alike.

Table 3–6. Common Oral Nutritional Supplements

Patient Population	Supplements
General supplements	Ensure Jevity Resource
Dairy intolerant	Nutren 1.5
Renal failure	Suplena Nepro
Diabetics	Diabetic Resource Glucerna
Malabsorption	Peptamen

- Nutrititional support is needed in settings of critical care, cancer, ICU, liver failure, renal failure, HIV, and short bowel syndrome.
- Key issues are if the patient is malnourished, if the disease causes malnutrition, and if improved nutritional status would benefit the prognosis or quality of life.
- If the answer is yes to all, decide whether nutritional requirements can best be met with oral supplements, an enteral feeding tube, partial parenteral nutrition, or TPN.
- If the patient needs short-term therapy, an NG tube for enteral and a peripherally introduced central vein catheter (PICC) or central venous catheter (subclavian or jugular) can be inserted.
- For long-term therapy, a PEG or PEJ tube is used for enteral feeding, whereas a Hickmann or Broviac catheter is required for parenteral nutrition.
- The disadvantages of enteral feeding include aspiration and diarrhea. The complications of parenteral feeding include infection, pneumothorax, and fluid overload. Patients on TPN should receive frequent monitoring of SMA-7, glucose, and liver function tests (LFTs).

Miscellaneous Facts in Nutrition

- Fat malabsorption (sprue, ileal resection) leads to deficiencies in vitamins A, D, E, and K.
- *Vitamin toxicities*:
  - Vitamin A (due to polar bear liver and faddism; symptoms include headache, increased intracranial pressure [pseudotumor cerebri], jaundice without scleral icterus, malaise, abdominal pain).
  - Vitamin D (overdose symptoms are the same as those of hypercalcemia).
  - Vitamin B_6 (overdose leads to neuropathy).
  - Vitamin C at very high doses rarely causes retinal hemorrhages; at such doses, it can treat Chédiak-Higashi syndrome.
  - Vitamin E at high doses can antagonize vitamin K.
- *Kwashiorkor*: This is protein malnutrition while caloric intake is still intact. It results in edema, especially ascites (pot-bellied babies in the Ethiopian famine of 1985), hypoalbuminemia, and preservation of subcutaneous fat.
- *Marasmus*: This is combined protein-calorie malnutrition, with severe wasting, growth failure, and loss of subcutaneous fat.

- *Flag sign*: A deficiency of protein intake during a recent period will cause a band of hypopigmented hair. Once the patient recovers, normal hair color will return, resulting in a striped appearance like a flag.
- *Merke's sign*: A protein deficiency also results in thin white bands on the fingernails.
- Table 3–7 lists the characteristics of different nutritional deficiencies.

Table 3–7. Specific Nutritional Deficiencies: Manifestations

Vitamin A	Xerophthalmia, night blindness, follicular hyperkeratosis, Bitot spots (foamy plaques on conjunctiva); severe xerophthalmia leads to corneal melting = keratomalacia
Thiamine (B_1) (alcoholics, polished rice eaters)	Wernicke's syndrome (ataxia, altered mental status, ophthalmoplegia, diplopia, nystagmus), Korsakoff's syndrome (psychosis, confabulation) Dry beriberi: peripheral neuritis, ataxia, foot drop, wrist drop Wet beriberi: congestive heart failure, edema, no albumin in urine
Riboflavin (B_2)	Angular stomatitis and cheilosis, magenta tongue
Niacin (B_3) (corn eaters; carcinoid tumors that use tryptophan, which requires niacin)	Pellagra (4 Ds = diarrhea, dermatitis, dementia, death)
Pyridoxine (B_6) (isoniazid)	Oxalate stones, polyneuritis, glossitis; high homocysteine
Cobalamin (B_{12}) (vegans, *Diphyllobothrium latum*, pernicious anemia/atrophic gastritis, intestinal bacterial overgrowth)	Subacute combined degeneration (posterior columns of spine leading to loss of sensation and lateral corticospinal tracts giving weakness) Megaloblastic anemia Dementia, atrophic glossitis
Folate (alcoholics)	Megaloblastic anemia. Don't give folate in such anemics without checking B_{12} (can mask deficiency); high homocysteine

Continued on next page

Table 3–7. Continued

Vitamin C (ascorbate)	Scurvy (capillary fragility, gumbleeds, petechiae, slow wound healing)
Vitamin D (calcitriol)	Rickets in kids (rachitic rosary in ribs, pigeon breast, bowing of long bones, knock-knees), osteomalacia in adults (spontaneous fractures)
	Hypocalcemia can cause tetany
Vitamin E	Possibly hemolysis
Vitamin K (antibiotics, poor diet)	Bleeding
Selenium	Congestive heart failure
Zinc (acrodermatitis enteropathica)	Poor wound healing
Biotin (overeating raw egg whites, which have avidin)	Perioral dermatitis, alopecia, ataxia
Essential fatty acids (too much fish in diet)	Perioral dermatitis, alopecia, ataxia

Items in parentheses in first column indicate etiologies.

4

Hematology

It is always with the best intentions that the worst work is done. —Oscar Wilde

Never cut what you can untie. —Joseph Joubert

ANEMIA

Quick Points
- Remember to take a careful history and perform a through physical examination.
  - Pay special attention to the family history, any history of bleeding, and diet.
  - On the physical, look for lymphadenopathy, hepatosplenomegaly, or any mucosal changes (a smooth tongue suggests megaloblastic anemia).
- Anemia is classified by whether there is decreased production, increased destruction, or splenic pooling. Another method of classification is based on cell size (which is what we commonly use).
- Anemia is defined as a numeric value below the normal range (hemoglobin [Hgb] < 13.5 g/dL in males, Hgb < 12 g/dL in females).
- The symptoms of anemia are usually due to poor oxygen delivery. How severe a patient's symptoms are depend on several factors: comorbidities, severity of anemia, rapidity of development, and how much a patient can compensate.

Initial Management
- If the patient is hemodynamically unstable, support with fluids and blood. Obtain evaluation concurrently and the following will be an overview of the evaluation process.
- *Remember to send off all of the appropriate tests prior to transfusion! A transfusion can wait as long as the patient is reasonably stable!*
- The CBC is the essential test. The first thing to make sure of is whether this process is confined to the erythroid line only. Pay spe-

cial attention to the mean corpuscular volume (MCV) and the mean corpuscular hemoglobin concentration (MCHC). A low MCHC indicates hypochromia, whereas an elevated level indicates the presence of spherocytes. The red cell distribution width (RDW) essentially reflects variation in red cell size (anisocytosis). A high RDW goes along with iron deficiency anemia (IDA). The reticulocyte count reflects production of new red cells. It is commonly expressed as a percentage, which is "uncorrected." It can be "corrected" by adjusting the percentage to a normal erythrocyte count as the denominator (reticulocyte values greater than 100,000 mcL are usually consistent with hemolytic anemia). There are three important values to look at: MCV (low is < 83, high is > 97), reticulocyte count, and WBC and platelet count (is it a pancytopenia?).

- Do not forget to review the blood smear (Table 4–1).

Table 4–1. Secrets of the Peripheral Smear/Bone Marrow

Finding	Condition
Nucleated RBCs	Hypoxia, myelofibrosis, hemorrhage, thalassemia
Teardrop cells	Myelophthisis (infiltration of marrow), thalassemia
Heinz bodies	Glucose-6-phosphate dehydrogenase deficiency
Howell-Jolly bodies	Asplenia
Auer rod	Acute myeloid leukemia
Schistocytes, burr cells, helmet cells	Thrombotic thrombocytopenic purpura, hemolytic-uremic syndrome, microangiopathic hemolysis

Further Discussion

- *Hypoproliferative anemia* is characterized by decreased production. There is decreased production of red cells in the bone marrow and therefore decreased reticulocytosis. Examples are renal failure, anemia of chronic disease, aplastic anemia, and red cell aplasia. Pure red cell aplasia is characterized by a bone marrow with very few erythroid precursors. This anemia can be normocytic or macrocytic and has a low reticulocyte count. No other cell line is affected. Pure red cell aplasia is seen with lymphoproliferative disease, thymoma, collagen vascular disorders, and certain drugs and with parvovirus B19 in sicklers.

- *Impaired hemoglobin synthesis* is seen in IDA, sideroblastic anemia, and other disorders. IDA is microcytic, and the RDW is usually elevated. Symptoms include koilonychia (nail spooning) and pagophagia (ice eating). Serum ferritin is a highly specific marker for IDA. The gold standard for IDA is the bone marrow aspirate. Keep in mind that ferritin is an acute phase reactant and can be elevated in inflammation and liver disease. Remember that a male, at any age, with IDA needs a GI evaluation. Menstruating females do not. Once they become postmenopausal, they require a GI evaluation. Iron deficiency is treated with oral iron. IDA without bleeding implies sprue. Plummer-Vinson (Paterson-Kelly) syndrome is a triad of iron deficiency, esophageal web, and esophageal adenocarcinoma. Bone marrow failure disorders are discussed below.

- *Sideroblastic anemia* may have multiple etiologies. A common cause of transient sideroblastic anemia is alcohol use. It can be due to a rare sex-linked hereditary defect in the first enzyme of hemesynthesis (treat with pyridoxine). The red cells are characteristically nucleated. Iron levels are elevated, with a high iron-binding capacity.

- *Anemia of chronic disease* can range from microcytic (15%) to normocytic. The Hgb is usually > 8, with MCV rarely below 75. In order to label a patient with anemia of chronic disease (ACD), there must be some sort of inflammatory response, and the condition must be chronic (> 1 month). Hyperthyroidism increases MCV. Patients with acquired immunodeficiency syndrome (AIDS), malignancies, or chronic inflammatory disease often have this disorder. These patients have a blunted erythropoietin response and impaired iron release to erythroblasts. Treat the underlying cause. Erythropoietin is an option. Distinguish this disorder from IDA. In ACD, total iron-binding capacity is decreased (vs. IDA).

- Renal failure causes diminished erythropoietin synthesis. These patients may also have other causes of anemia. The treatment is erythropoietin, with oral iron (if the ferritin is low).

- *Macrocytic anemias*:
  - Alcohol abuse and liver disease cause macrocytosis without anemia. Drugs such as zidovudine (AZT) also cause macrocytosis. Hypothyroidism elevates MCV.

- *Megaloblastic anemias* are primarily caused by cobalamin or folate deficiency. Rarer causes are drug effects or inborn errors of metabolism. It is important to identify the underlying disorder causing the vitamin deficiency. On peripheral smear, the characteristic finding is hypersegmented (six or more lobes) nuclei in neutrophils.
- *The first step in evaluation is measuring serum vitamin levels.* The problem is that 10% of elderly people have low cobalamin levels, without evidence of anemia. Approximately 5 to 10% of cobalamin-deficient patients have falsely normal serum cobalamin levels. Both vitamin B_{12} and folate are necessary in order to convert homocysteine to methionine using methionine synthase. Serum methylmalonic acid levels are elevated in B_{12} deficiency, not in folate deficiency. B_{12} deficiency is usually GI in etiology. The Schilling test should be done in B_{12}-deficient patients. Patients with bacterial overgrowth or ileal disease do not "correct" when given intrinsic factor. The most common cause of B_{12} deficiency is pernicious anemia, where there is not enough intrinsic factor secretion. The diagnosis of pernicious anemia can be made by testing for anti-intrinsic factor antibody. A serum gastrin level is also useful since 80% of patients with pernicious anemia have an elevated serum gastrin.
- *Folate deficiency* is usually dietary in origin (rare in B_{12}). Alcoholics are at high risk for folate deficiency. Malabsorption causes about 10% of folate deficiency. Treatment is aimed at repletion and treating the underlying cause if possible.

Hemolytic Anemias

There are several laboratory findings that point toward a hemolytic anemia: elevated reticulocyte count, elevated indirect bilirubin, elevated lactate dehydrogenase (LDH), and low haptoglobin.

- *Immune hemolytic anemia* is characterized by the presence of an antibody that destroys red cells. Patients have a direct Coombs' test, which is positive (antibody is on the cell surface). Approximately 70% of patients have warm autoantibodies (lymphoproliferative disease, systemic lupus erythematosus [SLE], ulcerative colitis [UC]), with 15% having the cold agglutinin syndrome (lymphoproliferative syndromes, *Mycoplasma,* infectious mononucleosis). About 10% of cases are secondary to drugs (third-generation cephalosporins). Hemolysis may improve with treatment of the underlying disease. Corticosteroids are used in patients with warm antibodies. Splenectomy is an alternative if steroids are not effective. Immunosuppressive agents may be of use.

- *Fragmentation hemolysis* includes artificial heart valves or microangiopathic hemolysis.
- Infections by *Babesia*, *Bartonella*, and *Plasmodia* (malaria) cause hemolysis.
- *Coombs' test*. A direct test mixes the patient's RBCs with Coombs' sera (anti-antibodies). If the patient's RBCs are coated, then the test will be positive (as in drug reactions, cold agglutinins, and SLE). An indirect test mixes patient's serum and normal RBCs (and implies autoantibodies).
- *Membrane disorders* include hereditary spherocytosis (high MCHC, no central pallor on smear, hemolysis, and splenomegaly) and hereditary elliptocytosis. Splenectomy is an option.
- *Enzyme disorders* include glucose-6-phosphate dehydrogenase (G6PD) deficiency and pyruvate kinase deficiency. G6PD deficiency is sex linked and can either be a mild chronic hemolysis or acute episodic hemolysis. The hemolysis is usually brought on by an acute illness. The smear contains "bite" cells (not specific) and Heinz bodies. G6PD deficiency is found in 10% of African-American men. In acute crises, deficient cells die, masking diagnosis, so a G6PD test is not done during crises. Patients must avoid certain drugs (sulfa) and exposure to mothballs and dyes. Those with the Mediterranean variant should avoid fava beans.
- *Hemoglobinopathies and thalassemia*:
  - *Sickle cell anemia* is characterized by chronic hemolysis, vascular occlusion (pain crisis), autosplenectomy, and infection. These patients are treated with oxygen, hydration, analgesia, folate, and hydroxyurea (increases the synthesis of HgbF). Bone marrow transplantation (BMT) is experimental.
  - *Thalassemia* is characterized by inadequate synthesis of the globin chains. These patients are microcytic. Beta thalassemia is characterized by an excess of alpha chains. In alpha thalassemia, there is an excess of beta chains. Hemoglobin electrophoresis is normal in alpha thalassemia because alpha globin is found in all of the hemoglobins. Beta thalassemia has an elevated Hgb A_2 and/or HgbF on

electrophoreseis. Heterozygous thalassemia is common in adults; homozygous patients have difficulty surviving to adulthood. The CBC of a patient with thalassemia minor is characterized by a microcytic anemia, high to normal erythrocyte count, and normal RDW.

- One alpha gene deletion is silent, two deletions cause alpha trait (low MCV, normal hemoglobin and hematocrit [H/H]), three deletions cause Hb H (beta tetramers, with low H/H), and four deletions cause hydrops fetalis.

HYPERCOAGULABLE STATES

Quick Points
- The hypercoagulable states consist of a group of prothrombotic disorders associated with an increased risk of thromboembolic events.
- The likelihood of discovering the cause of the hypercoagulable state in patients with a first DVT is 30%. This increases to 50% in patients with recurrent thromboembolic events or a positive family history.
- Many cases are due to stasis or direct vascular injury.

Hereditary Disorders

- All hereditary disorders are associated with venous thrombosis, except for homocysteinemia (also associated with arterial thrombosis).
- *Antithrombin III and protein C and S deficiency.* These are the "natural" anticoagulants, which limit thrombus formation at the site of vascular injury. Approximately 7% of patients with first thrombosis and 20% of patients with recurrent thrombosis have a hereditary defect in one of these factors. Most patients are heterozygotes (50% of factor levels). Homozygotes usually die in utero. These proteins are vitamin K dependent and irreversibly neutralize XIIa, XIa, Xa, and thrombin. There are two types: decreased synthesis of a normal molecule or a functional abnormality. Patients with these disorders and a history of thrombosis need long-term anticoagulation. Acute thrombosis decreases these factors, so you should test for these 2 to 3 months after an acute event.
- *Hereditary resistance to activated protein C (factor V Leiden).* This has been described recently. The etiology is a gene defect in coagulation factor V. This mutation prevents inactivation by protein C. There is a 7% carrier rate in the U.S. Homozygous incidence is 1/1,000.

Diagnostic tests include a plasma assay and polymerase chain reaction (PCR). This hereditary disorder is related to a mild hypercoaguable state. It is found in 20% of patients with first thrombosis and 50% of patients with recurrent thrombosis, especially in pregnancy and with oral contraceptives. It usually causes venous thrombosis (rarely arterial, so MI and CVA are rare). If risk factors are added, thrombosis is more likely. Estrogen use increases the risk for thrombosis with this disorder (35- to 50-fold). Anticoagulation is not indicated unless there is a history of thrombosis.

- *Homocystinemia* is associated with premature atherosclerosis and thrombosis and recurrent venous thrombosis. Increased homocysteine levels in the blood can damage vascular endothelium and promote thrombosis. Approximately 30% of young patients (< age 50) with MI, CVA, and peripheral vascular disease have elevated homocysteine levels. The prevalence of heterozygous disease is 1 in 70 in the general population. This disorder is secondary to an enzyme mutation in methionine remethylation and transsulfuration pathways. There is also a common defect in methylene tetrahydrofolate reductase (MTHFR) and cystathionine β-synthase. Homozygous individuals produce homocystinuria. Diagnosis is made by deoxyribonucleic acid (DNA) testing for MTHFR mutation. Another etiology of this disorder is inadequate dietary folate (this is associated with increased coronary artery disease ([CAD]) in the elderly). Who should be screened is unclear. Patients with premature atherosclerosis or DVT should be investigated. Treatment is folic acid 2 mg/d.
- Prothrombin gene mutation (recently reported) is associated with increased levels of plasma prothrombin and increased rates of venous thromboembolism. This disorder is present in 2% of otherwise healthy people and is associated with acute MI in young females with other risk factors (smoking, hypertension, hyperlipidemias).
- Hereditary dysfibrinogenemia is a rare cause of thrombosis (1%). These patients may need cryoprecipitate (source of fibrinogen) during surgery or after trauma.

Acquired Disorders

- *Antiphospholipid antibody* is associated with venous and arterial thrombosis, autoimmune thrombocytopenia, and fetal loss. There are two antibodies: anticardiolipin and the lupus anticoagulant. Both antibodies recognize protein phospholipid complexes. Common screening tests include "sensitive" activated partial thromboplastin time, Russell's viper venom (for diagnosis), kaolin clotting time (old), and hexagonal phospholipid neutralizing test (for diagnosis). The enzyme-linked immunosorbent assay (ELISA) is the most sensitive and specific for anticardiolipin antibody. Predictors of thrombosis include high antiphospholipid antibody levels, immune thrombocytopenia, Raynaud's disease, livedo reticularis, and a history of thrombosis. The cause of thrombosis is elusive. Patients with thrombosis may have clear evidence of SLE or may have no evidence (except a positive antinuclear antibody [ANA]). Treatment is anticoagulation (keep the international normalized ratio [INR] at 3.0). A catastrophic antiphospholipid syndrome requires IV cyclophosphamide, plasmapheresis, and IV immunoglobin with anticoagulation.

- *Heparin-induced thrombocytopenia* can be induced by full-dose heparin, prophlyaxis, or even heparin flushes. It manifests as a decreased platelet count and arterial and venous thrombosis and is associated with high mortality. The disorder is characterized by immune complex formation, which binds to circulating platelets, activating antibodies and promoting intravascular platelet aggregation. Diagnosis is made by the heparin-induced thrombocytopenia assay. This test is indicated when a patient receiving heparin has an acute drop in platelets (50%) in 24 to 48 hours. Therapy is to stop heparin. Remove all sources of heparin, even heparin-coated catheters. Danaparoid (low molecular weight heparin), hirudin, and argotroban (thrombin inhibitors) are treatments. All patients on heparin require a daily platelet count.

- *Myeloproliferative disorders* (polycythemia vera, essential thrombocytosis) have demonstrated an increased risk of venous and arterial thrombosis (especially the portal and mesenteric system). This can be the presenting system for these disorders. Treatment consists of anticoagulation and hydroxyurea (to decrease platelet counts).

- *Remember to obtain a family history from patients. If a patient has a hypercoagulable state, at least 50% of his or her first-degree relatives have the disorder.*

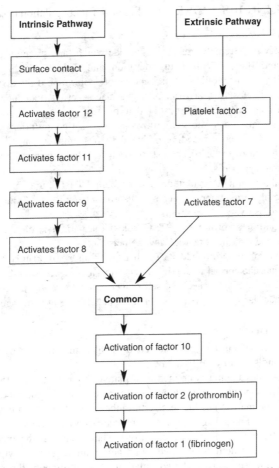

Figure 4–1. Coagulation cascade. Factor 4 = calcium (needed for vitamin K-dependent factors to work); factor 6 does not exist.

BLEEDING DISORDERS (see Fig. 4–1 for coagulation cascade)

Quick Points

- History is extremely important. Include which family member was affected, the site of bleeding, duration, and whether bleeding was localized or generalized. It is important to determine if the disorder is new in onset or has been lifelong. The severity, frequency, and location of the bleeding must be determined.
- Deep hematomas and hemarthrosis suggest a coagulation factor defect. Cutaneous bleeding or bleeding from mucous membranes suggests a disorder of hemostasis. Petechiae and purpura indicate thrombocytopenia.
- Initial screening tests include platelet count, PT/PTT, and fibrinogen. If the history supports a bleeding disorder, then further studies may be necessary.
- Evaluation of prolonged PT. Check if the patient is on warfarin (Coumadin). Check factor 7 level otherwise.
- Evaluation of prolonged PTT. Check PTT after 50:50 mix of the patient's and normal serum (if corrected, this indicates a factor deficiency; if not corrected, check Russell's viper venom time, which if normal indicates factor inhibitor and if abnormal indicates lupus anticoagulant).

Platelet Disorders

Qualitative defects can be assessed by a bleeding time or by a von Willebrand's factor (VWF) assay.

- Thrombocytopenia is defined as a platelet count less than 150,000. This may be due to decreased thrombopoiesis (no megakaryocytes in the bone marrow) or ineffective thrombopoiesis (normal to increased numbers of megakaryocytes in the bone marrow). Platelets can also be redistributed (splenic sequestration). There may also be increased platelet destruction, as is seen with autoimmune thrombocytopenia, disseminated intravascular coagulation (DIC), thrombotic thrombocytopenic purpura (TTP), infection, and mechanical trauma. Gestational thrombocytopenia (as low as 75,000) is benign.
- *Idiopathic thrombocytopenic purpura* (ITP) is a diagnosis of exclusion and is common, especially in young females. This disorder may be associated with underlying systemic disease (HIV, SLE, Hodgkin's).

Patients do not usually bleed until platelet counts are below 10,000. Bleeding is usually cutaneous, and rarely patients die from intracranial hemorrhage. Initial treatment is with corticosteroids in patients with counts less than 30,000 and patients with significant bleeding with counts from 30,000 to 50,000. Sustained remissions with steroids occur in 10 to 20% of patients. The next step is splenectomy. There are various chemotherapeutic regimens used for refractory patients. Platelet transfusions are only reserved for emergency situations. Patients with HIV are usually treated with IV immunoglobulin. Evans's syndrome is characterized by ITP and autoimmune hemolytic anemia.

- *Fragmentation anemia with thrombocytopenia:* Causes include mechanical valves, DIC, TTP, and hemolytic uremic syndrome (HUS). HUS may be due to toxin-producing *Escherichia coli* or *Shigella*. TTP is characterized by high fever, fluctuating mental status, proteinuria, abnormal urine sediment, and, of course, thrombocytopenia. The cause is unknown. Treatment includes plasma exchange and high-dose steroids. There is a 10 to 30% mortality.

- *Qualitative platelet disorders* may either be hereditary or acquired. von Willebrand's disease is common (1/100). Decreased or defective VWF causes a problem with adhesiveness. It is an autosomal-dominant disease (type 1 or 2) or a homozygotic or compound heterozygotic disorder (type 3). There is a severe deficiency in type 3 (< 5%). Type 1 patients have a mild to moderate deficiency of VWF activity. Common lab abnormalities are an increased PTT and bleeding time, but many patients have normal values. Treatment is with desmopressin acetate for types 1 and 2. An intrinsic platelet defect is Glanzmann's thrombasthenia. This is due to a defect in the glycoprotein IIb-IIIa fibrinogen receptor. Acquired defects are more common than hereditary defects. Acquired von Willebrand's disease is seen with B-cell lymphoproliferative disorders, myeloproliferative disorders, and autoimmune disorders. Other examples of acquired platelet disorders are uremia, monoclonal gammopathy, liver disease, and myeloproliferative disorders. Drugs can also affect platelet function.

- Table 4–2 lists diagnostics for bleeding disorders.

Table 4–2. Available Tests to Evaluate Bleeding Disorders

Test	Measured Parameter
Prothrombin time	Extrinsic and common pathway
Partial thromboplastin time	Intrinsic and common pathway
Platelet count	Self-explanatory
Bleeding time	Gross evaluation of platelet function
50:50 mix of patient's plasma with normal plasma	If PT/PTT is correct, this indicates factor deficiency; if there is no correction, then there is circulating anticoagulant
D-Dimer	Elevation implies clot formation, usually in disseminated intravascular coagulation
Thrombin time	Elevation implies presence of heparin or dysfibrinogenemia
Reptilase time (activates fibrinogen directly)	Prolongation implies fibrinogen deficiency or dysfibrinogenemia
Clot-urea solubility	Rapid dissolution of clot in urea implies deficient factor 13 (needed for clot stability)
Russell's viper venom (activates factor 10 directly)	Localizes defect to common pathway (eg, antiphospholipid antibody)

Hereditary Coagulation Disorders

- *Hemophilia* is the classic hereditary coagulation disorder.
- Specific factor assays are necessary to confirm deficiencies of factor VIII (deficiency causes hemophilia A; X-linked recessive), factor IX (deficiency causes hemophilia B or Christmas disease; autosomal recessive), and of other factors (rare).
- Treatment is with replacement of factor (usually recombinant factors given at this time).
- Factor 12 deficiency (Hageman's disease) causes high PTT but no bleeding problems.

Von Willebrand's disease is an autosomal-recessive disease of defective or deficient VWF, which is needed both for platelet aggregation and factor VIII transport in serum. Diagnose with platelet aggregation studies and VWF serum assay; note that factor VIII levels will be level in the presence of von Willebrand's disease. Treatment is with cryoprecipitate (containing VWF, fibrinogen, and factor VIII) or desmopressin (which stimulates the release of VWF from endothelium). Type 1 is a mild synthesis defect (low ristocetin-induced platelet aggregation [RIPA]); type 2a is defective endothelial release and impaired synthesis of large multimers (low RIPA); type 2b or pseudo von Willebrand's disease is due to increased affinity of VWF for platelet glycoprotein Ib, causing hypercoagulability (high RIPA), unlike true von Willebrand's disease; type 3 is total loss of synthesis (no RIPA).

Acquired Coagulation Disorders

- These often involve multiple factor deficiencies and/or thrombocytopenia.
- *Liver failure* results in decreased synthesis of all procoagulants. There may also be thrombocytopenia secondary to splenomegaly.
- *Vitamin K deficiency* is evidenced by a prolonged PT and sometimes a prolonged PTT. Vitamin K is necessary for carboxylation of factors 2, 7, 9, and 10. The result is the lack of γ-carboxyglutamic acid at the amino terminal of these factors. The causes of deficiency are warfarin, malabsorption, and antibiotic therapy. Patients with liver disease will have decreased vitamin K-dependent factors as well as factor V (made in the liver only).
- *Disseminated intravascular coagulation* is associated with infection, obstetric complications, trauma, tissue necrosis, malignancies, and shock. There is excessive thrombin production, causing a consumptive coagulopathy. DIC is characterized by thrombocytopenia, low fibrinogen, and elevated D-dimer. PT/PTT may be prolonged. Treat the cause.
- *Acquired inhibitors* are associated with severe bleeding. Coagulation tests fail to correct completely when normal plasma is added to the patient's plasma. Alloantibody to factor VIII is seen in hemophiliacs who have been transfused with factor VIII (seen in hemophiliacs transfused multiply with factor 8). Spontaneously acquired factor VII inhibitors occur in patients with autoimmune disorders. The majority respond to immunosuppressive therapy. The most common inhibitor of coagulation is the lupus anticoagulant. This results in a prolonged PTT, but there is associated thrombosis.
- *Massive transfusion* is the replacement of more than one blood volume (about 10 units) in 24 hours. Patients often have a coagulopathy and thrombocytopenia. There is no optimal management. Frequent

monitoring of platelet counts, PT/PTT, calcium, and fibrinogen are necessary. Replacement would use these values as guidelines.

TRANSFUSION MEDICINE

Quick Points

- Guidelines for blood transfusion recommend that blood should not be transfused prophylactically, except in those who are critically ill.
- They suggest that the threshold for transfusion should be a Hgb of 7.0 to 8.0 g/dL. It is important to assess for cardiac, pulmonary, or atherosclerotic disease.
- Perioperative transfusion is not recommended for young, healthy patients undergoing elective surgery with a Hgb of 8 to 9 g/dL. For patients at risk for myocardial or cerebral ischemia, a more optimal level may be necessary.
- Patients with chronic anemia have adapted to their low Hgb by a shift in the oxygen dissociation curve. Patients with known cardiac disease and chronic anemia usually do not require transfusion unless they are symptomatic (dyspnea, angina).

Blood Products

See Tables 4–3 and 4–4 for indications and risks.

- *Platelet transfusions* are usually not indicated unless patients are symptomatic or platelets fall below 20,000 (some physicians will use a cutoff of 10,000 or even 5,000 if patients are not infected, febrile, or in DIC). The recommendation for invasive procedures is a platelet count of at least 50,000. Remember that 1 "unit" of platelets is actually equal to 5 units of platelets. We usually use 1 unit for every 10 kg of body weight. This "unit" should increase the platelet count by 50,000. Post-transfusion platelet counts should be drawn within 1 hour (optimal). An adequate increase in platelet count is defined as 30% of the expected increase. Patients are considered "refractory" if they have received three platelet transfusions and are unable to raise their counts. Some patients may be alloimmunized and require human leukocyte antigen (HLA)-matched platelets.
- *Fresh frozen plasma* is used to correct factor deficiencies (eg, thrombin II, III, V, VII, IX, and XI or protein C or S).

Table 4–3. Indications for Blood Products

Product	Indication
Platelets	See text

Fresh frozen plama	Patients who are bleeding or at risk for bleeding with
	    Factor deficiency (see text)
	    Liver disease
	    Vitamin K deficiency
	    Warfarin use
	    Massive blood transfusions
	    Disseminated intravascular coagulation

Cryoprecipitate	von Willebrand's patients who cannot receive desmopressin and/or need acute replacement Fibrinogen-deficiency patients

Cytomegalovirus (CMV)-negative blood products	Prevent CMV infection in
	    Pregnancy
	    Bone marrow, stem cell, or solid-organ transplant
	        patients from CMV-negative donors
	    HIV-positive patients

Gamma-irradiated blood products	Prevent graft-versus-host disease in
	    Bone marrow or stem cell transplant patients
	    Patients on aggressive chemotherapy/radiation
	    Congenital immunodeficiency syndromes

Leukocyte-depleted blood products	Prevention of recurrent febrile, nonhemolytic transfusion reactions

Table 4–4. Risks of a Blood Transfusion

Hepatitis B	1/30,000–1/250,000
Hepatitis C	1/30,000–1/150,000
HIV	1/200,000–1/2,000,000
Acute hemolytic reactions	1/250,000–1/1,000,000
Bacterial contamination	1/500,000 (for RBCs) and 1/12,000 (for platelets)
Delayed hemolytic reactions	1/1,000
Acute lung injury	1/5,000

Transfusion Reactions

- The most common transfusion reaction is a febrile, nonhemolytic reaction. This is usually due to an antibody to donor leukocyte antigens or cytokines. Treat with acetaminophen (Tylenol).
- Fatal acute hemolytic reactions are due to erythrocyte ABO antigen incompatibility. These usually occur secondary to error (blood is given to the wrong patient) and cause intravascular hemolysis (lumbar pain, shock).
- Delayed hemolytic reactions are less severe and are due to an RBC antibody. These patients are Coombs' test positive. Extravascular hemolysis occurs 4 to 13 days post-transfusion.
- Other reactions that are immune mediated include anaphylaxis, urticaria, and noncardiogenic pulmonary edema.
- Patients may become volume overloaded from blood transfusions (think furosemide [Lasix] between your units, especially in patients with CHF).
- Massive transfusions of citrated blood can cause hypocalcemia.
- One complication of chronic transfusion therapy is iron overload. Iron is directly toxic to organs and can cause endocrine, liver, and cardiac dysfunction.

Apheresis

Apheresis is the removal of blood or one of its components from the body. Cytapheresis removes cells. Examples of uses for cytaphoresis include polycythemia vera, erythrocytosis, leukocytosis, and thrombocytosis. Plasmapheresis returns the cells and removes plasma. Table 4–5 shows several disorders where apheresis is indicated.

Table 4–5. Indications for Plasmapheresis

Thrombotic thrombocytopenic purpura

Cryoglobulinemia

Hyperviscosity syndromes

Guillain-Barré syndrome

Eaton-Lambert syndrome

Myasthenia gravis

Goodpasture's syndrome

Graft-versus-Host Disease

Acute graft-versus-host disease (GVHD) causes maculopapular rash (skin), diarrhea (GI), high LFTs, and fever. Chronic GVHD causes scleroderma-like rash, oral ulcers, and high bilirubin.

ACUTE LEUKEMIAS

Acute Myeloid Leukemia

Quick Points
- The median age of patients with acute myeloid leukemia (AML) is about 60. The incidence is equal between the sexes.
- Approximately one-third of patients will present with bruising or hemorrhage. One-quarter of patients will present with a serious infection. One-third of patients will have an elevated WBC count (typically, the absolute neutrophil count is low).
- AML is not limited to the bone marrow and blood. Rarely, patients may develop a granulocytic sarcoma.

Initial Management
- Cytogenetic analysis prior to starting therapy should be performed on all newly diagnosed patients. *The cytogenetic pattern may be the single most important prognostic factor* (see Table 4–6 for classification). The diagnosis of AML is established when 30% or more of all nucleated marrow cells are blast cells.
- The aim of therapy is to eradicate the neoplastic cells and restore normal hematopoiesis. The first step of therapy is remission induction. The two standard drugs are daunorubicin and cytarabine. Complete response rates of up to 80% have been observed in patients under age 20. All patients relapse unless postremission therapy is given. High-dose cytarabine has been used for consolidation therapy.
- Other strategies include intensive chemotherapy with allogeneic BMT (usually in patients younger than age 25). The use of autologous transplant has been tolerated in patients as old as age 60.
- The current recommended treatment for acute promyelocytic leukemia is all-*trans* retinoic acid (ATRA). Complete remission of up to 80% has been reported. Most patients treated with ATRA alone relapse. ATRA is often used sequentially with anthracycline-based

chemotherapy. ATRA can cause a transient increase in WBC, causing pulmonary leukostasis (treat with steroids and leukopheresis).

The French-American-British (FAB) classification has defined eight variants of AML:

- M0—large, agranular myeloblasts (2–3% frequency)
- M1—acute myeloblastic leukemia without maturation (20%)
- M2—acute myeloblastic leukemia with maturation. The translocation is usually associated. These patients have a high rate of remission (25–30%).
- M3 (acute promyelocytic leukemia)—leukemia cells with heavy azurophilic granulation (12%)
- M4—acute myelomonocytic leukemia with abnormal eosinophils (5%)
- M5—acute monoblastic leukemia
- M6—abnormal thrombocytopoiesis
- M7—marrow basophilia and fibrosis
- M2 and M3 have good prognosis; M4 is intermediate; the others are poor.
- Auer rods (cytologic finding) are pathognomonic of AML

Table 4–6. Acute Myeloid Leukemias

Type	Clinical Features	Markers
M0	Bleeding, infection	CD13+ CD33+
M1	Bleeding, infection	
M2	Splenomegaly, chloromas	t(8;21)
M3	Disseminated intravascular coagulation, bimodal age distribution	t(15;17)
M4	Involves gingiva, skin, and central nervous system	inv(16) or t(16;16)
M5	Gum, skin, and central nervous system involvement; hypokalemia	11q rearrangements
M6	Abnormal thrombocytopoiesis	
M7	Marrow basophilia and fibrosis	t(6;9)

Acute Lymphocytic Leukemia

Quick Points

- Acute lymphocytic leukemia (ALL) accounts for 20% of adult acute leukemias.
- Patients experience malaise, lethargy, fever, and night sweats for only a few weeks prior to diagnosis. Infection and hemorrhage are present in one-third of patients at the time of diagnosis. These patients may have lymphadenopathy, splenomegaly, and hepatomegaly (less common in AML). CNS involvement occurs in 5 to 10% of adult cases.

Initial Management

- Once again, there are two major phases of therapy: remission induction and postremission therapy. Vincristine and prednisone form the foundation of almost all ALL induction regimens.
- Approximately 33% of adults have the Philadelphia chromosome (t9;22). These patients are incurable when managed solely by chemotherapy. Allogeneic BMT represents the only possibility for cure.
- CNS prophylaxis is also an integral part of ALL adult treatment (cranial radiation with intrathecal methotrexate).

Further Discussion

The FAB classification divides ALL into three subtypes:

- L1 accounts for over 80% of all ALL in children and 30% in adults. It predominantly consists of small cells (2× diameter of a small lymphocyte).
- L2 accounts for most adult cases. Cells are larger than L1.
- L3 is the least common type. Morphology is identical to the neoplastic cells seen in Burkitt's lymphoma.

Approximately 5% of cases of ALL have the translocation t(4;11). Most of these cases have the L1 or L2 morphology. These patients often have splenomegaly and an elevated WBC count. The L3 morphology is characterized by the 8;14 translocation. These patients have a high rate of CNS involvement. T-cell ALL causes mediastinal masses and CNS disease. Poor prognostic features include t(9;22), t(4;11), and t(8;14).

CHRONIC LEUKEMIAS

Chronic Myelogenous Leukemia

Quick Points

- Chronic myelogenous leukemia (CML) accounts for 15% of all leukemias. It is a clonal disorder involving the pluripotent hematopoietic stem cell. The disease has an increased incidence in those with radiation exposure, but its etiology is unknown.
- The Philadelphia chromosome (t9;22) is the essential feature of CML. This translocation results in a chimeric *BCR-ABL* gene. The Philadelphia chromosome is present in 95% of cases of CML.
- CML is characterized by a chronic and an acute phase. The median age of CML patients is 50 years. Most patients present with fatigue, malaise, headache, weight loss, right upper quadrant fullness, and early satiety. Splenomegaly is common. High WBC, left shift, and basophilia are common.
- Patients in the chronic phase have 20% or less immature myeloid cells in the peripheral blood and 30% less in the bone marrow. Leukocyte alkaline phosphatase (LAP) is absent to low.
- Most patients undergo a gradual transformation from the chronic to the acute phase.
- The acute or blastic phase is characterized by the presence of circulating or marrow myeloblasts of 30% or more. Patients in the blastic phase present with fever, night sweats, weight loss, splenic pain, bone pain, fatigue, easy bruisability, and hepatosplenomegaly. The Hgb is usually < 10, WBC is > 50, platelet is < 100, and LAP is normal to elevated. The blast crisis is usually myeloid (60%). Use cytarabine plus daunorubicin in the blast phase. The median survival rate in this phase is 2 to 4 months.

Initial Management

- Busulfan, interferon-α (IFN-α), and hydroxyurea have been commonly used for chronic-phase patients. Allogeneic BMT has been shown to be curative. The best outcomes with BMT are in patients in the chronic phase, younger than age 30, or in the first year of diagnosis. In patients who are not candidates for BMT, IFN-α is used (which reduces the Philadelphia chromosome, increasing survival). The outlook for patients with acute-phase disease is poor, and they are usually treated with combination chemotherapy.

Further Discussion on Chronic Leukemias

Chronic Lymphocytic Leukemia

See Table 4–7 for staging.

- Chronic lymphocytic leukemia (CLL) accounts for 30% of the leukemias diagnosed in the U.S. Approximately 95% of the cases in the U.S. are B-cell CLL. There is an increased incidence with advanced age, and the disease is more prevalent in males (4:1). The cause of CLL is unknown.
- IgM is the most common surface immunoglobulin expressed in B-cell CLL. The most common cytogenetic abnormality is trisomy 12 (30%).
- *Diagnosis* is often incidental, when an elevated lymphocyte count is found on a routine CBC. Patients may be asymptomatic or have nonspecific symptoms such as fever and malaise. Physical examination may be completely negative or there may be lymphadenopathy, hepatomegaly, and splenomegaly. Most patients will have lymphadenopathy and splenomegaly during the disease.
- *Complications* of CLL include the following:
  - Hypogammaglobulinemia, which occurs in 50% of patients.
  - Impaired T-cell function.

Table 4–7. Rai Classification of CLL

Stage	Signs
0	Lymphocytosis (peripheral blood/bone marrow) only
1	Lymphocytosis and lymphadenopathy
2	Lymphocytosis with hepatomegaly and/or splenomegaly (± lymphadenopathy)
3	Lymphocytosis with anemia (Hgb < 11 g/dL) (± lymphadenopathy, splenomegaly, and/or hepatomegaly)
4	Lymphocytosis with thrombocytopenia (platelet count < 100) (± anemia, lymphadenopathy, splenomegaly, and/or hepatomegaly)

- Acquired autoimmune hemolytic anemia, which occurs in approximately 15% of patients.
- Infections, which complicate the disease in more than 75% of patients. Intravenous Ig can be used for patients with a low IgG or a history of recurrent bacterial infections.

- *Richter's syndrome* describes the evolution of CLL to a large cell lymphoma. Three to 10% of patients will transform. These patients present with fever, weight loss, decreased absolute lymphocyte count, bulky disease, and extranodal involvement.
- The two most important prognostic factors are the lymphocyte doubling time and the pattern of bone marrow infiltration.
- The median survival of CLL patients is approximately 4 to 6 years. Death is usually due to disease progression with infectious or hemorrhagic complications. For patients with low-risk disease (Rai 0), no cytotoxic therapy is recommended. Patients with intermediate disease (Rai I, II) are commonly treated with chlorambucil and prednisone. Patients who are high risk have a median survival of 1.5 years and are commonly treated with monthly chlorambucil and prednisone. Fludarabine is the preferred second-line treatment for stage 3 or 4 CLL, CLL with bulky nodes, or rapid WBC doubling.

Hairy Cell Leukemia

- Hairy cell leukemia (HCL) accounts for 1 to 2% of adult leukemias. Hairy cells must be present in the bone marrow in order to make the diagnosis. Hairy cells are B cells in mid- to late-stage differentiation.
- The bone marrow aspirate is normocellular to hypercellular, with increased reticulin. In more than 50% of cases, the bone marrow cannot be aspirated (dry tap).
- In both myelofibrosis and HCL, there is a dry tap. However, HCL will also cause neutropenia and fried-egg appearance on bone marrow biopsy.
- The median age of disease is the early 50s (ranging from age 20–90). There is a male predominance. Symptoms include weakness, fatigue, and splenic pain. Approximately 70 to 90% of patients have massive splenomegaly. Pancytopenia is present in 50% of cases at the time of diagnosis. Other symptoms include an autoimmune syndrome (25%), and, rarely, patients may present with lytic lesions of the axial skeleton.

- Pancytopenia is present in 50% of cases at the time of diagnosis. Cells contain tartrate-resistant acid phosphatase (TRAP positive).
- Two-thirds of patients suffer from infection. Infection is the major cause of death. One-third of infections are due to gram-negative organisms.
- HCL is a chronic disease. There is no curative treatment. Splenectomy will temporarily improve cytopenias and alleviate symptoms. IFN therapy also has a high response rate and decreases the frequency of infections. Systemic therapy should be used for HCL patients with a hypercellular marrow.

LYMPHOMAS

Non-Hodgkin's Lymphoma

Quick Points
- The average age at time of diagnosis is approximately 42 years.
- Several factors have been associated with the development of non-Hodgkin's lymphoma (NHL):
  - Prior Hodgkin's disease
  - Inherited and acquired immunodeficiency disorders
  - Collagen vascular diseases
  - Occupational and environmental exposure
- The most common presentation of lymphoma is adenopathy. In contrast to patients with Hodgkin's disease, most patients with NHL present with advanced stage III–IV disease. NHL involves unusual sites such as epitrochlear or popliteal nodes or Waldeyer's ring (nasopharynx). Sites that are rarely seen in Hodgkin's disease, but are seen in NHL, include the skin, thyroid, breast, GI tract, brain, ovaries, and testes. NHL often produces B symptoms (unexplained weight loss of > 10% of body weight, unexplained fevers with temperature > 38°C, and night sweats).

Initial Management
- Clinical evaluation should always begin with an H&P. Evaluation for the presence of B symptoms is important. Pay attention to the presence of any skin lesions, adenopathy, liver and spleen size, and the evaluation of Waldeyer's ring.

- Required studies are
  - Blood work: CBC with differential, peripheral smear, LDH, β_2-microglobulin levels, LFTs, renal function, and electrolytes (including calcium and uric acid). LDH and β_2-microglobulin levels correlate with the lymphoma's growth rate and invasive potential.
  - Bone marrow biopsies and aspirates
  - Radiology: CXR (PA + lateral), chest CT if the CXR is abnormal or the patient has pulmonary symptoms), CT scan of abdomen and pelvis, gallium scan (for intermediate to high-grade lymphomas)
  - When designing a plan for a patient with NHL, it is very important to take into account the patient's age, general health, extent of disease, and histologic subtype. Curative surgery is rare and is reserved for the patient with localized extranodal NHL. Surgery alone is never the sole treatment. Most patients should receive chemotherapy with or without radiation. Cyclophosphamide, Oncovin (vincristine), and prednisone (CHOP) are considered the standard for intermediate-grade disease.

Further Discussion

Table 4–8 is the Ann Arbor classification of NHL.

The most commonly used classification system is the Working formulation, sponsored by the National Cancer Institute in 1982. The lymphomas are divided into three prognostic groups:

- *Low grade:* Patients with indolent or low-grade lymphomas have a long history of disease that is slowly progressive over many years and

Table 4–8. Ann Arbor Classification of Non-Hodgkin's Lymphoma

Stage	Involved Area
I	Single lymph node region or extralymphatic site
II	Two or more lymph node regions with or without localized extralymphatic involvement on same side of diaphragm
III	As stage II but on both sides of diaphragm
IV	Disseminated (multiple extralymphatic sites with or without nodal involvement)

is usually asymptomatic. In 5 to 15% of cases, there are temporary "spontaneous remissions." Approximately 15 to 30% of cases convert to a more aggressive lymphoma. This is not related to therapy.

- The most common type is follicular, predominantly small cleaved cell. The common cytogenetic abnormality is the t(14;18) translocation. This involves dysfunction of the *BCL-2* oncogene (a gene that inhibits apoptosis). Approximately 80% of patients have bone marrow involvement (stage IV). For local disease, radiation is the treatment of choice. For patients with widespread disease, equal outcomes have been noted with single-agent chemotherapy, combination chemotherapy, or holding off on therapy until the disease progresses. The median survival is 10 years, and the disease is rarely curable.

- *Intermediate and high grade:* This type is more aggressive and rapidly growing. The B symptoms are more common in patients with aggressive lymphomas (40–50%). The International Index is a prognostic model that delineates clinical features that are independently associated with survival. They include age, LDH, performance status, stage, and number of extranodal sites.

  - The predominant cell type of the intermediate-grade lymphomas is the diffuse large cell type. Often, extranodal sites (GI tract, bone, skin, and brain) are involved. Patients with local disease (stage I/II) are treated with chemotherapy (CHOP) and radiation (70–90% cure rate). Patients with involvement of the paranasal sinuses, bone marrow, epidural area, and testicles have a higher incidence of leptomeningeal involvement. These patients may need prophylactic brain irradiation or intrathecal methotrexate.

  - The diffuse small noncleaved variant is included in the high-grade lymphomas. This tumor is aggressive, with greater than 50% of patients presenting with stage IV disease. All stages are treated with chemotherapy. Another variant is lymphoblastic lymphoma (high-grade T-cell lymphoma), which is common in young men. They present with a mediastinal mass. Burkitt's lymphoma (t 8;14) is also included in this subgroup.

New subtypes of lymphoma have been described, which don't fit into the working classification (eg, mucosa-associated lymphoid tissue lymphomas [MALT], Ki-1 large cell anaplastic lymphoma, and cutaneous T-cell lymphomas [mycosis fungoides and Sézary syndrome]).

Hodgkin's Disease

Quick Points
- The age distribution in Hodgkin's disease is bimodal (20s and 50s). Patients commonly present with cervical or supraclavicular adenopathy.
- Some patients may also experience B symptoms (essentially constitutional symptoms, eg, fever, night sweats, weight loss).
- Excision of the lymph node usually makes the diagnosis.
- The classic finding at pathology is the Reed-Sternberg cell (CD15+ and CD30+).

Initial Management
- Tests required for staging are as follows:
  - CBC, erythrocyte sedimentation rate (ESR), LFTs, LDH
  - CXR, chest CT, CT of abdomen/pelvis
  - Bone marrow biopsy
- Staging laparotomy is controversial. It is the most accurate way to evaluate the spleen. It is usually only done when radiation alone is going to be the treatment plan. If there is abdominal disease, this would alter the treatment.
- Staging is based on the Ann Arbor system (see NHL). Stage is the major predictor of survival. The following is a brief outline of currently used therapy:
  - Stage I, IIA, nonbulky—subtotal nodal irradiation (90% survival) or "mild" chemotherapy with radiation (without laparotomy).
  - Bulky disease (especially the mediastinum) or B symptoms—chemotherapy and extended field radiation.
  - Stage IIIA—combined chemotherapy and radiation.
  - Stage IIIB and IV—chemotherapy. Chemotherapeutic options include Adriamycin (doxorubiun), bleomycin, vinblastine, and daunorubicin (ABVD) (the standard) and alternating mechlorethamine (nitrogen mustard), Oncovine (vincristine), procarbazine, and prednisone (MOPP) and ABVD; MOPP alone is inferior. About 60% of patients with advanced disease are cured.

Further Discussion

- There are several histologic subtypes:
  - Nodular sclerosis (80%)
  - Mixed cellularity
  - Lymphocyte predominant
  - Lymphocyte depleted
- *Poor prognostic indicators* include age > 45 years, B symptoms, bulky mediastinal tumor, liver disease, marrow disease, extranodal involvement, anemia, high ESR, and high LDH. Most relapses are within the first 5 years. Patients relapsing in the first year are treated with high-dose chemotherapy with autologous bone marrow or peripheral blood stem cells.
- *Complications of treatment* include pneumococcal sepsis (after splenectomy). Patients are at increased risk for breast cancer, MI, hypothyroidism, and leg paresthesias (Lhermitte's sign) after mantle radiation. The cumulative incidence of AML with MOPP is 3 to 10%.

MULTIPLE MYELOMA

Quick Points

- Multiple myeloma (MM) is defined as the accumulation of malignant cells in the bone marrow. They usually produce an immunoglobin (monoclonal IgG or IgA).
- It is important to distinguish between MM and monoclonal gammopathy of undetermined significance (MGUS). MGUS is characterized by the presence of monoclonal IgG or IgA in the serum, without the presence of MM. Approximately 16% convert to MM, but it is not possible to predict whom. Close follow-up is necessary.
- There is an increased incidence of MM and MGUS in men, African Americans, and older populations.
- The most common clinical features of MM are
  - Osteolytic lesions (80% of patients) (as this is osteolytic, bone scan is not useful)
  - Anemia
  - Renal insufficiency (a common cause of death in MM)
  - Recurrent bacterial infections (a common cause of death in MM)
- If any of the above clinical features are seen with 10% atypical plasma cells in the bone marrow, light chains in the urine (seen with

renal failure), or serum monoclonal immunoglobins, the diagnosis of MM is high on the differential. Tumor mass is correlated with bone lesions, hypercalcemia, and anemia.
- In the past, myeloma often presented as overt disease. Currently, there is a shift in the presentation to more indolent or localized disease because of incidental detection on routine bloodwork.

Management
- Standard treatment is a combination of melphalan and prednisone. Use of high-dose melphalan with or without total body irradiation and BMT has been associated with a 30 to 40% chance of a dramatic decrease in tumor mass and clinical remission.
- Pamidronate is effective to reduce bone fractures and also seems to improve survival.
- Favorable prognostic indicators are the following:
  - Female sex
  - Low β_2-microglobulin concentration in the serum
  - Normal serum calcium

FURTHER DISCUSSION OF OTHER BONE MARROW DISORDERS

Aplastic Anemia

Quick Points
- Aplastic anemia is not only a disorder of the red cell, it is also a pancytopenia. The anemia can be normocytic or macrocytic.
- Mechanisms of marrow hypocellularity:
  - Direct marrow toxicity causing cell destruction—by chemicals (radiation, benzene) or infections (HIV, Epstein-Barr virus [EBV], TB)
  - Suppression of proliferation and maturation of stem cells—examples are idiopathic or drug induced. These patients may respond to immunosuppressive therapy with return of marrow function.
  - Another cause of aplastic anemia may be Fanconi's anemia. These patients often have a family history of leukemia and anemia.

Management

- A bone marrow aspiration and core biopsy are the key. Classically, the marrow is hypocellular, with a low reticulocyte count and decreased number of cells (fat-cell ratio of 9:1).
- Initial therapy is supportive, with transfusion therapy being the mainstay.
- Transfusions should be minimized and depleted of leukocytes in order to reduce sensitization (and decrease transplant rejection).
- BMT is usually considered in patients under 45 years of age. Transplantation can cure up to 80% of patients younger than 45 years old.
- Patients without a donor and with moderate anemia are treated with antithymocyte globulin and cyclosporine. Approximately 40 to 60% of patients respond within 2 to 3 months.

Paroxysmal Nocturnal Hemoglobinuria

Quick Points

- Paroxysmal nocturnal hemoglobinuria (PNH) is caused by an acquired mutation (*PIG-A* gene) in the stem cell that controls the synthesis of the transmembrane glycosyl phosphatidyl "anchor," which holds together a large number of proteins to blood cells. In PNH, complement inactivating proteins are not present, resulting in no membrane resistance to complements.
- Features include chronic intravascular hemolysis, unexplained abdominal pain, neutropenia, and thrombocytopenia. PNH is seen in 10 to 30% of cases of aplastic anemia. Patients with PNH can look very similar to patients with aplastic anemia.
- Serious complications include infection, renal failure, Budd-Chiari syndrome (hepatic vein thrombosis causing cirrhosis and leg edema), and leukemic transformation (rare).

Management

- The diagnosis of PNH used to be based on a positive Ham's test, which shows increased red cell susceptibility to complement mediated lysis at a low pH. This has largely been replaced by the more sensitive flow cytometry of erythrocyte and leukocytes.
- Treatment is usually supportive (transfusions, anticoagulation) or BMT.

Myelodysplastic Syndromes

Quick Points
- Myelodysplastic syndrome (MDS) presents with symptoms of pancytopenia (clotting abnormalities, anemia, infection).
- It occurs in patients who have received chemotherapy with or without radiation (secondary MDS) or in the elderly (primary MDS).
- In therapy-related MDS, there are often clonal chromosome abnormalities (loss of part or all of chromosomes 5 and 7 or chromosome 11 translocations) with multiple depressed cell lines.
- In the peripheral blood, there are immature myeloid cells with one- or bilobed mature neutrophils (Pelger-Huët) and abnormally shaped red cells.
- These patients do not have splenomegaly.
- The most significant complication of disease is transformation to AML.

Management
- Bone marrow biopsy is needed for diagnosis.
- The amount of blast cells in the marrow at diagnosis determines the severity of the disease.
- Most patients with MDS are treated with supportive measures (ie, granulocyte-macrophage colony-stimulating factor [GM-CSF], granulocyte colony-stimulating factor [G-CSF] and erythropoietin, transfusions, antibiotics).
- The only cure for MDS is bone marrow ablation followed by allogeneic transplantation.

Polycythemia Vera

Quick Points
- The classic patient with polycythemia vera presents with itching after a hot bath or shower.
- Other findings include a history of thrombotic (eg, Budd-Chiari) or hemorrhagic events, elevated H/H, leukocytosis and thrombocytosis, and splenomegaly (60–70% of patients).

- Most complications are from hyperviscosity; usually, the brain, heart, and lungs are at risk. Thrombosis or hemorrhage is common after surgery.
- Approximately 15% of patients will go on to a myelofibrotic or "spent phase." In less than 5% of patients, polycythemia vera transforms into an acute leukemia.

Initial Management
- The key to diagnosis is determining whether the polycythemia is primary or secondary. Erythrocytosis can be secondary to hypoxia (lung disease, right to left cardiac shunts, sleep apnea, hemoglobinopathy, smoking).
- Erythropoietin levels will be low in polycythemia vera and are usually elevated in cases of secondary erythrocytosis. The gold standard is increased in vitro spontaneous growth of erythroid stem cells (burst forming units-erythroid).
- If a patient with polycythemia vera needs surgery, bring hematocrit to < 45% and platelets < 500,000 preoperatively.
- In young patients, phlebotomy is the treatment of choice.
- If the platelet count is very high, it should be lowered (eg, with hydroxyurea).

Idiopathic Myelofibrosis

Quick Points
- Bone marrow is fibrotic, with ineffective extramedullary hematopoiesis.
- Symptoms include anemia, early satiety, splenomegaly, and left upper quadrant pain.
- It is believed that the primary defect in idiopathic myelofibrosis is a clonal stem cell proliferation of the megakaryocyte. The megakaryocyte secretes growth factors that cause a reactive fibrosis in the marrow.

Management
- Nucleated RBCs are present on peripheral blood smear.
- Patients are usually anemic, with other cell lines ranging from high to extremely low.

- Differential diagnosis: secondary fibrosis (occurs in HCL), infections, hyperparathyroidism.
- Treatment is mainly supportive; be wary of iron overload from multiple transfusions.

Essential Thrombocytosis

Quick Points
- This disorder is characterized by a markedly elevated platelet count. Approximately 50% of patients will also have a high WBC (10,000 to 25,000). Patients are often asymptomatic.
- Many cases are detected on routine CBC. Complications are thrombosis and hemorrhage.

Management
- Differentiate from masked polycythemia vera (polycythemia vera with IDA), CML, and reactive thrombocytosis (eg, infection, cancer, inflammation, surgery, hemolysis).
- Diagnosis is based on a sustained platelet count > 250,000 without another etiology. Confirm with a stem cell culture.
- Thrombosis should be treated with anticoagulation.
- Treat erythromelalgia (erythema and pain in the feet and hands from vessel occlusion) with aspirin (ASA).
- Some success has been reported with hydroxyurea (suppresses platelet production), anagrelide (suppresses platelet function), and IFN-α.

BIBLIOGRAPHY

Reviews

Armitage JO. Bone marrow transplantation. N Engl J Med 1994;330:827–38.

Beutler E. G6PD deficiency. Blood 1994;84:3613–36.

Bhatia R, et al. Autologous transplantation therapy for CML. Blood 1997; 89:2623–34.

Bick RL. DIC and related syndromes. Semin Thromb Hemost 1988;14:299–338.

Bordin JO, et al. Biologic effects of leukocytes present in transfused cellular blood products. Blood 1994;84:1703–21.

Bunn HF. Pathogenesis and treatment of sickle cell disease. N Engl J Med 1997;337:762–9.

Cohen AJ, Kessler CM. Treatment of inherited coagulation disorders. Am J Med 1995;99:675–82.

Deeg HJ. Delayed complications and long-term effect after BMT. Hematol Oncol Clin North Am 1990;4:641–57.

De Stefano V, et al. Inherited thrombophilia. Blood 1996;87:3531–44.

Engelfriet CP, et al. Autoimmune hemolytic anemia. Semin Hematol 1992;29:3–12.

Forman SJ. Myelodysplastic syndrome. Curr Opin Hematol 1996;3:297.

George JN, et al. Chronic ITP. N Engl J Med 1994;331:1207–11.

Goodnough LH, et al. Blood transfusion. N Engl J Med 1999;340:438–47.

Goodnough LT, et al. Erythropoietin therapy. N Engl J Med 1997;336:933–8.

Kearon C, Hirsh J. Management of anticoagulation peri-elective surgery. N Engl J Med 1997;336:1506–11.

Lind SE. The bleeding time does not predict surgical bleeding. Blood 1991;77:2547–52.

Lowenberg B, et al. Acute myeloid leukemia. N Engl J Med 1999;341:1051–62.

Mannucci PM. Hemostatic drugs. N Engl J Med 1998;339:245–53.

Messinezy M, Pearson TC. Apparent polycythemia: diagnosis, pathogenesis, and management. Eur J Hematol 1993;51:125–32.

Miller JL. von Willebrand's disease. Hematol Oncol Clin North Am 1990;4:107–28.

Olivieri NF, Brittenham GM. Iron-chelating therapy and the treatment of thalassemia. Blood 1997;89:739–61.

Petz LD. Drug-induced autoimmune hemolytic anemia. Transfus Med Rev 1993;7:242–54.

Pui CH, Evans WE. Acute lymphoblastic leukemia. N Engl J Med 1998;339:605–15.

Rothenberg ME. Eosinophilia. N Engl J Med 1998;338:1601–7.

Sawyers CL. Chronic myelogenous leukemia. N Engl J Med 1999;340:1330–40.

Shapiro SS. The lupus anticoagulant/antiphospholipid syndrome. Ann Rev Med 1996;47:533–53.

Steinberg MH. Management of sickle cell disease. N Engl J Med 1999;340:1021–31.

Tefferi A. Myelofibrosis with myeloid metaplasia. N Engl J Med 2000;342:1255–65.

Toh BH, et al. Pernicious anemia. N Engl J Med 1997;337:1441–8.

Topper AH, Gorson KC. Neuropathies associated with paraproteinemia. N Engl J Med 1998;338:1601–6.

Weitz JI. Low molecular weight heparins. N Engl J Med 1997;337:688–99.

Weller PF, Bubley GJ. The idiopathic hypereosinophilic syndrome. Blood 1994;83:2759–79.

Young NS, Maciejewski J. The pathophysiology of acquired aplastic anemia. N Engl J Med 1997;336:1365–72.

Guidelines

Edwards CQ, Kushner JP. Screening for hemochromatosis. N Engl J Med 1993; 328:1616–20.

Goodnough LT, et al. Indications and guidelines for the use of hematopoietic growth factors. Transfusion 1993;33:944–59.

Moll S, White G. Treatment of the hemophilias. Curr Opin Hematol 1995;2:386–94.

Rintels PB, et al. Therapeutic support of the patient with thrombocytopenia. Hematol Oncol Clin North Am 1994;8:1131–57.

Studies and Trials

Anemias

Carmel R. Prevalence of undiagnosed pernicious anemia in the elderly. Arch Intern Med 1996;156:1097–100. (*A prospective survey in the elderly showed that 2% had undiagnosed pernicious anemia.*)

Charache S, et al. Effect of hydroxyurea on the frequency of painful crises in sickle cell anemia. N Engl J Med 1995;332:1317–22. (*A randomized controlled trial [RCT] of sicklers with frequent recurrences (> 3/year) who had fewer crises and blood transfusions if given hydroxyurea.*)

Platt OS. Mortality in sickle cell disease. N Engl J Med 1994;330:1639–44. (A prospective study that showed that acute chest syndrome, renal failure, seizures, low hemoglobin F, and a baseline WBC > 15,000 were risk factors for early death.)

Rockey DC, Cello JP. Evaluating the GI tract in iron deficiency. N Engl J Med 1993;329:1691–5. (*This prospective study found that iron deficiency was explained by endoscopy in 62%.*)

Serjeant GR, et al. Painful crisis of sickle cell disease. Br J Haematol 1994; 8:586–91. (*A prospective study finding that skin cooling is a common precipitant of crises and that noninfectious fever is frequent even in mild crises.*)

Bleeding Disorders

Hylek E. Acetaminophen and other risks for excessive warfarin anticoagulation. JAMA 1998;279:657–62. (*Regular acetaminophen use [not overdose] increased INR.*)

Rock GA, et al. Comparison of plasma exchange with plasma infusion in the treatment of TTP. N Engl J Med 1991;325:393–7. (*An RCT showing that plasma exchange was superior to plasma infusion for TTP.*)

Bone Marrow Disorders

Hillmen P, et al. Natural history of PNH. N Engl J Med 1995;33:1253–8. (*PNH patients had high rates of thrombosis [39%], death from thrombosis or hemorrhage [58%], aplastic anemia [29%], and spontaneous remission [15%].*)

International Chronic Granulomatous Disease Study Group. A controlled study of IFN-gamma to prevent infections in chronic granulomatous disease. N Engl J Med 1991;324:509–16. (*This RCT showed that IFN-γ effectively reduces infections in chronic granulomatous disease.*)

Negrin RS, et al. Treatment of the anemia of myelodysplastic syndrome using recombinant human G-CSF in combination with erythropoietin. Blood 1993;82:737–43. (*Use of G-CSF with erythropoietin was effective in treating MDS and did not increase rates of acute leukemia.*)

Tichelli A. Late hematological complications in severe aplastic anemia. Br J Haematol 1988;69:413–8. (*Twenty percent of patients who received antilymphocyte globulin developed leukemia or myelodysplasia, whereas none who underwent BMT did.*)

Hypercoagulability Disorders

Khamashta MA, et al. The management of thrombosis in the antiphospholipid-antibody syndrome. N Engl J Med 1995;332:993–7. (*An RCT showing that warfarin therapy targeted for an INR of 3 was more effective than low-intensity warfarin, aspirin, or placebo.*)

Ridker PM, et al. Mutation in the gene coding for coagulation factor V and the risk of MI, stroke, and venous thrombosis in apparently healthy men. N Engl J Med 1995;332:912–7. (*Factor V leiden was found in 6.1% of the subjects in the Physicians' Health Study, and the relative risk of spontaneous DVT was increased by 3.5. In those over 60, the relative risk was increased by 7.0. There was no association with MI or CVA.*)

Schulman S, et al. A comparison of 6 weeks with 6 months of oral anticoagulant therapy after a first episode of venous thromboembolism. N Engl J Med 1995; 332:1661–5. (*An RCT showing that 6 months of therapy is far superior to 6 weeks of anticoagulation for proximal DVTs.*)

Simioni P, et al. The risk of recurrent DVT in patients with factor V leiden. N Engl J Med 1997;336:399–403. (*Factor V leiden doubled the risk of recurrence and was found in one-sixth of unexplained DVTs.*)

Leukemias

Clift RA. Marrow transplantation for CML. Blood 1994;84:2036–43. (*An RCT showing that CML can be cured with high-dose chemotherapy and BMT.*)

Ohnishi K, et al. A randomized trial comparing interferon-alpha with busulfan for newly diagnosed CML in chronic phase. Blood 1995;86:906–16. (*IFN-α prolonged survival relative to busulfan in this RCT.*)

5

Infectious Diseases and Antibiotics

This science is formed slowly, but it preserves every principle which it has acquired. —Joseph Fourier

There are two ways of meeting difficulties: you alter the difficulties or you alter yourself to meet them. —Phyllis Bottome

This chapter is divided into three parts: Common Issues and Entities, Antibiotics, and Finer Points of Clinical Microbiology. The first two are the most pertinent for day-to-day management. The last should be read in your down-time on the floor (when you have nothing else to do), for it is more geared for context and grilling sessions.

COMMON ISSUES AND ENTITIES
See Tables 5–1 and 5–2 for bacterial classification and treatment courses of bacterial infections.

Indications for Precautions
- Airborne (eg, measles, TB)
- Contact: *Clostridium difficile,* methicillin-resistant *Staphylococcus aureus* (MRSA), vancomycin-resistant *Enterococcus*
- Airborne + contact: varicella-zoster virus (VZV) (although contact is an unlikely mode of transmission of VZV)
- Droplet: meningococcus

Vaccines
1. Most people born between 1957 and 1980 need a booster measles vaccine, which you should give as an outpatient. Don't give it if the patient is or is planning to become pregnant, if he or she has an egg allergy, or if he or she is immunocompromised.

2. Everyone should get a flu vaccine, especially those over 65, the immunocompromised, diabetics, patients with multiple comorbidities (especially heart/lung disease), and, drumroll please, you.
3. If you haven't had chickenpox and/or are seronegative for the antibody (85% of those who are negative by history are antibody positive), get the vaccine (coming from personal experience).
4. Remember diphtheria and tetanus boosters every 10 years and basically anytime someone has a dirty skin wound and doesn't remember their tetanus status.

Table 5–1. Classification of Clinically Relevant Bacteria

	Gram Positive	*Gram Negative*
Cocci (spheres)	*Staphylococcus* (clusters) *Streptococcus* (chains) *Stretpococcus pneumoniae* (pneumococcus, lancet-shaped diplococci) *Enterococci* (one of the bacteria in the former *Strep.* group D)	*Neisseria* (diplococci) Gonorrhoeae (gonococcus) Meningitidis (meningococcus)
Bacilli (rods)	*Corynebacterium* *Bacillus*	*Pseudomonas* *Haemophilus* (pleomorphic coccobacillus) *Enterobacteriaceae* Escherichia coli Enterobacter Klebsiella Proteus Serratia Acinetobacter Helicobacter
Anaerobes	*Clostridium* (rod) *Peptostreptococcus* (oral coccus)	*Bacteroides* (rod)

Don't confuse *Enterococcus* (a gram-positive coccus), *Enterobacter* (a gram-negative rod), and *Enterobacteriaceae* (a family of gram-negative rods in the gut).

Pseudomonas, Escherichia coli, Serratia, Citrobacter, Klebsiella, and *Enterobacter* have all been reported to manifest in vitro sensitivity to antibiotics to which they are resistant in vivo.

Table 5–2. Treatment Courses of Bacterial Infections

Infection	Treatment Course
Cellulitis	1 wk
Septicemia	2 wk
Staphylococcal septicemia	3 wk
Septic arthritis	2 wk
Meningitis	2–3 wk
Left endocarditis	4–6 wk
Right endocarditis	4 wk
Urinary tract infection	5–7 days
Pneumonia	10 d to 3 wk (highly variable depending on course)
Upper respiratory infections	1 wk (or none at all)
Osteomyelitis	6 wk
Intra-abdominal abscess	2–4 wk (drainage is critical)

5. Rabies vaccine is needed for animal bites except for rats or squirrels.
6. Travel to endemic areas (eg, Africa) requires appropriate vaccines.
7. Typhoid vaccine is effective.
8. Meningococcal vaccine covers serotypes A, C, Y, and W-135 but not type B, which causes half of the cases of meningococcal meningitis. Give it to those going to sub-Saharan Africa.
9. Cholera vaccine is useless.
10. Japanese B encephalitis vaccine is recommended for travelers going to rural Indochina or Asia for more than a month.
11. *Haemophilus influenzae* type b (Hib) vaccine does not prevent meningitis (which is usually due to nontypable *H. influenzae*).
12. Pneumovax is now 23-valent.

Management of Immunocompromise

Neutropenics

Quick Points
- Traditional neutropenic precautions (reverse isolation) do not affect outcome. Patients with a WBC of 0.0 walk around on the wards at certain hospitals without untoward effect. Neutropenics get infections

from their own flora (gram negatives) and from lines. However, if you have a cold, we recommend that you not cough on these patients.

- The main pathogens are gram-negative rods, *Pseudomonas, Staphylococcus, Streptococcus, Candida*, and *Aspergillus*.
- Avoidance of fresh fruits and vegetables that can't be peeled is probably a good idea.
- Handwashing is essential.
- Panculture fever (although most of these cultures will turn out negative). Be aggressive in ordering diagnostic procedures of suspicious sites (early bronchoscopy of pulmonary infiltrates).

Initial Management

- The traditional antibiotic regimen is double coverage with a broad-spectrum beta-lactam (piperacillin, ticarcillin-clavulate [Timentin]) and aminoglycoside (gentamicin, tobramycin). Some recent studies have shown equivalent results with monotherapy using ceftazidime, cefepime, or imipenem (but there are serious questions about engendering resistance with that approach). If the patient is allergic to penicillin, alternates include vancomycin + ceftazidime, ciprofloxacin, and/or gentamicin. Cover everything, and double cover *Pseudomonas*.
- This is essentially the same approach used for possible sepsis patients.
- If the patient is not responding within 48 hours, add vancomycin (consider it earlier if the patient has a line infection or other risk factors for MRSA or *Enterococcus*).
- If the patient is still febrile after 1 week, consider amphotericin B.
- Ciprofloxacin or trimethoprim-sulfamethoxazole (TMP-SMX) prophylaxis is effective in reducing gram-negative infections in patients with expected duration of neutropenia > 1 week.
- Colony-stimulating factors (G-CSF/GM-CSF) are recommended for prophylaxis in patients with a 40% chance of getting neutropenia (risk is based on the chemotherapy regimen).

B-Cell (Humoral) Dysfunction

Quick Points
- Occurs in asplenic patients (postsplenectomy, CLL, MM).
- Watch out for encapsulated organisms (especially *H. influenzae* and pneumococcus) and traditional pyogenic organisms (*Staph., Strep., Pseudomonas*). IV gammaglobulin may be of benefit, especially in Bruton's agammaglobulinemia.

Initial Management
- Vaccinations (Pneumovax, Hib, meningococcus) are key but unfortunately often don't yield an antibody response.
- Chronic penicillin prophylaxis may be used in splenectomized patients.

See Chapter 17 for more information.

Cellular Dysfunction

This occurs in AIDS, leukemia, Hodgkin's disease, and patients on steroids. Watch out for protozoa (*Pneumocystis carinii* pneumonia [PCP], toxoplasmosis), TB, and viruses (CMV, VZV). See Chapters 4 and 11 for management of these disorders.

Diabetes

Watch out for urinary tract infections (UTIs) (especially with *Candida, Torulopsis*), mucormycosis (rhinocerebral), malignant external otitis (*Pseudomonas*), and cellulitis/osteomyelitis (anaerobes, *Pseudomonas*).

Fever of Unknown Origin

- Pay close attention to H&P, especially travel and animal exposure.
- Differential includes TB, HIV, ehrlichiosis, brucellosis, tularemia, endocarditis, lymphoma, sarcoidosis, Lyme disease, and lupus.
- CT should be done to rule out intra-abdominal abscess.
- A gallium scan can also be done, but it is not commonly helpful in detecting occult sites of infection.

Lymphadenopathy

1. *Characterize by location* (axillary, cervical, inguinal), tender versus nontender, discrete versus matted, mobile versus fixed, acute versus chronic, and texture (firm, hard, or fluctuant).
2. *Lymphadenopathy* occurs in many infections and neoplasias. Cervical nodes are easier to biopsy than groin nodes.
3. *Buboes* (groin) occur with plague, lymphogranuloma venereum (due to *Chlamydia*), and *Calymmatobacterium granulomatis* (granuloma inguinale), also a sexually transmitted disease (STD).
4. Test questions focus on
   - *Cat-scratch disease* (due to *Bartonella henselae*), which presents first as a small papule ~ 5 days after infection at the scratch site. Nodes occur 1 to 8 weeks after the papule (neck, head, and arms; epitrochlear nodes are characteristic). Diagnosis is on biopsy (stellate abscesses, direct visualization of organisms). Treat with tetracycline or erythromycin.
   - *Diphtheria*, which causes cervical nodes, pharyngeal pseudomembrane, and myocarditis.
   - *Kikuchi's disease*, which is characterized by benign cervical nodes and is self-limited.
   - *Castleman's disease*, which is characterized by generalized nodes, hepatosplenomegaly, and anemia; biopsy shows angiofollicular hyperplasia; there is no good treatment.
   - *Kawasaki's disease*, which is characterized by scarlatiniform rash, fever, periungual desquamation, and vasculitis in children; coronary artery aneurysms occur in 25%. ASA and IV gammaglobulin reduce the aneurysm rate.

Skin/Soft-Tissue Infections

Quick Points
1. *Staphylococcus aureus* is a frequent cause of
   - Furuncles (deep-seated necrotic infection of a hair follicle, with fever and constitutional symptoms), requiring drainage.
   - Carbuncles (deep infection of contiguous follicles), requiring surgical drainage.

- Bullous impetigo (perioral crusting and bullae).
- Cellulitis.
- Psoas abscesses (which are seeded hematogenously or from vertebral osteomyelitis).
- Toxic shock syndrome (TSS) (mediated via *Staph.* toxins): an acute, life-threatening complex of fever, hypotension, erythematous rash, desquamation, diarrhea, hypocalcemia, and multiorgan dysfunction. One of the first major outbreaks occurred due to tampon use in menstruating women. With postsurgical toxic shock, any implanted device should be removed immediately (the same goes for tampons). *Staph.* TSS blood cultures are usually negative.
- *Staph.* scalded skin syndrome (termed Ritter's disease in newborns and toxic epidermal necrolysis in adults), which occurs in neonates and patients with renal failure or immunosuppression. It consists of erythematous rash, fever, and sloughing of epidermis (with Nikolsky's sign; see Chapter 17) and bullae. There is a higher mortality rate in adults than children. Treat with antibiotics, fluids, and skin care (such patients are often kept in burn units).

2. *Streptococcus* causes several skin syndromes (usually due to *S. pyogenes*, which mediates its effects through M protein, which helps resist phagocytosis):
- Scarlet fever (due to toxins), which consists of pharyngitis and sandpaper rash (often with Pastia's lines, accentuation of rash in skin folds). Circumoral palor and strawberry tongue also occur.
- Impetigo (usually in children).
- Cellulitis (especially erysipelas, characterized by involvement of legs, cheeks, nose, with erythematous peau d'orange skin that is sharply demarcated).
- Lymphangitis (red streaks that extend proximally along superficial lymphatics).
- Deep infections including necrotizing fasciitis (flesh-eating disease), which can occur even after minor trauma. Symptoms include severe pain (often out of proportion to findings) and fever progressing to numbness, dusky erythema, edema, and shock. Surgery is vital; antibiotics are adjunct.

- Myositis can occur with *Strep.* as well (surgery is essential).
3. Gas gangrene occurs due to *C. perfringens*, which causes aggressive myofasciitis when released after trauma to the GI tract.
4. *Vibrio vulnificus* causes skin infection and hemorrhagic bullae. Risk factors include sea water exposure, alcoholism, and splenectomy. Treat with ceftriaxone or ciprofloxacin.
5. *Pseudomonas* causes hot tub folliculitis and ecthyma gangrenosum (hemorrhagic, necrotic skin lesions that often occur in patients with burns or neutropenia).

Management
- Diagnosis is clinical (aspiration of leading edge is insensitive).
- With group A *Strep.*, remember that skin infections can cause late sequelae of rheumatic fever and glomerulonephritis (whereas strep throat only causes rheumatic fever).
- Antibiotics for *Staph./Strep.* infections include cefazolin (Ancef or Kefzol) 1 g IV q8h or nafcillin 1 to 2 g IV q4h; use vancomycin 1 g IV q12h if methicillin resistance is a concern.
- For necrotizing fasciitis, prompt surgical débridement is vital.
- *Clostridium* treatment: hyperbaric oxygen chamber (controversial) + surgery + antibiotics (penicillin G + clindamycin)
- *Vibrio* treatment: ceftriaxone or ciprofloxacin

Bites

1. *Staph.* and *Strep.* are common.
2. *C. tetani* can occur in any wound contaminated with organic matter (tetanus, also known as lockjaw, presents with diffuse muscular spasm due to neuromuscular toxin).
3. *Pasteurella* occurs in 25% of dog bites and 55% of cat bites. Treat with doxycycline or amoxicillin/clavulanate (Augmentin).
4. Use irrigation and elevation of the affected extremity. Do not suture the wound initially, except in the face, which is highly vascular and needs cosmesis.
5. Tetanus shot is mandatory.
6. Consider rabies vaccine (not needed in rat bites).

7. Human bites:
   - These are the worst of all. They include *Staph., Strep.*, anaerobes, *Eikenella,* and *Haemophilus.*
   - Clenched fist injuries should be referred to a hand surgeon.
   - Consider a baseline x-ray.

Differential of Skeletal Infections and Manifestations

- Septic hip: groin tenderness and pain on passive hip motion; diagnose by aspiration and bone scan.
- Sacroiliac osteomyelitis: buttock pain, pain on hip compression; diagnosis on CT.
- Psoas abscesses: groin tenderness, pain on hip extension, flank and thigh pain (due to femoral nerve compression) (psoas sign). Predisposed by Crohn's disease, renal abscess, sacroiliac/vertebral osteomyelitis. Seen on x-ray or CT.
- Vertebral osteo: localized spine tenderness; pain on straight-leg raising; diagnose on MRI (x-ray shows late changes).

Osteomyelitis

Quick Points
- *Staph.* is the #1 cause.
- In sicklers, *Staph.* is still #1 (*Salmonella* is #2; this is a classic medical student trap).
- If the bone can be probed in a diabetic foot through an ulcer, osteomyelitis is present until proven otherwise. You must take care of neuropathic and vasculopathic contributing factors in diabetics.
- In nail puncture wounds (especially those through tennis shoes), *Pseudomonas* is the classic pathogen.

Management
- X-rays are rarely useful. A bone scan or MRI is needed. Bone scan and x-ray are not good in diabetics.
- Vancomycin is often needed (if you are sure that MRSA is not involved, you can use cefazolin [Ancef]). In diabetics, you need clindamycin and ciprofloxacin to cover anaerobes and *Pseudomonas.*
- For infected prosthetic joints, surgery is required.

Respiratory Infections

Upper: Pharyngitis, Otitis Media, Sinusitis

Quick Points and Management
- *S. pyogenes* is indicated in pharyngitis by a temperature >100°F, tender cervical nodes, and exudative tonsils. Hoarseness goes for viral disease or diphtheria. Give the patient penicillin. Streptococcal pharyngitis causes both rheumatic fever and poststreptococcal glomerulonephitis (PSGN); streptococcal impetigo causes only PSGN.
- Diphtheria (*Corynebacterium*) causes pharyngeal pseudomembrane, sore throat, and fever. Its toxin causes myocarditis, CHF, and polyneuritis. Treat with erythromycin/penicillin and antitoxin (the latter is more important).
- MRSA carriers. Mupirocin (Bactroban) nasal ointment and rifampin can eradicate nasal carriage and diminish transmission.
- *Peptostreptococcus* and *Streptococcus viridans* are responsible for most oral and dental infections. Clindamycin is effective.
- Necrobacillosis. *Fusobacterium* infection causes pharyngitis, progressing to jaw infection, *S. pneumoniae*, internal jugular thrombosis, sepsis, and death.
- For otitis media or sinusitis, the main pathogens are, *H. influenzae,* and *Moraxella*. The mainstays of treatment are cefuroxime 500 mg PO bid, clarithromycin (Biaxin) 500 mg PO bid, and TMP-SMX (Bactrim) 1 tablet PO bid, for 10 to 14 days. Bullous myringitis is due to *Mycoplasma pneumoniae* (macrolide is needed). Perform sinus puncture sinusitis if there is no response after 2 weeks of antibiotics.

Lower: Pneumonia, Tracheobronchitis

See Table 5–3 for the epidemiology of pneumonia.

Quick Points and Management
- *S. pneumoniae* is one of the most common respiratory pathogens, capable of causing pneumonia, otitis, and sinusitis. Meningitis occurs more commonly with concurrent pneumonia than pharyngitis or otitis. Treat with cefuroxime 500 mg PO qid or 750 mg IV q8h.

- *Moraxella* (formerly *Branhamella*) is more prone to occur in the immunodeficient or patients with COPD. Treat with cefuroxime 500 mg PO qid or 750 mg IV q8h.
- *Legionella* can cause pneumonia and is transmitted by aerosol. Like *Mycoplasma pneumoniae*, CXR is worse than an examination. *Legionella* can cause pneumonia, disseminated disease, or Pontiac fever (flu-like illness). Clues are diarrhea or CNS changes prior to or in addition to pneumonia. Treat with erythromycin 500 mg PO qid.
- *Bordetella pertussis* (gram-negative coccobacillus) causes whooping cough, prolonged paroxysmal cough, and lymphocytosis. Treat with erythromycin 500 mq PO qid.

Initial Management

1. For community-acquired pneumonia, the standard has long been cefuroxime (500 mg PO bid or 750 mg IV q8h). Due to resistance, ceftriaxone may be used as first-line treatment depending on specific local sensitivities. Add erythromycin (500 mg PO/IV q6h) if atypicals (*Legionella, Mycoplasma*) are a concern (in young patients, in cases of "walking pneumonia," and in those for whom CXR is much

Table 5–3. Epidemiology of Pneumonia

Group	Pathogens
Infants < 6 mo	Respiratory syncytial virus, *Chlamydia trachomatis*
Children 6 mo–5 yr	*H. influenzae*
Young adults	*Mycoplasma* and *Chlamydia pneumoniae*, *S. pneumoniae*
Elderly	*Legionella, Moraxella, H. influenzae*, Pneumococcus
Neutropenics	*S. pneumoniae, Staphylococcus aureus, Aspergillus*, gram negatives
Asplenia or hypogammaglobulinemia	*S. pneumoniae, H. influenzae*
Nosocomial	Gram negatives, *Staphylococcus aureus*, anaerobes
Aspiration	Anaerobes
Alcoholics	Anaerobes, *Klebsiella pneumoniae*

worse than an examination). For cefuroxime-allergic patients, erythromycin 500 mg PO qid, clarithromycin (Biaxin) 500 mg PO bid, and TMP-SMX (Bactrim) 1 tablet PO bid are alternatives.

2. For high-level pneumococcal resistance and nosocomial pneumonia, use ceftriaxone (1 g IV q12h) instead of cefuroxime.

3. For aspiration pneumonia, use ceftriaxone (1 g IV q12h) and clindamycin (600–900 mg IV q8h).

4. For alcoholics who aspirate, *Klebsiella* is a major concern as well (causes Friedlander's pneumonia [high level of fibrosis]), so use ceftriaxone and clindamycin or ticarcillin-clavulate (Timentin) (1 g IV q8h–q12h, depending on renal failure).

5. *Pneumocystis carinii* pneumonia (PCP) occurs in HIV, Hodgkin's disease, and BMT patients.

6. In terms of duration of IV antibiotics, a patient with pneumonia can be treated as an outpatient if he or she is not toxic, has few or no comorbidities, and is reliable. Once admitted, you do not need a full 2 weeks. As soon as the patient is clinically better and afebrile, and the WBC is coming down, you may switch to po and discontinue.

7. Empyema is an infected pleural effusion accompanied by severe pleuritic pain and chest wall tenderness. The old adage is "Never let the sun rise or set on an empyema."

   • Etiologies include anaerobes, *S. aureus*, TB, group A *Streptococcus*, and *S. pneumoniae*.

   • It is diagnosed on thoracentesis showing gross pus, pH < 7.0, pleural glucose < 50, or positive pleural Gram's stain/culture.

   • Treatment involves drainage with a chest tube and antibiotics.

   • Not all parapneumonic effusions are infected (perform thoracentesis if free fluid separates the lung from the chest wall by more than 1 cm on decubitus CXR, if there are loculations, or as the clinical situation dictates).

   • If loculated, urokinase or streptokinase can be injected to break up loculations, or thoracoscopy can be performed.

Meningitis

Quick Points
- Lumbar puncture (LP) is essential (high protein and low sugar [normal CSF sugar is two-thirds that of serum] implies bacterial etiology; viral meningitis usually has high protein and normal sugar). Send studies for India ink, Gram's stain, culture, and others as indicated.
- *Listeria* risk factors are lymphoma, leukemia, neonates, the elderly, and pregnant women. (For a reason that is unclear, *Listeria* is not seen much in AIDS patients.)
- Meningococcus risk factors are complement or humoral deficiencies. Meningococcemia presents with purpura fulminans, DIC, Waterhouse-Friderichsen syndrome (adrenal hemorrhage), and shock. Because it is easily transmissible, most meningitis patients are in respiratory isolation until it has been ruled out.
- See Table 5–4 for age-based classification.

Table 5–4. Meningitis Etiologies by Age Group

Age Group	Pathogens
Neonates	Group B *Streptococcus* (*agalactiae*) E. coli, Listeria
Young children	*H. influenzae*, meningococcus, *Pneumococcus*
Teenagers/adults	Meningococcus type B, *H. influenzae*, *Pneumococcus*
Elderly	*Pneumococcus*, meningococcus, *Listeria*

Initial Management
- The basic approach is ampicillin and ceftriaxone (ampicillin for *Listeria*, ceftriaxone for the others).
- You can eschew ampicillin in older children and adults.
- Finally, add vancomycin if resistant pneumococcus is a concern. IV should be continued for 2 weeks (you may get the patient a PICC line and discontinue once he or she is stable).

- For *Listeria*, use ampicillin and gentamicin if it is severe (although it doesn't penetrate the CSF well). Use vancomycin/TMP-SMX for penicillin-allergic patients.
- For meningococcus, treat with high-dose IV penicillin G.
- For meningococcal prophylaxis for close contacts, treatment used to be with rifampin; now ciprofloxacin is the mainstay.

Endocarditis

See Table 5–5 for classification of endocarditis and Chapter 12 for further discussion.

Table 5–5. Endocarditis Classification

Type	Pathogens	Risks/Associations	Therapy
Subacute	Viridans, enterococci	Valve/congenital heart disease	Penicillin/ampicillin + gentamicin
Acute	*Staphylococcus, Streptococcus,* enterococci	New-onset congestive heart failure, valve regurgitation	Vancomycin/nafcillin + gentamicin
Early prosthetic (< 2 mo postoperatively)	*S. aureus* and *epidermidis*; *Candida, Aspergillus*		Vancomycin + gentamicin + rifampin Amphotericin B + 5-flucytosine + surgery
Late prosthetic (after 2 mo)	Viridans, enterococci		Penicillin/ampicillin + gentamicin
	S. aureus and epidermidis		Vancomycin + gentamicin + rifampin
Culture negative		Vegetation on echo	Vancomycin + gentamicin
	HACEK	Symptoms > 3 mo	Ceftriaxone
	S. bovis	Gastrointestinal cancer	Penicillin G + gentamicin
	C. septicum		Penicillin G/ tetracycline/ clindamycin

HACEK = *Haemophilus, Actinobacillus, Cardiobacterium, Eikenella,* and *Kingella.*

Quick Points

- Do three sets of cultures in the first 24 hours.
- In subacute endocarditis, hold cultures for 3 to 4 weeks to rule out *Haemophilus, Actinobacillus, Cardiobacterium, Eikenella,* and *Kingella* (HACEK).
- An echocardiogram is essential; TEE is 90% sensitive, whereas transthoracic echocardiogram is only 60 to 80% sensitive.
- TEE is indicated in aortic valve and prosthetic valve endocarditis to detect extension and complications.
- For injection drug users (IDUs), MRSA, *Pseudomonas*, and enterococci are common; right-sided endocarditis is common in IDUs.
- *S. epidermidis* should be treated as a pathogen in patients with prosthetic valves.
- Change or remove any lines that may be involved, especially in those with fungi and gram-negative infections.

Initial Management

1. Vancomycin is the main alternative to penicillin/nafcillin in patients with gram-positive organisms (*Staph., Strep.,* viridans, enterococci).
2. Consider avoiding aminoglycosides in the elderly and those with ear or renal disease; you can stop after a few days in endocarditis anyway.
3. Injection drug users with right-sided endocarditis can have a shorter course of antibiotics (only 2 weeks).
4. Antibiotics can be given on an outpatient basis (portable pumps, PICC lines).
5. Have follow-up blood cultures in 5 to 7 days to look for persistent bacteremia.
6. You must remove the Hickmann/Broviac and central lines for fungus, *Pseudomonas*, and vancomycin-resistant enterococcus (VRE).
7. Indications for surgery are as follows:
   - Refractory CHF
   - Uncontrolled infection
   - More than one serious systemic embolic event (eg, stroke)
   - Severe valve dysfunction (especially aortic regurgitation) or local extension (quantitated by echocardiogram)
   - Mycotic aneurysms

- Most prosthetic valve endocarditis
- Candidal endocarditis
- Pseudomonal endocarditis

Prophylaxis

- Given to patients with a history of endocarditis or structural heart disease (left valve insufficiency or regurgitation, mital valve proplapse [MVP], idiopathic hypertrophic subaortic stenosis, aortic coarctation).
- Given for dental procedures, cystoscopy, drainage of abscesses, procedures breaking mucosa.
- Not needed for bronchoscopy, cesarean section, or vaginal delivery.
- Give 1 hour before the procedure and no longer than 6 hours later.
- If the patient had rheumatic fever and is already getting long-term penicillin, give clindamycin as prophylaxis for procedure.

Myocarditis

This is usually due to coxsackie group B (there is no good treatment). Endomyocardial biopsy is needed to

- Monitor allograft rejection;
- Assess toxicity from doxorubicin, daunorubicin, or idarubicin; or
- Rule out trypanosomiasis (Chagas' disease) or trichinosis.

Corynebacterium diphtheriae causes cardiac failure secondary to diphtheria toxin; antibiotics do not prevent cardiac disease. Management is supportive care.

Rheumatic fever (due to group A *Strep.*) can cause carditis, with subsequent mitral stenosis and CHF. Diagnosis is by Jones criteria (Table 5–6) and requires evidence of preceding streptococcal infection (eg, cul-

Table 5–6. Jones Criteria for Rheumatic Fever

Major	Minor
Carditis	Arthralgia
Erythema marginatum	Fever
Migratory polyarthritis	Prolonged P-R interval on EKG
Subcutaneous nodules	Rising C-reactive protein
Sydenham's chorea	

ture, rising antistreptolysin O titer, rapid antigen test) plus either two major Jones criteria or one major and two minor Jones criteria.

Treat acute rheumatic fever with oral penicillin V 500 mg PO bid for 10 days, followed by benzathine penicillin 1.2 million U IM monthly indefinitely. Salicylates (up to 2 g qid) are useful for arthritis, whereas both NSAIDs and steroids benefit severe carditis.

Gastroenteritis

1. *Bacillus cereus* causes gastroenteritis, as can *Staph.*, both by way of toxins. Treat with clindamycin or vancomycin.

2. Botulism (due to *C. botulinum*) also occurs classically after eating spoiled canned food; botulin is the most potent toxin. Therapy revolves around antitoxin more than antibiotics.

3. *Salmonella* typhoid fever is usually from contaminated water. Risk factors include gallstones, sickle cell anemia, and asplenic patients. It causes fever, leukopenia, and rose spots (1 week after fever). Ciprofloxacin or TMP-SMX are mainstays; ampicillin and chloramphenicol are alternatives. If you give ampicillin, give probenecid as well to decrease clearance of ampicillin. *Salmonella* are often spread by poultry, eggs, turtles, pets younger than 6 months, and Caesar salad dressing. Nontyphi *Salmonella* cause diarrhea.

4. Cholera is secretory diarrhea (toxin blocks cyclic adenosine monophosphate [cAMP]), whereas viral diarrhea is osmotic (usually affects epithelium).

5. Cholera and travelers' diarrhea (enterotoxic *E. coli*) are not invasive bacteria; enteroinvasive *E. coli*, *Shigella*, *Salmonella*, *Campylobacter*, and *Yersinia* are enteroinvasive, causing bloody diarrhea.

6. Note that *Shigella* is the most potent (only 10 bacteria are needed to cause disease).

7. *Campylobacter* is associated with subsequent Guillain-Barré syndrome.

8. For travelers' diarrhea, ciprofloxacin and TMP-SMX are effective.

Sexually Transmitted Diseases

General

- Screen young, sexually active men and women.
- For men, Gram's stain of urethral discharge is the best test for gonorrhea (95% sensitive, 98% specific).

- For women with urethral discharge, a culture and DNA probe are needed.
- Because of co-infection, anyone with gonorrhea (a gram-negative diplococcus) should be treated for chlamydia and vice versa.
- Treat with ceftriaxone 1 g IM × 1 + doxycycline 100 BID × 1 week; the alternative is a single dose of azithromycin (Zithromax) (2 g PO), which ensures compliance.

Pelvic Inflammatory Disease

Quick Points
- Infertility after the first episode of pelvic inflammatory disease (PID) is 10%, which doubles after each additional episode; long-term sequelae (eg, ectopic pregnancy, chronic pain) occur in 25%.
- Risk factors for PID are youth, promiscuity, and intrauterine devices (IUDs). PID occurs in one-eighth of sexually active teenagers.
- Signs and Symptoms:
  - Chronic lower abdominal pain ranging to acute peritonitis, adnexal tenderness, and cervical motion tenderness
  - Pustules and arthralgia in young women indicate gonorrhea (disseminated gonorrheal infection) until proven otherwise.
  - Pyuria and dysuria without bacteriuria in young women imply chlamydia.
  - *Fitz-Hugh-Curtis syndrome:* perihepatitis (peritoneal violin-string adhesions and increased LFTs) due to PID (usually due to gonorrhea, sometimes chlamydia)

Initial Management
- Clinical sensitivity is only 65%, so the threshold for empiric treatment should be low.
- For outpatients, use ceftriaxone 250 mg IM × 1 and then doxycycline 100 mg bid × 2 weeks.
- Hospitalize for uncertain diagnosis, possible abscess or peritonitis, vomiting, if the patient has HIV or is pregnant, and poor compliance (eg, adolescents).
- For inpatients, use cefoxitin + doxycycline or clindamycin + gentamicin. Partners must be treated.

Genital Herpes

Counsel patients to use condoms at all times and to abstain during recurrences to minimize transmission. Transmission during birth is high (33–50%) in the first episodes and low (3%) in patients with a history. Acyclovir is given for the first episodes and severe recurrences. Use long-term suppression for those with frequent recurrences; famciclovir (Famvir) and valacyclovir (Valtrex) are easier to use because a less frequent dosing is needed. For resistant viruses (fairly common in HIV patients), use foscarnet or cidofovir.

Syphilis *(due to* **Treponema pallidum***)*

Quick Points
- Stages:
  - Primary—painless chancre and regional nodes. Chancre resolves in 2 to 6 weeks.
  - Secondary—rash (centrifugal), generalized nodes. Lasts for 3 to 12 weeks and then goes into latency.
  - Tertiary—occurs in one-third of untreated cases. The main targets are the CNS and aorta.
- In the CNS, the patient can get tabes dorsalis (demyelination of posterior columns leading to loss of proprioception, causing broad-based gait, footdrop, and Romberg's sign) and chronic dementia/meningitis.
- Aortitis leads to aneurysms of the aortic arch (always rule out syphilis and Marfan syndrome when the ascending aorta has an aneurym; syphilitic aneuryms do not dissect due to infarction of vasa vasorum, unlike aneuryms due to cystic medial necrosis).
- Gummas (granulomas of various size) occur in any organ, especially the skin and skeleton. In the genital area, they are condyloma lata.
- Transmission to a newborn causes snuffles (rhinitis) and Hutchinson's teeth (notched, widely spaced, peg-like upper incisors), among other things.
- Diagnosis: screen by venereal disease reactive laboratory/reactive plasma reagin (VDRL/RPR) and confirm with fluorescent-treponemal antigen (antibodies) (FTA-Abs).
  - FTA-Abs, once positive, will always be positive.
  - VDRL will decline with therapy and time.

Initial Management
- Treat with penicillin (*Treponema* is exquisitely sensitive).
- A demented patient with positive CSF VDRL should be treated as having tertiary syphilis (CSF FTA-Abs is very insensitive and unnecessary).
- Patients with latent syphilis with positive LP should receive daily procaine penicillin 1.2 million U IM.
- Patients with latent syphilis with negative LP should receive benzathine penicillin 1.2 million U every month.

Chancroid

Chancroid is caused by *H. ducreyi* (causes painful ulcer—different from syphilis). Treat with ceftriaxone or erythromycin.

Human Papilloma Virus

Types 6 and 11 cause most condylomata acuminatum. Types 16 and 18 cause 80% of cervical cancer, as well as anal and penile cancer. Recurrence is 25% at 3 months with any therapy (laser, cryotherapy).

Genitourinary Tract

Quick Points
- *S. saprophyticus* causes UTIs in young women
- *S. agalactiae* causes UTIs in pregnant women, postpartum endometritis, and bacteremia.
- Enterococci cause UTIs and often cause sepsis after TURP. BPH increases *Enterococcus* infection.

Initial Management
1. Includes ampicillin 500 mg PO bid, TMP-SMX 1 tablet PO bid, and ciprofloxacin 500 mg PO bid. Three-day courses are effective for uncomplicated UTIs.
2. TMP-SMX penetrates the prostate very well.
3. For pyelonephritis (WBC casts in urine, CVA tenderness, fever), use ciprofloxacin for at least 10 days.

ANTIBIOTICS

Sulfonamides were the first antibiotics in modern times. Made by the Germans, they are bacteriostatic agents and are seldom used now, except in combination (Bactrim/Septra = trimethoprim-sulfamethoxazole [used for PCP]; Fansidar = pyrimethamine-sulfadoxine [used for toxoplasmosis]) or in the eye (Bleph-10 = sulfacetamide; used for conjunctivitis and blepharitis).

Penicillins, Relatives, and Cephalosporins

Penicillins

To counter the German monopoly on antibiotics (which would have been a strategic advantage in World War II), the Briton Alexander Fleming developed, as we all know, penicillin, a cell-wall bacteriocidal antibiotic. Due to resistance, its indications are now fairly limited:

- Syphilis
- Actinomycosis
- Penicillin-sensitive *S. Pneumoniae*
- *S. pyogenes* pharyngitis
- Known meningococcal meningitis
- Penicillin prophylaxis for dental procedures in patients with splenectomy, rheumatic heart disease, and sickle cell anemia

Penicillin G is parenteral; penicillin V is oral. Procaine and benzathine penicillin are long-acting (1 week and 1 month, respectively). The main toxicities are allergy, interstitial nephritis, and seizures (the latter at extremely high doses).

However, the penicillin family is vast and highly effective. The following are a few that you will see in common practice. The development of the penicillins has essentially paralleled the development of bacterial resistance.

Amoxicillin and ampicillin were the first two penicillins developed for wide use. They are fairly broad spectrum, with some activity against gram-positive and gram-negative and some anaerobic organisms. They have similar activity spectrums. The only difference is that ampicillin is sometimes used for *Salmonella* (in which case, it can lead to a carrier state) and for UTIs. Ampicillin can be given intravenously or orally (whereas amoxicillin is only oral). Ampicillin is a mainstay against *Enterococcus* UTIs. Ampicillin/amoxicillin + allopurinol cause increased rash. Ampicillin decreases atenolol's absorption.

Due to beta-lactamase development by bacteria, beta-lactamase inhibitors were developed. Sulbactam combined with ampicillin is Unasyn (IV only), whereas clavulanic acid combined with amoxicillin is Augmentin (PO only). Unasyn is often used for cholecystitis, whereas

Augmentin is commonly used for pharyngitis/otitis and as the oral antibiotic that is switched to after a ticarcillin-clavulanate (Timentin) course. Augmentin often causes a lot of diarrhea.

For gram positives that were resistant to the above extended-spectrum penicillins, methicillin (IV) and oxacillin (PO/IV) were developed. Newer agents with similar properties are nafcillin (IV) and dicloxacillin (PO), which have better side-effect profiles than their older counterparts. They are exclusively gram-positive agents, with activity against just about only *Staph.* and *Strep.* They are quite effective as long as the organism is not methicillin resistant (in which case, you would need to use vancomycin; see below). Dicloxacillin antagonizes warfarin.

Broad-spectrum penicillins include ticarcillin, piperacillin, and mezlocillin. These have excellent activity against most organisms, including *Pseudomonas* and anaerobes. Ticarcillin combined with clavulanic acid is Timentin, and piperacillin combined with tazabactam is Zosyn. Different institutions use each of these differently: some hospitals are ticarcillin-clavulanate hospitals, whereas others are piperacillin or mezlocillin hospitals. These agents do not cover methicillin-resistant organisms and are of limited use against *Enterococcus.* They should also not be used singly against *Pseudomonas.* Watch out for the high salt load of ticarcillin-clavulanate in CHF patients.

Penicillin Relatives

Compounds related to penicillin include imipenem and meropenem of the carbapenem family and aztreonam, a monobactam. The carbapenems are extremely powerful antibiotics and can resist most beta-lactamases. In fact, imipenem's nickname is "Gorillacillin." Points to remember include that imipenem always comes in combination with cilastatin, which blocks renal dihydropeptidase (which would otherwise metabolize imipenem). Again, don't use imipenem alone against *Pseudomonas*; remember also that it is only static against *Enterococcus* and not active against MRSA. Meropenem, which is newer, has the advantages of causing fewer seizures, being more active against *Pseudomonas*, and not needing cilastatin.

Aztreonam, which is active only against gram-negative aerobes, is used mainly in the context of penicillin allergy. It is highly unlikely for patients to be allergic to aztreonam. Aztreonam can synergize with ciprofloxacin against *Pseudomonas* but has no synergy with other beta-lactams.

Cephalosporins

Like penicillins, these are cell-wall agents. There are so many of these that one is tempted to throw one's hands up when trying to learn them. In fact, lecturers have often made up fake cephalosporin names that their audiences did not know were fake. Below are listed just those seven or eight in common use.

First generation. This group is just against gram positives, especially *Staph.* and *Strep.* The main agents here are cephalexin (Keflex, PO) and cefazolin (Kefzol/Ancef, IV). They are used principally for skin coverage (are commonly used to provide coverage for clean surgical wounds). They do not enter the CSF.

Second generation. This is first generation + coverage against *H. influenzae, Neisseria,* and *Moraxella.* The main agent here is cefuroxime (Zinacef/Kefurox IV, Ceftin, PO). Cefuroxime has become the workhorse for community-acquired pneumonia, covering *S. pneumoniae*, *H. influenzae*, and *Moraxella.* Cefaclor (Ceclor) is often used for children with otitis media.

Second generation + anaerobic coverage. This is self-explanatory. Cefoxitin is the principal agent; cefotetan is also in this group but has side effects (see below). The arena for use is bowel surgery (skin, some gram negatives, anaerobes).

Third generation. This group basically covers gram negatives. Ceftriaxone is the main agent here. Its indications include nosocomial pneumonia, community pneumonia in areas of high penicillin-resistant pneumococcus, gonorrhea, and sepsis. It can cause intrahepatic cholestasis. Cefotaxime is used mostly in pediatric meningitis cases. Although some may tell you that ceftriaxone covers gram-positives as well, it is not really useful or indicated in those infections.

Third generation + Pseudomonas. This is self-explanatory. Ceftazidime is the main agent here.

Fourth generation. Cefepime is the latest addition to the family. It covers third generation + *Staph.* and *Strep.*

Notes

1. There is at least a 10% cross-reactivity of cephalosporins with penicillin allergy. Thus, the consensus is to use them in these patients except in cases of known anaphylaxis of the patient to penicillins.

2. Some cephalosporins have an *N*-methylthiotetrazolium (NMTT; the name's not important) side chain. This NMTT causes two toxicities: first, an increase in PT (by blocking vitamin K metabolism), and, second, a disulfiram-like reaction on exposure to alcohol. As such, most of these have been taken off the market or out of common use. The only widely used NMTT cephalosporin is cefotetan (this is ironic, as one would think that surgeons would not want to raise the PT of their patients). Other cephalosporins with NMTT include cefamandole, cefmetazole, and cefaperazone.

Aminoglycosides

This family targets gram-negative aerobes by attacking their ribosomes. They can also be used against *Mycobacteria* or *Staph.* in synergy with other antibiotics. Toxicities are to the kidneys and ears. The renal toxicity of aminoglycosides is increased by vancomycin, amphotericin, NSAIDs, cyclosporine, contrast, and furosemide. Levels must be monitored in general, and doses need to be adjusted for renal failure. Once-daily dosing is coming into favor for all uses except endocarditis and neutropenic fever. Once-daily dosing is done by injecting 5 to 7 mg/kg, checking the level at 6 to 14 hours, and then adjusting the frequency (not the dose) to q24h, q36h, or q48h, based on the graph below (Figure 5–1). Note that renal function does not enter this process at all.

Development of aminoglycosides, like other antibiotic families, has been a battle against ever-increasing bacterial resistance. In order of entry, the aminoglycosides are streptomycin, kanamycin, gentamicin, tobramycin, amikacin, and netilmicin. The first two are generally not used much anymore except for second-line treatment against TB. Gentamicin and tobramycin are the workhorses. Tobramycin can be used as an ophthalmic ointment. Amikacin and netilmicin are reserved for highly resistant organisms.

Macrolides

Erythromycin is the prototype. This bacteriostatic family targets bacterial ribosomes as well. Erythromycin use is now generally as a back-up for

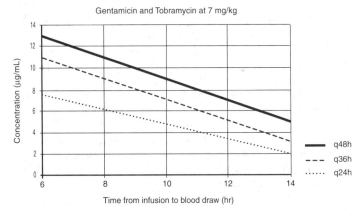

Figure 5–1. Nomogram: once-daily dosing.

patients who are allergic to penicillin, in bacterial conjunctivitis, and against atypical pneumonia (*Legionella, Chlamydia, Mycoplasma*). Toxicity is generally mild, with GI upset as the principal problem. However, interactions with earlier antihistamines (terfenadine [Seldane] and astemizole [Hismanal]) cause torsades de pointes by prolonging the QT. This eventually led to Seldane being pulled off the market. Erythromycin also has a lot of interactions with other drugs, as it is metabolized in the P-450 system (eg, it increases theophylline and carbamazepine [Tegretol]). IV erythromycin causes reversible deafness.

The new macrolides clarithromycin (Biaxin) and azithromycin (Zithromax) have a broad spectrum. Clarithromycin can be used as a single agent for mild community-acquired pneumonia. Both also work against *Mycobacterium avium-intracellulare* complex (MAC). Azithromycin also works against *H. influenzae*, gonococcus, and *Chlamydia*. The advantage of azithromycin is that it can be given every week for MAC and as a single dose for many STDs (see above). These new agents also cause less GI toxicity.

Quinolones

This highly effective, generally safe, bacteriocidal class targets gram-negative aerobes by inhibiting bacterial DNA gyrase. Ciprofloxacin is the prototype. Quinolones also have excellent GI absorption and hence should be given enterally unless the gut is malfunctioning. The newer agents (levofloxacin, sparfloxicin, trovafloxacin) are broad-spectrum agents (gram positives and anaerobes), and their proper niches are still being defined. Antacids (aluminum, magnesium), iron, and sucralfate reduce the absorption of quinolones.

Toxicities

- There are interactions with other drugs that are metabolized by P-450 (eg, ciprofloxacin increases theophylline).
- They are bad for pregnant women and children (they block fetal development and children's cartilage formation).
- They cause photosensitivity.
- Trovafloxacin is hepatotoxic.

Miscellaneous Antibiotics

Tetracycline, a static agent, has limited uses (basically against weird bugs, *Chlamydia, Rickettsia*). It is perhaps more important to remember its toxicity of causing bluish tooth discoloration when used in children or in pregnant women (the teeth of the baby are affected, not the mother). Antacids (aluminum, magnesium), iron, and sucralfate reduce its absorption. Tetracycline may have activity against VRE and MRSA. It causes photosensitivity and increases digoxin.

Clindamycin, also static, works only against gram positives and anaerobes. It is ironic that its use often leads to colitis from *C. difficile* (a gram-positive anaerobe). Metronidazole (Flagyl) is used against anaerobes as well and certain protozoa (*Trichomonas, Entamoeba, Gardnerella*). It is accepted that patients with anaerobic infections above the diaphragm (tooth infections, aspiration pneumonia) should receive clindamycin, and those with infections below the diaphragm (abdomen) should receive metronidazole. Metronidazole causes a metallic taste, increases warfarin, and causes a disulfiram-like reaction if alcohol is ingested. Phenytoin and barbiturates decrease metronidazole.

Chloramphenicol is highly effective. However, its toxicities of gray baby syndrome and aplastic anemia (both of which are very rare) have banished it to the netherworld of treating strange bugs (*Rickettsia* and company).

Vancomycin is the big gun, the gold standard, for gram-positive infections (*Staph., Strep.*, etc). Toxicities are to the ear and kidney. Vancomycin frequently causes red man syndrome (erythema of the face and neck), which is not a true allergy. All that needs to be done is to slow the infusion rate (it is probably a good idea to order vancomycin infusion over 1 hour). Diphenhydramine can also be used for symptomatic relief. Since vancomycin resistance in a pathogen like *Staph.* would be a very bad thing, use vancomycin sparingly, only if there is proven or strongly suspected methicillin resistance (eg, lines, severe or nonresponding infections).

The combination of TMP and SMX (Bactrim, Septra) is very useful. Both elements block different steps in bacterial folate metabolism and hence the synergy that arises from the combination. It is quite effective for a variety of gram-positive and gram-negative agents. Its primary indications are for community-acquired pneumonia, UTI, and protozoal infections (especially PCP and toxoplasmosis). TMP-SMX has some activity against MRSA. Trimethoprim causes hyperkalemia (it is a potassium-sparing diuretic). TMP-SMX increases warfarin, phenytoin, and sulfonylureas and lowers cyclosporine. It can cause renal failure through interstitial nephritis; however, a simple rise in creatinine without a corresponding rise in blood urea nitrogen (BUN) is just an artifact of TMP-SMX competing with creatinine for secretion (ie, the glomerular filtration rate is unaffected in such a scenario and is thus okay). The other main toxicity of TMP-SMX is allergy (very common in AIDS patients). It can also cause Stevens-Johnson syndrome (erythema multiforme major, with erosion of multiple mucous membranes).

Synercid (quinupristin-dalfopristin) (streptogramin class) and teicoplanin may be good against VRE and VRSA. Synercid was recently approved by the U.S. Food and Drug Administration (FDA) (fall 1999). Zyvox (linezolid) was approved in April 2000 for efficacy against VRE; it can cause thrombocytopenia.

FINER POINTS OF CLINICAL MICROBIOLOGY

Bacteriology

The meat of bacteriology has been covered in the Common Entities section. What follows is a combination of appetizer and frosting.

Lyme Disease

Quick Points and Management
- Lyme disease is caused by *Borrelia burgdorferi*. The vector is the *Ixodes* tick.
- There are three stages of Lyme disease:
  1. Early: erythema chronicum migrans (bull's eye rash); spirochetemia
  2. Middle: cardiac involvement (atrioventricular block, mild pericarditis, mild CHF), syncope, neurologic symptoms (lymphocytic meningitis, multifocal radiculoneuritis, facial palsy)
  3. Late: arthritis (large joints, mono- or oligoarticular), chronic neurologic changes, acrodermatitis chronica atrophicans
- Diagnosis: ELISA serology, confirmed by Western blot, or PCR
- The management of Lyme disease is shown in Table 5–7.

Table 5–7. Management of Lyme Disease

Early disease	Doxycycline 100 mg PO bid × 3 wk
Facial palsy	Doxycycline 100 mg PO bid × 3 wk
Other neurologic disease	Penicillin G 20 million U daily
First-degree atrioventricular block	Doxycycline 100 mg PO bid × 3 wk
Other cardiac disease	Ceftriaxone 1 g IV q12h × 2–4 wk
Arthritis	Doxycycline 100 mg PO bid × 1 mo

Other Spirochetes

1. *Borrelia recurrentis* causes relapsing fever.
2. *Treponema pallidum* causes syphilis (see the STD section above). Nonvenereal treponemal diseases include yaws, pinta, and bejel (found mostly in the Third World).
3. Leptospirosis is transmitted by water and infected animals and causes aseptic meningitis and Weil's syndrome (hepatitis, renal failure, and hemorrhage). Note that the bilis are increased out of proportion to other LFTs. Treat with penicillin/doxycycline.

Acid-Fast Bacteria (Stained by Ziehl-Neelsen)

- *Mycobacterium* is a large and nefarious genus.
- TB will be discussed in Chapter 7. Note that disseminated TB can masquerade as almost any organ pathology. Questions on Pott's disease (vertebral TB osteomyelitis) are frequently asked on tests and rounds. Extrapulmonary TB should be considered when there are neutrophils and monocytes but no growth on culture (eg, sterile pyuria, CSF with polymorphonuclear neutrophil leukocytes [PMNs] but no bacteria).
- *M. scrofulaceum* causes large cervicofacial nodes that fistulize and drain (it is thought that men started wearing ties and collars to cover their neck fistulas). Treatment is surgical.
- *M. kansasii:* Midwest origin, AIDS, IDUs; causes lung cavities, abdominal nodes, and pulmonary and GI disease.
- *M. marinum* is the fishtank bacillus, spread by handling fish or fishtanks; it causes nonhealing skin ulcers and strings of lesions along lymphatics. Treat with ethambutol and rifampin.
- *M. avium-intracellulare* complex is discussed in the section on HIV.
- *M. leprae* causes leprosy. Diagnosis is in biopsy or culture in armadillos (the only other host). Treat with clofazimine.
- *Nocardia asteroides* starts as a lung infection (thin-walled cavity) but can cause focal brain abscesses and chronic neutrophilic meningitis. Asteroid bodies can be seen on biopsy. Treat with TMP-SMX or, in immunodeficient patients, amikacin + imipenem.
- *Actinomyces*, which is anaerobic, is given away by the presence of sulfur granules. It causes cervicofacial fistulas (often after dental infections), PID after IUD, and chronic neutrophilic meningitis. Treat with penicillin or ampicillin.

Intracellular Parasites

Chlamydia are intracellular parasites. Three species are pathogenic: *psittaci, trachomatis*, and *pneumoniae* (formerly known as TWAR):

1. *C. psittaci*, found in bird droppings (especially poultry), causes psittacosis and is manifested by pneumonia, splenomegaly, and high fevers. (Note that histoplasmosis, with similar symptoms, is found in bird and bat droppings.)

2. *C. pneumoniae* causes community-acquired pneumonia (clues are bronchospasm and a CXR worse than a physical examination).

3. *C. trachomatis* causes STDs and trachoma (chronic corneal infection [keratitis] with development of cataract). In endemic areas, it is transmitted eye to eye via fomites, hands, and flies, causing trachoma, whereas in nonendemic areas, it can be given to newborns (causing pediatric trachoma, inclusion conjunctivitis, and neonatal pneumonia) by infected mothers. In endemic areas, erythromycin ointment is given to all children to control trachoma. Specific serotypes of trachoma also cause lymphogranuloma venereum (see above). Treatment can be with tetracycline or erythromycin ointment or oral azithromycin.

Rickettsia are also intracellular parasites:

1. *R. rickettsii* (transmitted by ticks) causes Rocky Mountain spotted fever (but this is actually more common in Virginia and Long Island). Symptoms include rash, fever, arthralgias, diarrhea, and abdominal pain. Rash is characterized by a centrifugal nature (spreading from the palms and soles inward; only Rocky Mountain spotted fever and syphilis have a centrifugal rash). Diagnosis is on skin biopsy.

2. *R. typhi* (spread by fleas) causes endemic typhus.

3. *R. prowazekii* (spread by lice) causes epidemic typhus (high fever, severe headache, photophobia, skin necrosis, gangrene, confluent maculopapular rash sparing face, palms, and soles) and has a 40% fatality if untreated. Brill-Zinsser disease is recrudescent epidemic typhus, which is milder and occurs years after acute disease in the elderly or immunosuppressed.

4. *R. tsutsugamushi* (spread by chiggers) causes scrub typhus.

5. *R. akari* (spread by mites of mice) causes rickettsialpox (vesicle turning to eschar, followed by macular rash).

6. *Coxiella burnetii* (transmitted by livestock) causes Q fever.

7. Treatment for rickettsiae includes chloramphenicol, tetracycline, and quinolones.

Ehrlichiosis is an intracellular pathogen (targeting neutrophils or monocytes) transmitted by *Ixodes* and *Dermacentor*, often in the Rocky Mountains (often called spotless Rocky Mountain fever). Symptoms are constitutional signs, leukopenia, thrombocytopenia, and high LFTs. Diagnosis is by serology. Treat with doxycycline.

Miscellaneous Bacteriology and Weird Bugs

1. *Corynebacterium jeikium* is a big problem in BMT units, causing line infections. Vancomycin and ciprofloxacin are the main therapies.

2. *Bacillus anthracis* (gram-positive rods) causes anthrax. Ninety-five percent of cases are cutaneous; 5% are pulmonic. It is often called woolhandler's disease. It starts as a painless papule, becomes a vesicle, ulcerates, and then becomes an eschar (all painless). Treat with penicillin G; alternatives are erythromycin or tetracycline.

3. *Francisella* (or *Pasteurella*) *tularensis* causes tularemia (rabbit fever). As a zoonosis, it often affects hunters. Signs and symptoms include irregular ulcer at the site of inoculation, fever, rash, and nodes. Diagnosis is by aspirating nodes and culture (not a biopsy). Treat with gentamicin or tetracycline.

4. *Brucella* is transmitted by the milk and cheese of goats and cattle, causes abortions in cattle, and is part of a fever of unknown origin work-up. Serology, like syphilis, can have a prozone effect (very high antibody titer limits cross-linking and precipitation and causes a false negative); thus, serum may need to be diluted to turn up positive.

5. *Yersinia pestis* causes plague. The reservoir is rodents, and the vector is fleas. Two types include bubonic (buboes are large regional suppurative nodes) and pulmonic. Both can lead to death. Plague is differentiated from tularemia as the latter has a rash. Diagnose plague by aspirating nodes and doing a culture (not a biopsy). Treat with streptomycin, tetracycline, or chloramphenicol.

6. *Erysipelothrix schenckii* occurs in fishhandlers. Symptoms include cellulitis and adenopathy along lymphatics. Treat with penicillin.

7. Hib causes serious infections (orbital cellulitis, epiglottitis, meningitis). Nontypable *H. influenzae* causes pneumonia, otitis, and sinusitis (which is why these infections have not decreased following the introduction of the vaccine for Hib).

8. *E. coli* serotype 0157:H7 causes HUS about 1 week after ingestion of uncooked meat (eg, the 1993 Jack-in-the-Box hamburger outbreak in children). It causes hemorrhagic colitis, renal failure, vomiting, and fever.

9. *Bartonella* (formerly *Rochalimaea*) *quintana* and *henselae* are small gram-negative rods. *Bartonella quintana* causes relapsing fever (trench fever). In the Andes mountains (Peru, etc), it is transmitted by sand-

flies, causing Oroya fever, which is febrile hemolytic anemia. *Salmonella* is often a co-infection. *B. henselae*, spread by cats and their fleas, causes cat-scratch disease (fairly common in children) and bacillary angiomatosis in AIDS patients. Bacillary angiomatosis and peliosis hepatis occur in AIDS patients infected by either *B. henselae* or *quintana*. Symptoms include purplish vascular papules (in differential of Kaposi's sarcoma); it is diagnosed on biopsy. Treat with erythromycin ± gentamicin/rifampin. It can also cause endocarditis, the treatment for which is gentamicin + ceftriaxone/doxycycline for 4 weeks.

Fungi
See Table 5–8 for classification of fungi.

Table 5–8. Morphologic Characteristics of Fungi

Morphology	Organisms
Yeasts	*Candida, Cryptococcus*
Molds	Dermatophytes
Dimorphs (can be yeast or mold)	*Histoplasma, Coccidioides, Blastomyces*
Nonseptate hyphae	*Mucor*
Branching hyphae	*Mucor, Aspergillus*

Candida

Quick Points
- Risk factors for candidemia:
  - Instruments: ventilators, Swan-Ganz and Foley catheters
  - Use of multiple antibiotics or prolonged use
  - *Candida* from other sites
  - Renal failure
- Candidemia can cause three lethal syndromes:
  - Septic peripheral thrombophlebitis (needs to be resected)
  - Septic thrombosis of great veins (edema of upper body; candidemia after removal of lines) (needs surgical evaluation)

- Hepatosplenic candidiasis (especially in febrile leukemics with negative cultures). This presents as fever, right upper quadrant pain, and increased alkaline phosphatase as neutropenia ends.
- Other common candidial infections include vaginitis and esophagitis (thrush).

Initial Management

1. Efficacy of amphotericin B is equal to fluconazole in nonimmuno-compromised patients (Mycoses Study Group). It is vital to remove or replace fungally infected lines.
2. Candidemia requires a retinal examination (retinitis can progress even on systemic therapy).
3. Non-albicans *Candida* is usually resistant to fluconazole (Diflucan).
4. See the antifungal section below for the dosing of antifungals.
5. Vaginitis can be treated with topical clotrimazole or miconazole (see Chapter 18 for more information).
6. Esophagitis can be treated with systemic fluconazole or amphotericin or oral amphotericin B (see Chapter 11 for more information).

Coccidioides

Coccidioides is often in the Southwest (Arizona is the classic question on tests). It causes valley fever. Symptoms include focal lung disease, nodes, meningitis, or diffuse lung disease and dissemination. It can cause erythema nodosum. Diagnose on complement fixation. Treat with amphotericin for severe disease and fluconazole for less severe disease and maintenance in HIV patients. For coccidioidal meningitis, fluconazole is the treatment of choice.

Histoplasma

Histoplasma is usually in the Ohio Valley. Involved organs include the lungs, liver, spleen, nodes, marrow, GI tract, and CNS. Splenomegaly, palate ulcers, and interstitial pneumonia are characteristic. Diagnose by screening for urine histoplasma antigen; definite diagnosis is on biopsy and/or culture. Treat with amphotericin and then itraconazole for maintenance.

Blastomyces

Blastomyces is common in the Southeast. It causes crusted skin lesions and involves the lungs.

Sporothrix schenckii

Sportothrix schenckii causes sporotrichosis (no kidding!). It usually affects gardeners pricked by a (rose) thorn. Cutaneous and lymphangitic forms are treated with potassium iodide. Pulmonary and disseminated forms need amphotericin B.

Penicillium

Penicillium is focused in Southeast Asia. This fungus causes chronic wasting and skin lesions resembling molluscum. It is sensitive to most antifungals except fluconazole.

Aspergillus

Aspergillus is a big problem in transplant patients. There are four kinds of aspergillosis:

1. Tracheobronchitis. Often this is a prelude to dissemination.
2. Allergic bronchopulmonary aspergillosis. This is generally benign; think of this in patients with asthma and eosinophilia. Treat with steroids and itraconazole.
3. Aspergilloma. This is more commonly known as a fungus ball and occurs in patients with old TB cavities.
4. Disseminated/invasive. This kind has a high mortality rate, as *Aspergillus* can cause a lot of vascular invasion and necrosis. Surgery can be done to resect lesions in BMT patients. CNS involvement is virtually always lethal.

Notes

1. *Aspergillus* gives a halo sign on CT.
2. High-dose lipid suspended amphotericin B is good for *Aspergillus.*
3. Nodular or hemorrhagic skin lesions and lung infiltrates in immuno-compromised patients imply infection with *Aspergillus* or *Nocardia.*
4. *Aspergillus* causes stridor and pseudomembrane in tracheobronchitis.

Cryptococcus

See Chapter 11. Know that Hodgkin's disease increases the risk of *Cryptococcus meningitidis.*

Mucor/Rhizopus is found in diabetics, the immunocompromised, patients with acidosis, and those on desferoxamine. It spreads rapidly. If the patient has sinus or orbital involvement, rapid surgical intervention is essential, or infection will spread to the brain. Amphotericin B is also essential, as is treatment of any acidosis that is present. In diabetics with orbital cellulitis or purulent sinus drainage, think of this and rule this out.

Umbilicated nodular skin lesions in HIV occur due to molluscum, *Cryptococcus*, histoplasmosis, and *Penicillium* (the latter is found in Thailand and China).

Antifungals

1. Amphotericin B is the big gun of antifungal therapy. It has a lot of toxicity, especially to the kidneys, and it is vital to monitor potassium and magnesium during therapy. See Chapter 11 for more information.
2. Fluconazole (Diflucan) is used for the Cs: *Candida, Coccidioides*, and *Cryptococcus*. It has excellent GI absorption. The dose is 100 to 400 mg PO qd.
3. Itraconazole (Sporanox) is used for *Histoplasma* and *Aspergillus*, *Blastomyces*, and onychomycosis (nail fungus).
4. Ketoconazole is cheaper than these drugs but more toxic (to liver and adrenals), and there are more drug interactions (rifampin, cyclosporine, P-450–affecting agents).
5. Ketoconazole and itraconazole need gastric acidity to be absorbed, so avoid them in patients on Pepcid/Prilosec or with atrophic gastritis.
6. Nystatin, griseofulvin, terbinafine, clotrimazole, miconazole, and terconazole are the main topical agents for skin or mucosal (oral, vaginal) infections.

Parasites

See Table 5–9 for classification of parasites.

Other Protozoa

Cryptosporidium, Isospora, Microspora, and *Cyclospora* are common in HIV patients and also occur in healthy people too. Diarrhea (chronic in HIV) and malabsorption (of fat, vitamin B_{12}, carbohydrates, and D-xylose) occur. *Cryptosporidium* may be benefited by paromomycin (Humatin), *Microspora* by albendazole and metronidazole, and *Cyclospora* by TMP-SMX.

Table 5–9. Classification of Parasites

	Protozoa			Helminths	
Ameba	Sporozoa	Flagellates	Nematodes	Cestodes (Tapeworms)	Trematodes (Flukes)
Entamoeba	*Toxoplasma*	*Giardia*	*Trichinella*	*Diphyllo-*	*Schistosoma*
	Crypto-	*Trichomonas*	*Toxocara*	*bothrium*	*Clonorchis*
	sporidium	*Trypanosoma*	*Wuchereria*	*Taenia*	*Opsothorchis*
	Isospora	*Leishmania*	*Onchocerca*	*Echinococcus*	
	Pneumocystis		*Loa*		
	Babesia		*Dracunculus*		
	Plasmodium		*Strongyloides*		
			Pinworms		
			Hookworms		
			Whipworms		
			Roundworms		

Ringworm is actually fungi, not worms.

Cryptosporidium, Isospora, and *Cyclospora* are all acid fast. *Cryptosporidium* are small and round. *Isospora* are large and oval. *Cyclospora* are large and round.

Entamoeba histolytica occurs by contaminated food; it usually occurs in the institutionalized, immigrants, and homosexuals. It can cause enteritis and hepatic abscesses, which, when drained, look like anchovy paste. Abscesses show neither ameba nor PMNs. Diagnosis is on stool ova and parasites. Treat with metronidazole (generally surgery isn't needed, even for abscesses).

Giardia lamblia usually affects campers, travelers (to the western U.S.; clusters are reported around Vale, Colorado), daycare children, homosexuals, and those with IgA deficiency and/or hypogammaglobulinemia. Symptoms include flatulence and watery diarrhea. Diagnose on stool ova and parasites. Chronic cases may need to be diagnosed with the string test (patient swallows a string, which is taken out and checked for trophozoites, which look like happy faces. Treat with metronidazole.

Leishmania donovani is spread by the sandfly (there are three other species, but these are of interest only to infectious disease and tropical medicine specialists). Kala-azar (visceral form) has hepatosplenomegaly,

GI symptoms, fever, pancytopenia, and hyperglobulinemia. Skin involvement is characterized by leonine facies. Diagnose on buffy coat smear and culture. Treat with antimonials (stibogluconate).

Trypanosomiasis is caused by *T. brucei* and *T. cruzi*. *Trypanosoma brucei* (found in Africa) is transmitted by tse-tse fly and causes sleeping sickness. Symptoms include fever, leukocytosis, anemia, and CNS involvement (lethargy, listlessness). A classic early finding is Winterbottom's sign (enlargement of posterior cervical triangle nodes). Diagnose on smear (buffy coat, marrow, node aspirate). Treat with suramin or pentamidine. *Trypanosoma cruzi* (found in Latin America) is transmitted by the reduvid bug and causes Chagas' disease, which basically involves loss of the nervous system of the heart and GI tract, leading to heart blocks, CHF, achalasia, and megacolon. The classic sign is chagoma, which is the area of erythema and edema where the parasites entered. If chagoma is around the eyes, this is called Romaña's sign. Diagnose on buffy coat smear. Treat with nifurtimox (works only 50% of the time and only for acute disease; chronic disease patients may go to heart transplant); benznidazole is an alternative.

Malaria

Quick Points

- The vector is the *Anopheles* mosquito.
- Four species of *Plasmodium* protozoa are the cause:
  - *P. falciparum*: the severest; no carrier; continuous random fevers; causes almost all deaths and has widespread chloroquine resistance.
  - *P. vivax* and *P. ovale*: carrier; fever q48 hours (tertian malaria).
  - *P. malariae*: no carrier state; fever q72 hours (quartan malaria).
- Diagnose on thick blood smears (look for intra-RBC parasite).
- Banana gametophyte implies *P. falciparum*.
- *P. malariae* most commonly causes nephrotic syndrome.
- *P. vivax* attaches to Duffy RBC antigen.

Cerebral malaria (due to *P. falciparum*) occurs in 10% of hospitalizations and causes 80% of deaths. Retinal hemorrhages, congestion, and edema are poor prognostic signs, as are coma and respiratory distress. Pentoxifylline seems to improve survival and shorten coma when used with quinine, possibly by increasing capillary flow. Do exchange transfusion for patients with altered mental status and > 10% parasitemia.

Initial Management
- Prophylaxis. The standard regimen in areas without resistance (which are few and decreasing) is chloroquine (500 mg PO qwk). In areas of resistance, you can use doxycycline (daily), mefloquine 250 mg PO qwk (which is safe in pregnancy), or primaquine 26.3 mg PO qwk.
- Treatment:
  - The standard regimen is quinine 650 mg PO tid or quinidine 324 mg PO bid if there is any question about resistance, with the addition of clindamycin 900 mg IV q8h for severe cases. Toxicities of quinine/quinidine include cinchonism (tinnitus, nausea, postural hypotension), hypoglycemia, and long QT interval.
  - Halofantrine is rapid (but causes QT prolongation and is not available in the U.S.).
  - Artesunate is great for mefloquine-resistant malaria.
  - For self-treatment of malaria, use pyrimethamine-sulfadoxine (Fansidar) (when you're stranded on safari without access to parenteral medication).
  - Use primaquine 26.3 mg PO qd for carrier state (1 dose 6 weeks after treatment is completed).
  - Remember that Fansidar and primaquine can cause favism (hemolytic anemia in G6PD-deficient patients), so screen patients prior to using them.

Babesiosis

Babesia microti is transmitted by the *Ixodes* tick (the same tick that transmits Lyme disease and ehrlichiosis). It is found in Long Island, California, Washington, and Africa. Symptoms include fever, hemolysis (like malaria, it infects RBCs), and hemoglobinuria. It is more severe in asplenic or immunocompromised patients. Diagnose on peripheral smear (higher yield if taken during chills) (you can see a Maltese cross from the intra-RBC tetrad, as opposed to malaria, which has a ring form). Treat with clindamycin or quinine (both in HIV patients).

Worms

General

- Worms don't replicate in the body, but they do cause eosinophilia (opposite in both cases from protozoa).
- Worms occur especially in patients who travel to and from the Third World.
- Treat with mebendazole or albendazole in general for intestinal worms.

Intestinal Nematodes

1. *Ascaris* (roundworm) (fecal-oral transmission) can cause pneumonitis and bowel and biliary obstructions/perforations.
2. *Necator/Ancylostoma* (hookworm) penetrate the skin (purported to be the reason why Southerners, who often used to walk barefoot, used to have a reputation for not being as mentally gifted as their Northern brothers) and chronically cause GI blood loss and iron deficiency.
3. *Strongyloides* is the only helminth that can replicate in the body (because it is "Strong"). Symptoms can include GI and respiratory distress and eosinophilia. Because of the ongoing life cycle and recurrent penetration of bowel mucosa, recurrent bacteremias can occur. Treat with thiabendazole or albendazole; use ivermectin in AIDS patients.
4. *Trichuris* (whipworm) is usually asymptomatic. It can cause rectal prolapse and growth retardation in children.
5. *Enterobium* (pinworm) causes rectal itching in kids. Diagnose by a Scotch tape test. It can be treated with niclosamide.
6. *Trichinella* (found in uncooked pork or beef, eg, steak tartar) causes diarrhea, fever, eosinophilia, periorbital edema (heliotrope rash, like dermatomyositis), and muscle invasion (myalgias, myocarditis). Steroids may be useful for myocarditis, but there is no treatment once organisms are encysted (so cook your meat, or else).

Tissue Nematodes

1. *Toxocara canis* or *cati* (transmitted by ingestion of dog or cat feces in soil [don't wonder how]) causes visceral larva migrans (hepatosplenomegaly, eosinophilia, invasion of any organ) and ocular larva migrans (which can

be mistaken for retinoblastoma and cause unnecessary enucleation). Disease is usually self-limited.

2. *Ancylostoma braziliense* causes cutaneous larva migrans (very itchy); treat with thiabendazole.

Filariae

1. *Wuchereria bancrofti* causes filariasis (elephantiasis) by invading lymphatics after being transmitted by mosquitoes (*Culex, Aedes*, or *Anopheles*). Diagnose on nocturnal blood smear. Symptoms include massive lymphedema. Treat with lymphedema management (stockings, elevation, etc.) and diethylcarbamazine (DEC).

2. *Onchocerca volvulus* migrates into the eyes, leading to corneal scarring, chorioretinitis, and optic atrophy. This is known as river blindness (the vector is located along rivers in Africa). Diagnose on biopsy. Treat with surgical removal and ivermectin.

3. *Loa loa* causes loaiasis, manifested by Calabar swellings (localized angioedema + erythema). Diagnose on blood smear. Treat with DEC.

4. *Dracunculus* (guinea worm) is of interest because the worm emerges from the skin and is removed by a matchstick, the use of which is one story of the origin of the caduceus, the symbol of medicine.

Tapeworms

1. *Taenia saginata* (beef tapeworm) causes mild GI symptoms and passage of proglottids in the stool. Diagnose on stool. Treat with praziquantel; second-line treatment is niclosamide.

2. *T. solium* (pork tapeworm) causes GI symptoms but also cysticercosis (larva in brain and muscles), leading to seizures, hydrocephalus, and myositis. Treat with praziquantel (second-line treatment is niclosamide) and surgery if needed. Give steroids during therapy.

3. *Diphyllobothrium latum* (fish tapeworm) causes diarrhea and vitamin B_{12} deficiency. Treat with praziquantel and B_{12} if needed.

4. *Echinococcus* (transmitted by dog feces in soil) can cause hydatid cysts in the liver, peritoneum, or lung. If they rupture, they can cause anaphylaxis or at least the spread of new cysts. Treat with en bloc removal by surgery (a recent *N Engl J Med* study showed that alcohol instillation was also effective). Albendazole may also be used.

Trematodes

1. *Schistosomiasis* is due to three species, including *Schistosoma mansoni*, *japonicum*, and *haematobium* (the first two affect the liver; the last affects the bladder). Acute infection leads to swimmer's itch and Katayama fever (fever, nodes, diarrhea). Liver involvement leads to cirrhosis, varices, glomerulonephritis, and pulmonary (yes, pulmonary) HTN. Bladder involvement causes hemorrhagic cystitis and predisposes to late bladder cancer. Treat with praziquantel.
2. *Clonorchis* is the Chinese liver fluke, and *Opsothorchis* is found in Indochina. They lead to cholangiocarcinoma after prolonged infection. Treat with praziquantel.

Virology

Herpes Viruses

Herpes Simplex Virus
- A DNA virus, herpes simplex virus (HSV) has two types. HSV-1 is responsible for most oral herpes, whereas HSV-2 causes most (75%) genital herpes. Both cause vesicular lesions on an erythematous base.
- Diagnose on Tzanck smear (scraping of lesion that shows multinucleated giant cells).
- HSV-1 also causes keratitis, and meningoencephalitis (the characteristics of which are temporal lobe predilection [which causes temporal lobe seizures, the signs of which include abnormal behavior and smelling of burning rubber], and blood in the CSF).
- Treat with acyclovir (indicated in the first episodes to reduce the frequency of later recurrences and also as maintenance to suppress infection to reduce frequency of recurrences in people with very frequent or very severe recurrences). For HSV resistant to acyclovir, use foscarnet.

Varicella-Zoster Virus
- This causes chickenpox mostly in children, but also in nonimmune adults (in whom it is worse, with a 20% chance of varicella pneumonia). In the elderly, it causes shingles (zoster), the hallmark of which is a dermatomal distribution.
- Acyclovir and prednisone do not reduce the frequency of post-herpetic neuralgia, although acyclovir does shorten the course of acute disease.

- Famciclovir (Famvir) does reduce the frequency of post-herpetic neuralgia.
- For post-herpetic neuralgia, topical capsaicin and amitriptyline are also of benefit.

Notes

- In immunosuppressed patients or those with severe disease (HSV or VZV), use IV acyclovir.
- Use varicella-zoster immune globulin in immunosuppressed patients exposed to VZV within 4 days of exposure.
- ASA should not be given to children with chickenpox (or influenza) because it can cause Reye's syndrome, which causes CNS damage, hypoglycemia, renal failure, and hepatic dysfunction (fatty liver) without jaundice. Treat Reye's with glucose, mannitol, and fresh frozen plasma.
- VZV can cause Ramsay Hunt syndrome (infection of the geniculate ganglion of the facial nerve, leading to facial palsy, vesicles in the ear canal (very painful), and hypogeusia (loss of taste on the anterior two-thirds of the tongue).
- VZV can also infect the nasociliary nerve (branch of V1), leading to Hutchinson's sign, which causes vesicles on the tip of the nose as well as keratitis (corneal involvement), as the nerve supplies both.

Cytomegalovirus. See Chapter 11 for a full discussion.

- This ubiquitous herpes virus can cause an acute mononucleosis-like syndrome in the immunocompetent patient. Serious disease occurs in immunocompromised patients (ie, AIDS or transplant patients). This includes pneumonitis, retinitis, encephalitis, hepatitis, colitis, and adrenalitis; however, retinitis does not occur in BMT patients.
- Diagnose by inclusion bodies on tissue biopsy or culture of buffy coat but not by serology (remember, almost everybody's been infected, so the presence of antibodies is not diagnostic of acute or active infection).
- Treat with foscarnet, ganciclovir, or cidofovir.

Epstein-Barr Virus

This virus is responsible for mononucleosis, Burkitt's lymphoma (especially in Africa), oral hairy leukoplakia (in AIDS patients), and nasopharyngeal carcinoma (especially in China). Diagnose on monospot (heterophile antibody). There is no specific therapy.

RNA Viruses

Measles.
- Also called rubeola (vs. rubella), the symptoms of measles include the three C's (cough, coryza, and conjunctivitis), as well as malaise and fever. Koplik's spots (white spots on an erythematous base) occur on the buccal mucosa 2 to 3 days before the rash (which starts from the head and goes down).
- Note that many people born between 1957 and 1980 received the measles, mumps, rubella vaccine, which requires a second booster that many have not received. You should give it to these patients as long as they are not allergic to eggs and are not pregnant or planning to be pregnant in the next 3 months.

Mumps. Mumps causes parotitis, meningoencephalitis, and orchitis.

Rubella.
- Rubella is also known as "German measles." In children, it causes centripetal rash, often accompanied by posterior auricular and cervical nodes.
- Fifty percent of exposed fetuses develop congenital defects, including cataract, heart disease, deafness, retardation, diabetes, and pulmonic stenosis. The earlier the infection occurs in the pregnancy, the worse it is in terms of frequency and severity of congenital defects.

Picorna. These are small (pico) RNA viruses and include the rhinoviruses (which cause colds), the enteroviruses (eg, coxsackie A and B (hand-foot-and-mouth disease; myocarditis]), and polio, which causes asymmetric paralysis and decreased deep tendon reflexes (DTRs) (vs. Guillain-Barré syndrome, which is symmetric and has intact DTRs). Rhinoviruses are inactivated in the stomach, whereas enteroviruses are not.

Slow Viruses and Miscellaneous

Parvovirus B19.
- This causes a slapped cheek appearance known as erythema infectiosum ("fifth" disease [first four rash diseases are measles, rubella, scarlet fever, and rheumatic fever]).
- Parvovirus B19 also causes aplastic anemia in sicklers (it infects marrow stem cells; normal people are asymptomatic due to the long half-

life of RBCs, but sicklers have a short half-life of RBCs, so even a transient drop in production causes decompensation).

Influenza A and B.
- These cause epidemic influenza.
- Give influenza vaccine to anyone over 55, people with lots of comorbidities (especially heart disease, COPD, and diabetes), and health care workers (including *yourself*).
- Amantadine and rimantidine confer protection against influenza A (indicated, for example, in nursing homes at the beginning of an outbreak).
- Use ribavirin for influenza B and Respiratory Syncytial virus (RSV).
- Neuraminidase inhibitors (oseltamivir [Tamiflu], zanamivir [Relenza]) seem to prevent and treat influenza well if given within the first 48 hours.

Rabies.
- This is found in bats, dogs, raccoons, skunks, and foxes but not squirrels or rats.
- Rabies causes hydrophobia, encephalitis, and death.
- When treating bites from unknown-status animals, give both immune globulin and vaccine (administer in different sites, give vaccine at five intervals: days 0, 3, 7, 14, and 28).
- Don't forget a tetanus shot in bitten victims.

Miscellaneous. RSV causes pneumonia in infants and sometimes in adults.

Papovavirus in HIV patients causes progressive multifocal leukoencephalopathy (PML).

Subacute sclerosing panencephalitis is a rare late complication of measles presenting with dementia, myoclonus, and seizures around age 10 in children who had measles before age 2. It is fatal.

Kuru occurs via cannibalism in New Guinea, whereas Creutzfeld-Jakob disease is transmitted by corneal transplants and cadaveric growth hormone injections. Both are due to the scrapie prion. Symptoms include dementia and myoclonus. Electroencephalogram of Creutzfeld-Jakob disease shows generalized slowing interrupted by bilaterally synchronous sharp wave complexes. Bovine spongiform encephalopathy (mad cow disease) and fatal familial insomnia (you do not want this disease) are related.

Lymphocytic choriomeningitis is transmitted by mice, hamsters, and rats (look for it in the homeless, gerbil/hamster owners, and those with frequent exposure to rodents).

Dengue fever is transmitted by the *Aedes aegypti* mosquito and causes breakbone fever (headache, back pain, petechiae). One serotype can cause hemorrhagic fever and shock. It occurs in the tropics and the southern U.S.

Arboviral encephalitides include Japanese, La Cross, St. Louis, and Eastern and Western equine types. They are transmitted by insects. These occur generally in summer and early fall. Treatment is supportive.

Lassa fever, yellow fever, Ebola virus, and dengue fever can all cause hemorrhagic shock. They usually occur in Third World countries. Yellow fever is also transmitted by *Aedes aegypti*.

BIBLIOGRAPHY

Reviews

Artinian MA, et al. Vertebral osteomyelitis. N Engl J Med 1993;329:399.

Balfow HF. Antiviral drugs. N Engl J Med 1999;340:1330–40.

Bisno AL, Stevens DL. Streptococcal infections of the skin and soft tissues. N Engl J Med 1996;334:240–5.

Caputo GM, et al. Assessment and management of foot disease in patients with diabetes. N Engl J Med 1994;331:854–60.

Cohen M, et al. STDs in the AIDS era. Parts I and II. Infect Dis Clin North Am 1993;7:739–899; 8:751–825.

de Marie S, et al. Clinical use of liposomal and lipid-complexed amphotericin B. J Antimicrob Chemother 1994;33:907–16.

deShazo RD, et al. Fungal sinusitis. N Engl J Med 1997;337:254–9.

Durack DT. Prevention of infective endocarditis. N Engl J Med 1995;332:38–44.

Emori TG, Gaynes RP. An overview of nosocomial infections. Clin Microbiol Rev 1993;6:428–42.

Hirshman JV. Fever of unknown origin. Clin Infect Dis 1997;24:291–302.

Hoofnagle JH, Bisceglio AM. The treatment of chronic viral hepatitis. N Engl J Med 1997;336:347–56.

Humar A, Keystone J. Evaluating fever in travelers returning from tropical countries. BMJ 1996;312:953–6.

Lee WM. HBV infection. N Engl J Med 1997;337:1733–45.

Lemon S, Thomas DL. Vaccines to prevent viral hepatitis. N Engl J Med 1997;336:196–204.

Lew DP, Waldvogel RA. Osteomyelitis. N Engl J Med 1997;336:999–1007.

McCormack W. Pelvic inflammatory disease. N Engl J Med 1994;330:115–9.

Murray BE. Vancomycin-resistant enterococcal infections. N Engl J Med 2000; 342:710–21.

Pizzo PA. Management of fever in patients with cancer and treatment-induced neutropenia. N Engl J Med 1993;328:1323–32.

Quaglierello VJ, Schold WM. Treatment of bacterial meningitis. N Engl J Med 1997;336:708–17.

Rosen FS, et al. The primary immunodeficiencies. N Engl J Med 1995;333: 431–40.

Schwartzman WA. Infections due to *Rochalimaea*. Clin Infect Dis 1993;17: 612–24.

Steckelberg JM, Wilson WR. Risk factors for infectious endocarditis. Infect Dis Clin North Am 1993;7:9–19.

Stevens DL. Streptococcal toxic shock syndrome. Emerg Infect Dis 1995;1: 69–78.

Stout JE, Yu VL. Legionellosis. N Engl J Med 1997;337:682–7.

Tibbles PM, Edelsberg JS. Hyperbaric oxygen therapy. N Engl J Med 1996; 334:1642–8.

Wheeler AP, Bernard GR. Treating patients with severe sepsis. N Engl J Med 1999;340:207–24.

Guidelines

American Diabetes Association. Foot care in patients with diabetes mellitus. Diabetes Care 1996;19:S23–4.

American Diabetes Association. Standards of medical care for patients with diabetes mellitus. Diabetes Care 1996;19:S8–15.

American Heart Association. Preventing bacterial endocarditis. JAMA 1997; 277:1794–801.

Centers for Disease Control. STD treatment guidelines. MMWR Morb Mortal Wkly Rep 1993;42:1–102.

del Brutto OH, et al. Therapy for neurocysticercosis. Clin Infect Dis 1993; 17:730–5.

Garner JS. Guidelines for isolation precautions in hospitals. Infect Control Hosp Epidemiol 1996;17:53–80.

Hospital Infection Control Practices Advisory Committee. Recommendations for preventing the spread of vancomycin resistance. Am J Infect Control 1995;23:87–94.

Larson EL. Guidelines for hand washing and hand antisepsis. Am J Infect Control 1991;19:8–15.

Wilson WR, et al. Antibiotic treatment of adults with infective endocarditis. JAMA 1995;274:1706–13.

Studies and Trials

Bacterial Infections

Arrendo JC, et al. Oral clindamycin and ciprofloxacin vs. intramuscular ceftriaxone and oral doxycycline in the treatment of mild to moderate PID. J Infect Dis 1997;24:170–8. (*An RCT showing that 2 weeks of oral clindamycin [600 tid] + oral ciprofloxacin [250 bid] was equivalent to the traditional regimen of IM ceftriaxone [250 mg] + PO doxycycline [100 bid]. Note that this may not apply to the real world, where compliance is a big issue.*)

Ericsson CD, et al. Ciprofloxacin or TMP-SMX as initial therapy for travelers' diarrhea. Ann Intern Med 1987;106:21–20. (*An RCT showing that both ciprofloxacin and Bactrim decreased diarrhea's duration and were well tolerated.*)

Genc M, Mardh PA. Cost-effectiveness analysis of screening and treatment for *Chlamydia trachomatis* infection in asymptomatic women. Ann Intern Med 1996;124:1–7. (*Screening was cost effective if the incidence of asymptomatic chlamydial infection was 6% or more. A single dose of azithromycin [1 g] was equivalent to 7 days of doxycycline.*)

Hatala R, et al. Once-daily aminoglycoside dosing in immunocompetent adults. Ann Intern Med 1996;124:717–25. (*A meta-analysis that showed that once-daily aminoglycoside dosing is safe and effective in immunocompetent patients with normal renal function. There are insufficient data to comment on neutropenic patients and in those with renal failure.*)

Marrie TJ, et al. Ambulatory patients with community pneumonia: frequency of atypical agents. Am J Med 1996;101:509–15. (M. pneumoniae *accounted for 22.8% of community cases and* C. pneumoniae *for 10.7%.*)

Ribera E, et al. Effectiveness of cloxacillin with and without gentamicin in short-term therapy for right-sided *Staphylococcus aureus* endocarditis. Ann Intern Med 1996;125:969–74. (*Cloxacillin efficacy was equivalent to cloxacillin + gentamicin in an RCT.*)

Scholes D, et al. Prevention of PID by screening for cervical chlamydial infection. N Engl J Med 1996;334:1362–6. (*An RCT showing that screening and treating women at risk for chlamydial infection significantly reduced the incidence of PID.*)

Shapiro ED, et al. A controlled trial of antimicrobial prophylaxis for Lyme disease after deer-tick bites. N Engl J Med 1992;327:1769–73. (*Antibiotics are not indicated if the tick is engorged but may be indicated if the tick is engorged.*)

Fungal Infections

Rex JH, et al. A randomized trial comparing fluconazole with amphotericin B for the treatment of candidemia in patients without neutropenia. N Engl J Med 1994;331:1325–30. (*An RCT showing that fluconazole had similar efficacy to amphotericin B for treatment of candidemia in non-neutropenic patients.*)

Rex JH, et al. Intravascular catheter exchange and duration of candidemia. Clin Infect Dis 1995;21:994–6. (*Removal of catheters in patients with candidemia reduced duration to 2.6 versus 5.6 days and correlated with clinical improvement.*)

Stevens DA, et al. Randomized trial of itraconazole in allergic bronchopulmonary aspergillosis. N Engl J Med 2000;342:756–61. (*Itraconazole improves symptoms in patients with steroid-resistant allergic bronchopulmonary aspergillosis.*)

Parasitic Infections

Albonico M, et al. A randomized control trial comparing mebendazole and albendazole against *Ascaris, Trichuris,* and hookworm infections. Trans R Soc Trop Med Hyg 1994;88:585–9. (*The two drugs were equal in efficacy [97% cure rate] for* Ascaris. *Albendazole was better for hookworm [57% vs. 22% cure]. Neither was good for* Trichuris *[< 15%]).*

Khuroo MS, et al. Percutaneous drainage compared with surgery for hepatic hydatid cysts. N Engl J Med 1997;337:881–7. (*Percutaneous drainage [with intracystic alcohol instillation] and oral albendazole treatment was as effective as surgery and had a lower length of stay.*)

Nosten F, et al. Mefloquine prophylaxis prevents malaria during pregnancy. J Infect Dis 1994;169:595–603. (*An RCT showing that mefloquine conferred 86% protection from malaria, with no adverse effects on the pregnancy or fetus.*)

Weiss WR, et al. Daily primaquine is effective prophylaxis against falciparum malaria in Kenya. J Infect Dis 1995;171:1569–75. (*Daily primaquine, with an 85% efficacy, was comparable or superior to doxycycline, mefloquine, or chloroquine + proguanil.*)

White AC, et al. Paramomycin for cryptosporidiosis in AIDS. J Infect Dis 1994;170:419–24. (*An RCT showing that paramomycin decreased stool weight and frequency by 50% in this population.*)

Viral Infections

Diaz MF, et al. Oral famciclovir for the suppression of recurrent genital herpes. JAMA 1998;280:1256–63. (*Famcicloivir is safe and effective for suppression of HSV in those with frequent recurrence.*)

Hayden FG. Use of oseltamivir in experimental human influenza. JAMA 1999;282:1240–6. (*Oseltamivir, an oral neuraminidase inhibitor, inhibited development of and reduced symptoms of clinical influenza in this RCT.*)

Wald A, et al. Suppression of subclinical shedding of HSV-2 with acyclovir. Ann Intern Med 1996;124:8–15. (*A double-blind, crossover trial that showed that acyclovir reduced asymptomatic viral shedding by up to 94%, but not completely. Thus, the authors recommended that patients with HSV-2 use condoms at all times.*)

THE WARDS

6

Cardiology

It's better to ask a dumb question than to correct a dumb mistake. — John Madden

Good judgment comes from experience; experience, that comes from bad judgment! — Mark Twain

CHARACTERIZE HISTORY

Chest Pain: Onset, time, duration, intermittent versus constant, getting worse or better, quality (pressure vs. sharp vs. dull), radiation (to shoulder, arm, jaw, neck, or back), activity at time of onset, course over hours, days, weeks. Be mindful of anginal equivalents (SOB; abdominal, neck, and back pain; nausea) and that they can change after revascularization.

Inferior MI: Diaphragmatic/vagal irritation (nausea or vomiting, epigastric pain, diaphoresis, hiccuping)

Associated Symptoms: SOB, dyspnea on exertion (DOE), paroxysmal nocturnal dyspnea (PND [does the patient need to open a window at night?]), orthopnea (does the patient get SOB on lying flat), nausea and vomiting, lightheadedness (always clarify dizziness), palpitations, syncope, diaphoresis

Risk Factors: HTN, diabetes mellitus (DM), hypercholesterolemia (not obesity per se), smoking, male sex, postmenopausal, family history (of MI under 55), homocysteinemia

Negative Risk Factor: Elevated high-density lipoprotein (HDL) (> 60)

KEY POINTS TO THINK ABOUT ON PHYSICAL

General description, hemodynamic status

Neck: Jugular venous distension (JVD) (defined as distension of external jugular [EJ] distended at 45 degrees > 2 cm above the sternoclavicular notch)

Bruits

Jugular venous pulse: a (atrial), c (closure of tricuspid), and v (ventricular) waves

- Cannon a waves (asynchronous with pulse) occur in atrioventricular dissociation or tricuspid stenosis (atria contracting against closed valves)
- Cannon v waves (synchronous with pulse) occur in tricuspid regurgitation

Chest: Lung edema, cardiac asthma, Ewart's sign—pericardial fluid with left subscapular dullness

Heart: Rate, regularity, heart sounds, point of maximal impact, murmurs, rubs (see below)

S3: (ventricular gallop), heard after S2 (due to rapid ventricular filling), physiologic in young, but sign of CHF in old

S4: (atrial gallop), heard before S1 (due to stiff ventricle), occurs in aortic stenosis (AS), left ventricular hypertrophy (LVH), HTN

S2 splitting is due to A2 coming before P2; splitting increases with inspiration as more venous return to right heart leads to later P2

Paradoxical S2 splitting is when inspiration reduces splitting (occurs when A2 is late, eg, AS, aortic regurgitation [AR], hypertrophic obstructive cardiomyopathy/idiopathic hypertrophic subaortic stenosis [HOCM/IHSS], left bundle branch block [LBBB], ventricular pacemaker).

Fixed splitting occurs in atrial septal defect (ASD) or right ventricle (RV) dysfunction.

Atrial flutter sometimes manifests as heart sounds going faster than the pulse.

Abdomen: Hepatic congestion, hepatojugular reflux

Extremities: Edema, pulses, capillary refill

Neurology: Focal deficits, inner ear signs in cases of syncope

LABS

- CXR, EKG (see below); WBC is often acutely elevated post-MI.
- CPK-MB q8h × 3 (false chronic elevations occur in cases of renal failure and cardiomyopathy).
- Troponins seem to enable earlier and more sensitive diagnosis and provide prognostic information as well.
- Cholesterol/lipoprotein levels may be artifactually lower after acute events.

CORONARY CIRCULATION

Always try to correlate coronary circulation with EKG findings.

Right coronary artery (RCA) and left main (LM) artery come off the aorta. The LM divides into the left anterior descending (LAD) and left circumflex (Lcx). RCA and Lcx go around the antrioventricular groove, while LAD goes anteriorly over the septum. The RCA gives off branches to the sinoatrial and atrioventricular nodes, while the Lcx gives off obtuse marginals. LAD gives off septal perforators (which supply the lower part of the atrioventricular node and bundle of His), diagonal branches, and ramus. RCA and Lcx join to become the posterior descending artery (PDA), which goes posteriorly over the septum (whichever gives more to PDA determines right vs. left dominance) (Figure 6–1).

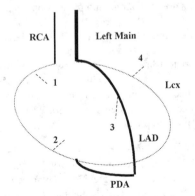

1. **Sinoatrial nodal artery**
2. **Atrioventricular nodal artery**
3. **Septal perforators, diagonal branches, ramus**
4. **Obtuse marginals**

Figure 6–1. Coronary circulation - the two-hoops model. LAD = left anterior descending; Lcx = left circumflex; PDA = posterior descending artery; RCA = right coronary artery.

ELECTROCARDIOGRAM READING

The electrocardiograms referred to in this chapter appear in Appendix H.

Note Well

1. EKG reading is a sport (drink it up!). But, seriously, it takes 1,000 EKGs to be good at them. So read every tracing you can get your hands on and, most importantly, have your resident, attending physician, or any available EKG master take you through the EKG stacks on the telemetry floor (for soft rule out MIs and occasional goodies) and critical care unit (CCU) (for *real* EKGs) at least two or three times a week. Every medicine resident should do a Cardiology elective sometime, on which the attending physician should read ~50 EKGs with you a day, getting you to your benchmark of 1,000. You must dedicate time to this art.

2. Dynamic changes are easier to read and more important than static changes, so *always* get the old EKG and *always* get a repeat EKG. Also, extrapolate patterns across the precordium with lead placement changes.

3. If you ever have to use an old-fashioned machine to hook up leads by yourself, remember, "Christmas tree below the knee, green means go (right knee), red means stop (left), and above the arm, white is right" (and suction cup across the precordium).

4. *Don't* look at the computer interpretation (but *do* use the numbers) and *never, ever trust another doctor over the phone* (too many people just read the computer version).

5. Suspect arm lead reversal if there is a tall R wave in aVR, especially if there is no tall R in V1.

6. Signal-average EKGs (which detect late potentials) show regions of slowed intraventricular conduction associated with the presence of spontaneous, inducible, sustained monomorphic ventricular tachycardia (VT): the idea is to recognize post-MI patients at risk for VT (negative predictive value = 90%, positive predictive value = 25%).

Distribution versus Circulation

- Distribution: anterior (I, aVL, V2–6), inferior (II, III, aVF), septal (V2–3), lateral (I, L, V5–6), posterior wall (interpret indirectly: reverse changes of anterior wall MI [AWMI] on leads V1–3; ie, tall R [R > S] with ST depression in V1–3; hold EKG backwards and upside down).

- RCA supplies the inferior wall, posterior wall, sinoatrial node (ischemia can manifest as bradycardia), atrioventricular node (manifests as first degree or Wenckebach's block), and RV (manifests as hypotension, right heart failure, without pulmonary edema) (*EKG 1 —inferior MI*).
  - In inferior/posterior wall MI (IWMI/PWMI), always check right-sided EKG (look for ST elevation in V1 or rV4).
  - Significance of right ventricle MI (RVMI): treat with lots of fluids to maintain preload and avoid nitrates/morphine, which reduce preload; RVMIs heal better than left ventricular MI (LVMI).
- LAD does anterior dose lateral wall (infarction of which really cuts left ventricular function [LVF]) and can cause hypotension, shock, pulmonary edema, and mural thrombi), supplies lower bundle of His (causes Mobitz II blocks), and apex (site of aneurysm formation and free wall ruptures) (*EKG 2—anterior MI*).
- Lcx supplies the lateral wall, sometimes the posterior wall, and the papillary muscle of the mitral valve (thus, Lcx infarction [LWMI/PWMI] can lead to acute mital regurgitation [MR], a surgical emergency).

Interpretation

Normal Variants

- Isolated Q in III
- Q and inverted T in V1/aVR
- Early repolarization (elevated J point) in young adults (don't confuse with ST elevation)
- Check P waves (best leads are II and V1, which is right over the right atrium)
- Ectopic pacemaker (inverted Ps in II) and wandering pacemaker (multimorphic Ps) are benign.
- Multifocal atrial tachycardia (MAT) (tachycardic multimorphic P waves), usually due to COPD or pulmonary disease
- If there are no P waves, then it may be atrial fibrillation (irregular baseline; irregularly irregular rate) (*EKG 3*), junctional rhythm (regular rate), or ventricular rhythm (wide complexes) (*EKG 4*). Atrial flutter has a sawtooth baseline due to the high atrial rate (*EKG 5*).
- Relationship of P to QRS: 1:1, P-R interval > 200 ms means first-degree block. Dropped beats mean second-degree block (Mobitz I or Wencke-

bach [often due to IWMI, digoxin toxicity] is successive P-R prolongation leading to dropped beat, whereas Mobitz II is dropped beats with
fixed P-R intervals). No relationship between P and QRS ("Ps marching
through" = atrioventricular dissociation) is complete block; if there's a
pattern, it's not complete. If there are dropped beats but it's not Mobitz
I or II, it's high-degree atrioventricular nodal block.

- Pacemakers should be placed quickly in Mobitz II and complete heart
  block (*EKG 6—complete heart block*).
- Mobitz II is worse as the block is lower in the atrioventricular node or
  in the bundle of His; hence, the escape rhythm is ventricular (more
  unstable), whereas escape in Mobitz I is junctional.
- Junctional rhythm: no P wave (low junctional rhythm can give invert-
  ed P after QRS due to retrograde conduction)
- Left atrial enlargement (LAE): biphasic or negative P wave (1 mm^2) in
  V1; gives bifid, long P in II (occurs with left ventricular hypertrophy
  [LVH], CHF, MR, and mitral stenosis [MS]) (*EKG 7—LAE*)
- RAE: tall, peaked P in II (occurs with CHF, right ventricular hyper-
  trophy [RVH], tricuspid regurgitation [TR], COPD)

Ions

- Low calcium, magnesium prolong QT; high calcium shortens QT;
  high potassium increases T, prolongs QRS; low potassium causes flat
  T and appearance of U wave
- Hypertrophy: LVH (due to HTN, AS, IHSS); RVH (due to COPD/pul-
  monary HTN)
  - LVH (*EKG 8*): concept is tall Rs in left chest leads and deep Ss in
    right chest leads
    - R in V5/V6 > 25 mm
    - R in V5/V6 + R in V1 > 35 mm
    - R in aVL > 11 mm
    - In vertical heart (when QRS in aVR and aVL are both downgo-
      ing; often normal variant or due to COPD), R in aVF > 1 mm
    - Strain pattern—ST depression/T wave inversion in V4–6 (not
      ischemia; now called "repolarization abnormality")
    - Tall Rs laterally without deep Ss in V1–3 can occur in left
      mastectomy

- RVH: R in V1 > 19 mm; can cause "strain pattern"—T wave inversion in V1–3
- IHSS: LVH, "septal" Qs in aVL, V2–6, and inferiorly ("pseudoinfarction")

Ischemia/Infarction

- Q means > 1 mm width (not depth) or wider than one-third of QRS (*EKGs 7, 9*), except in V2, where any initial downward deflection is a Q (*EKG 10*)
- ST depression (*EKG 11*): "scooped" = digoxin toxicity; downslope or flat = ischemia; upslope = nonspecific
- Infarction: hyperacute T waves, ST elevation (if large, called "tombstones," for obvious reasons), biphasic Ts, inverted Ts, and then Qs (tracing rises, then descends) (*EKGs 1–2, 6–7, 12–13*)
- Global ST elevation—pericarditis (specific signs are pulmonic regurgitation depression in II and ST elevation in aVR)
- Prolonged ST elevation—recurrent infarction; if > 7 days, consider aneurysm formation

Wide-Complex Tachycardia: Need to differentiate VT from supraventricular tachycardia (SVT) with aberrancy

- Cardiac history, old age, structural heart disease go for VT (*EKG 14*)
- AV dissociation (on EKG or jugular cannon a waves/varying S1 on examination) and concordance (all precordial complexes going in same direction) go for VT
- QRS > 140 or QRS shorter in tachycardia than in sinus rhythm implies VT
- Right rabbit ears taller than left (rsR) favors SVT
- Right bundle branch block (RBBB), deep Q in V6, slow first phase of QRS favor VT
- Ashman's phenomenon: short, long, short R-R intervals prior to tachycardia favor SVT
- VT: initial premature ventricular contraction (PVC), R on T, fusion (of normal and PV) beat, capture beat (normal beat in run of tachycardia)
- Do not give verapamil to wide-complex tachycardia (kills the patient and the doctor).

Bundle Blocks (usually due to ischemia or fibrosis): Key is right versus left

- Normal QRS < 100 ms; incomplete bundle > 100 ms; complete bundle > 120 ms
- *In leads where QRS complexes are up, it is part of the bundle block to have depressed STs and inverted Ts (not ischemia); where QRSs are down, you can have ST elevation (not infarction).*
- In RBBB, QRSs are upgoing in right chest leads (V1–3) (*EKG 15*).
- In LBBB, QRSs are upgoing in left chest leads (1, L, V5–6) (*EKG 5*).
- Other elements of RBBB: RSR pattern in V1–2; S waves in I, L, V5–6.
- Ventricular pacemakers produce an LBBB pattern as they are in RV (*EKG 16*).
- If criteria for both left and right BBB are present, it is called nonspecific intraventricular conduction delay.
- In RBBB, the first half of QRS is affected, not affecting the STs as much, so it is easier to interpret signs of infarction (RSR patterns can still Q out, giving qR patterns), whereas LBBB limits the ability to call ischemia/infarction (unless there is obvious ST elevation in leads where there should be depression).
- RBBB PVCs (come from LV) have a worse prognosis than LBBB PVCs (from LV).
- QT is artificially prolonged by excess of QRS over 100 ms (correct accordingly).

Hemiblocks (fascicle blocks)

- The left bundle has two fascicles (anterior and posterior), so you can have left anterior fascicular block (LAFB) or left posterior fascicular block (LPFB).
- Fascicular blocks do not prolong QRS per se.
- Criteria for LAFB: qR pattern in I, L, and rS pattern in II, III, F; left axis deviation (*EKG 10, 12*); S in III > S in II; R wave in aVR comes after R wave in aVL (specific).
- Criteria for LPFB: rS pattern in I, L, and qR pattern in II, III, F; right axis deviation; S in I, Q in III (remind you of something?)
- *LAFB can be very hard to call in the presence of IWMI.*
- *LPFB can only be called in the absence of pulmonary disease.*

- LAFB is much more common than LPFB and thus more common in bifascicular block (BFB); however, LPFB almost always occurs in association with RBBB because it is anatomically next to it.
- RBBB + LAFB often indicate ostium primum ASD (often with first-degree block as well)

Causes of Axis Deviation

- Left axis deviation: LVH, LBBB, LAFB, IWMI (Q and loss of R wave in III)
- Right axis deviation: COPD, PE, LPFB, RVH
- RBBB does not cause right axis deviation per se (only if LPFB is present).
- It is sometimes difficult to differentiate RBBB with LPFB from PWMI or RVH.

Four Fascicles of Conduction System: LAF, LPF, RB, atrioventricular node

- More fascicles blocked, higher risk of complete heart block
- In a new trifascicular block, especially in setting of ischemia, most would put in a pacemaker.
- Trifascicular block: first-degree atrioventricular block + (LBBB or RBBB + LAFB or RBBB + LPFB) or alternating left and right BBB

Tamponade

Electrical alternans (alternating up and down QRSs due to motion of heart in pericardium) and low voltage in all leads (vs. low voltage in limbs with normal or high voltage across precordial leads, which goes for cardiomyopathy)

Prolonged QT

- < 440 ms = normal; 440–460 = borderline; > 460 = abnormal
- In a slower heart rate, it is okay for QT to be longer—hence QTc, which is QT corrected by formula $QTc = QT/(R\text{-}R)^{\frac{1}{2}}$
- Causes: low calcium/magnesium, quinidine, procainamide, tricyclics, or phenothiazines
- Causes sine wave and torsades de pointes (rotation of baseline of arrhythmia) (*EKG 17*)
- Treatment: IV magnesium sulfate; transvenous pacing

CARDIAC DIAGNOSTICS

- *Echocardiogram*: assesses structural heart disease, wall motion, LVF
- *Stress echocardiogram*: treadmill and/or dobutamine as stressor
- *MUGA (nuclear medicine scan)*: gives specific number for ejection fraction (EF); used especially prior to doxorubicin therapy to get baseline
- *Stress test*: test for ischemia (adding thallium improves sensitivity and gives information on perfusion)
- *Dipyridamole* (Persantine) thallium is done if the patient can't walk (dipyridamole dilates coronary arteries, stealing blood and thus stressing blocked arteries that can't dilate due to fixed obstruction).
- Specific chemical tracers are constantly changing and can't be remembered.
- When doing a stress test, it is critical that the heart reach at least 85% of the maximal predicted heart rate (which is 220 − age [yr]); if the patient isn't cooperative or is on beta-blockers, you lose the sensitivity of the test.
- *Catheterization*: gives anatomy; with ventriculogram, you also get wall motion and EF
- Positron emission tomography (PET): assesses perfusion and viability
- MRI: wave of the future (could replace all tests except echocardiography and catheterization)
- Viability studies differentiate hibernating from dead myocardium
  - Rest-rest thallium: check thallium perfusion after initial injection and 6 hours later; delayed perfusion to initially unperfused areas indicates viability
  - Dobutamine echocardiogram: low-dose dobutamine stimulates hibernating (but not dead) areas to contract
  - PET: measures fluorodeoxyglucose uptake (living tissues will take it up)
- Viability studies are needed if there is a question as to the benefit of revascularization therapy (the classic case is the patient with three-vessel disease and poor EF; surgeons don't want to perform a coronary artery bypass graft (CABG) because they think the LV is already beyond salvage). See Table 6–1 for a description of myocardium in injury.

Table 6–1. Myocardium in Injury

Myocardium	Function	Perfusion	Viability
Normal	+	+	+
Stunned	−	+	+
Hibernating	−	−	+
Dead	−	−	−

Coronary Artery Disease (Including Unstable Angina and Myocardial Infarction)

Quick Points
- Managing coronary ischemia focuses on maximizing perfusion, which depends on the heart's time in diastole (thus, the slower the rate, the better, as time in systole per beat is fixed) and the gradient of diastolic pressure between the aorta and the LV end-diastolic pressure (thus lower preload is better).
- A second principle is reducing thrombus in the artery.
- Prinzmetal's (variant) angina (occurs at rest with transient ST elevation; diagnose with ergonovine provocation test) is due to spasm, not thrombus; calcium blockers are better than beta-blockers for this.
- The initial evaluation focus is on to admit or not to admit (ie, does the patient have an acute coronary syndrome, such as unstable angina or MI) and to emergently reperfuse or not (is it acute MI?).

Initial Management
1. ASA 325 mg PO × 1 (most important) + oxygen (basic)
2. Beta-blockers (↓ chronotropy and inotropy; ↑ time in diastole and ↓ oxygen demand): metoprolol (Lopressor) 5 mg IV q5 min × 3 down to a rate of 60
3. Nitrates (sublingual) 0.4 mg × 3 and morphine 2–4 mg SQ (both reduce pain and preload)
4. Angiotensin converting enzyme (ACE) inhibitors (within 24 hours of MI and post-MI, they increase survival, especially if EF < 40%): enalapril (Vasotec) 1.25 mg IV × 1; see below for more

5. Heparin (standard of care in unstable angina; controversial in MI—generally give it unless the patient has brain metastases or another severe contraindication, as blood can be replaced but not the heart): 5,000 U IV bolus, followed by 25,000 U/250 cc D_5W at 10 cc/hr (titrate PTT to 60–80)
6. Abciximab (ReoPro): monoclonal antibody against glycoprotein IIb-IIIa platelet receptor (impairs platelet aggregation)—target receptor is defective in Glanzmann's thrombasthenia
7. On admitting H&P, comment on the need or use of ASA, nitrates, heparin, and beta-blocker

Revascularization

During an acute event, this should be done within 6 to 12 hours.
1. Thrombolytics
2. Catheterization (stents have fewer restenoses than standard percutaneous transcoronary angioplasty [PTCA] and reduce death, reinfarction, and recurrent ischemia)
3. CABG (main indications are three-vessel or left main disease; rarely done emergently)

Notes

- Catheterization may have a slight mortality benefit over thrombolytics in meta-analyses.
- Morbidity of catheterization (groin hematoma/infection; contrast nephropathy; rarely, coronary dissection, etc) is less than that of thrombolytics (hemorrhagic stroke, GI bleed, allergy, etc)
- Post-stent patients are put on ASA 325 mg PO qd and ticlopidine (Ticlid) 250 mg PO bid to prevent restenoses (latter can be tapered in a month; remember that ticlopidine can cause agranulocytosis; follow absolute neutrophil count every week).
- The decision to catheterize is based not just on medical need but also the institutional setting and time of day (is there a 24-hour catheterization lab available?).
- Tissue plasminogen activator (TPA) has a short half-life and thus needs concomitant heparin to prevent reocclusion, unlike streptokinase (which, however, has more problems with anaphylaxis).

- Contraindications to thrombolytics:
  - Absolute: history of intracranial bleed or tumor, allergy, CVA or head trauma in last 6 months, active internal bleeding
  - Relative: GI bleed in last month, BP > 200/110, surgery/trauma in last 2 weeks, age > 80

Postmyocardial Infarction Issues

Quick Points
1. Risks are recurrent ischemia, CHF/cardiogenic shock, arrhythmias (causing sudden death), and free wall rupture (usually 1 week after large infarcts).
2. Subendocardial (non–Q wave) versus transmural (Q wave): the former has better short-term prognosis, but more events over the next several months lead to a similar long-term prognosis; non–Q-wave MI may also benefit from diltiazem (Cardizem) (decreased reinfarction in hospitalization).
3. To catheterize or not to catheterize: at many hospitals, basically everyone gets catheterized post-MI; however, a sound argument can be made to decide on catheterization based on a low-level stress test in patients with uncomplicated transmural infarcts.
4. Left ventricular function is the most important prognostic factor.
5. Other prognosticators include the Killip classification of hemodynamic status at the time of MI, age > 65, and female sex. DM, HTN, prior unstable angina/MI, reinfarction, and VT are bad prognosticators.

Initial Management
- Start at a low dose with short-acting medication and then maximize, and then switch to long-acting medications.
- Beta-blockers:
  - Most commonly used one (at least in our neighborhood) is metoprolol (Lopressor)
  - IV dose: metoprobol 5 mg × 3 (target heart rate for 60s)
  - PO dosage: start at 25, then maximize (can go up to 100 bid)
  - Reduces mortality of sudden death post-MI and helps with angina
- ACE inhibitors:
  - Start captopril (Capoten) (short acting) with 6.25 test dose; can maximize to 50 mg PO tid or enalapril (Vasotec) 20 bid.

- Watch BUN/creatine (especially postcatheter contrast and in patients with very low EF).
- Cough is also a big side effect.
- Anyone with a low EF or segmental wall dysfunction should be on these.
- Angiotensin II receptor blockers; at this time, they are used in those who don't tolerate ACE I.
- Losartan (Cozaar): start at 50 qd.
- Doesn't have bradykinin effect of ACE I, so there is less coughing.
- Calcium blockers:
  - Rule of thumb: *Procardia is bad* (tends to reflex tachycardia, increasing ischemia).
  - Verapamil (80–120 mg PO tid) and diltiazem (Cardizem) (60–180 mg PO bid) are useful in those with angina + HTN who can't tolerate beta-blockers.
  - Amlodipine (Norvasc) (5–10 mg PO qd) is coming into favor and is good for coronary spasm.
- Digoxin:
  - Used for rate control for atrial fibrillation and for symptomatic relief of CHF.
  - Digitalization: 0.25 mg q6h × 4 (less in renal failure or small patients), then 0.125 mg PO qd
  - Toxicity: bradycardia, AV block, any kind of arrhythmia (paroxysmal supraventricular tachycardia [PSVT] + block is classic), xanthopsia (everything looks yellow)
  - Low potassium/magnesium; drugs (see below) potentiate digoxin toxicity

Congestive Heart Failure

Quick Points
- Principal causes are HTN, ischemia, cardiomyopathy (alcohol, beriberi, etc).
- Ask about exacerbating factors (stress, infection, noncompliance with medication/diet).

- Signs and symptoms include SOB, dyspnea on exertion, PND, orthopnea, S3, S4, rales, JVD, hepatojugular reflux, and edema.
- Clarify in your mind diastolic versus systolic dysfunction and right versus left failure.

Initial Management
- Echocardiography is essential.
- Symptomatic CHF:
  - Digoxin (if EF is low, digitalize as above)
  - Nitrates to reduce preload (common starting medication isosorbide dinitrate [Isordil] 10–40 mg PO tid, then switching to Ismo 20 mg PO bid or Imdur 30–60 mg PO qd [the last two are long-acting forms of isosorbide mononitrate])
  - Diuresis (furosemide 40–100 mg PO or IV as often as indicated)
- Survival enhancers:
  - ACE inhibitors of proven benefit (see above discussion on ACE inhibitors)
  - The recent MERIT trial showed extended-release metoprolol (start 25 mg/d and increase up to 200 mg/d) to reduce mortality and hospitalizations for CHF
  - Carvedilol (increases short-term morbidity, with unclear long-term survival benefit)
- For diastolic dysfunction, beta-blockers are still useful; some cardiologists use calcium blockers (diltiazem [Cardizem], amlodipine [Norvasc]) as well.

Other Cardiology Issues

Syncope

1. Rule out MI, arrhythmia, structural heart disease, and CNS vascular insufficiency. (NB: CVA and transient ischemic attack [TIA] don't cause syncope unless they are massive or are in basilar circulation.)
2. Standard tests include rule out MI work-up, echocardiogram, monitor, and carotid Doppler (consider head CT).
3. In vasovagal cases, consider a tilt-table.
4. In elderly men with BPH, think of micturition syncope (you can treat BPH medically).

5. Many, if not most, telemetry syncopes wind up with no diagnoses.

Cocaine-Induced Myocardial Ischemia

- Avoid beta-blockers (will cause unopposed α-receptor stimulation).
- Benzodiazepines, nitrates, alpha-blockers are good.

Pulmonary Hypertension

- Treat treatable causes as soon as possible.
- Procardia may be of benefit (first dose should be given in ICU with Swan monitoring).
- Prostaglandins may be of benefit.

Hyperlipidemia

Table 6–2 lists types of hyperlipidemias.

> Quick Points
> 1. Low-density lipoprotein (LDL) = total cholesterol − HDL − (triglycerides ÷ 5) (shows up on test questions).
> 2. Very-low-density lipoprotein (VLDL) = triglycerides; IDL = intermediate-density lipoproteins.

Table 6–2. Hyperlipidemias

Hyperlipidemia	Type/Defect	Lab	Signs and Symptoms
Familial lipoprotein lipase deficiency	I: Lipoprotein lipase	↓ Chylomicrons	Pancreatitis, eruptive xanthomas, lipemia retinalis; no CAD
Familial hypercholesterolemia	IIa: LDL receptor, apoB	↓↓ LDL	CAD, tendon xanthoma
Combined hyperlipidemia	IIb	↓ VLDL, LDL	CAD, tuberous xanthoma
Dysbetalipoproteinemia	III: apoE	↓ VLDL, IDL	Palmar/tuberous xanthoma, CAD
Familial hypertriglyceridemia	IV	↓ VLDL	Eruptive xanthoma, CAD
Familial apoCII deficiency	V: apoCII	↓ VLDL, chylomicrons	Pancreatitis, eruptive xanthoma, CAD

apo = apoprotein; CAD = coronary artery disease.

Initial Management

1. Stepladder of 30s: In patients with CAD, the goal of therapy is to lower LDL to < 100 (start medcations at 130). In patients with more than two risk factors, the goal is 130 (start medications at 160); in patients with less than two risk factors, the LDL goal is 160 (start medications at 190). Start diet and exercise therapy if the LDL is over the goal level.
2. Treat low HDL (< 35) with drugs if there are associated LDL or triglyceride abnormalities.
3. Niacin treats both LDL and triglycerides. Toxicity includes flushing, GI upset, glucose intolerance, PUD, and pruritus (many of which are avoided by Niaspan, a new long-acting formulation).
4. Statins are the workhorse of the modern era. Lovastatin (Mevacor), simvastatin (Zocor), pravastatin (Pravachol), and fluvastatin (Lescol) are all basically the same in treating high LDL. A new drug, atorvastatin (Lipitor), treats LDL, increases HDL, and decreases triglycerides. Toxicity includes myositis and transaminitis. There is an increased risk of myositis with niacin, gemfibrozil, erythomycin, and cyclosporin.
5. Gemfibrozil treats triglycerides only and also increases HDL.
6. Probucol and bile resins are not used much anymore.

Arrhythmias

Indications for Electrophysiologic Studies

1. Patients with syncope + RBBB, LBBB, or BFB
2. Patients with 2:1 atrioventricular block (need to differentiate Mobitz I from II)
3. Patients with complete heart block
4. Recurrent/refractory tachyarrhythmias (for ablation of autonomous foci or re-entry pathways)

Atrial Fibrillation/Flutter

Quick Points
• Diagnosis: idiopathic, thyrotoxicosis, mitral stenosis, CHF, ethanol (holiday heart), MI.

- New-onset atrial fibrillation generally gets ruled out for MI.
- Atrial fibrillation is bad because of risk of stroke (rarely PE as it is the left atrial appendage that is clot conducive), loss of atrial kick (with consequent risk of CHF), and rapid rate.

Initial Management
- Management decisions revolve around decisions on cardioversion, rate control, and anticoagulation.
- Atrial flutter is unstable, meaning only that it usually converts to fibrillation or normal sinus rhythm.
- Rate control:
  - Digoxin (vagotonic, slow effect, good in CHF patients)
  - Beta-blockers (metoprolol 5 mg IV prn; switch to 25–50 mg PO bid)
  - Diltiazem (15–25 mg IV as often as needed; switch to 30 mg PO qid and increase up to a maximum of 360 mg a day [you can give long-acting diltiazem (sustained release) 180 mg PO bid once the patient is stable]
  - Vagal maneuvers: carotid massage (unilateral, please), Valsalva's, ice-water face immersion
- Convertors:
  - Electric
  - Medications: sotalol, procainamide, amiodarone
  - Leave the decision on modality to the electrophysiologic specialists
  - Most drugs are better for fibrillation than flutter.
- Ibutilide (Corvert) 1 mg IV slow infusion × 1; can be repeated, better for flutter than fibrillation.
- Anticoagulate 2 weeks prior to conversion of long-standing (> 48–72 hours) atrial fibrillation (unless TEE documents absence of a clot) and always for 2 weeks after conversion (atrial mechanical conversion is delayed after electrical conversion).

Wolff-Parkinson-White Syndrome (EKG 18)
- Accessory pathway is from RA to RV, leading to re-entry SVT.
- Delta wave (slurred upstroke), short pulmonic regurgitation interval (< 120 ms), and prolonged QRS are the key signs.
- Traditional management of SVT (slow atrioventricular node with beta- or calcium blockers, digoxin, or adenosine) is bad because the

slowing atrioventricular node leaves the accessory pathway as the sole conduction pathway and that is unstable, easily degenerating into ventricular fibrillation.

- Thus, use procainamide.

Bradyarrhythmias

- Decide on sinoatrial node versus atrioventricular disease; consider atropine and a pacemaker if unstable.
- For calcium blocker overdose, use calcium.
- For beta-blocker overdose, epinephrine is ineffective (receptors already blocked), so use glucagon (bypasses straight to the cAMP pathway).
- For digoxin overdoses (classic arrhythmias are sinus bradycardia, nonparoxysmal junctional tachycardia, or PSVT with block), use Digibind (FAB fragment antibodies they artifactually prolong digoxin levels on lab tests) and/or phenytoin (good for digoxin arrhythmias).

Ventricular Arrhythmias and Antiarrhythmics

- Conceptually, arrhythmias are divided into re-entry (which can be controlled by shock or slowing atrioventricular node) and automaticity (from drug [digoxin, theophylline] toxicity, severe cardiopulmonary disease, and ion imbalances), in which the cause needs to be treated. See Table 6–3 for classification and Table 6–4 for indications for antiarrhythmics.
- CAST study: prophylactic suppression of post-MI PVCs in an effort to curb sudden death with certain antiarrhythmics actually increases mortality. Hence, when a nurse tells you about runs of VT, start medications only for hemodynamic instability or sustained VT (> 30 seconds, not 30 beats).
- As procainamide is metabolized to *N*-acetyl procainamide when given orally, it is not good to suppress VT.

Key Toxicities

- Ibutilide: prolonged QT
- Sotalol: pulmonary fibrosis
- Procainamide: lupus, prolonged QT
- Quinidine: prolonged QT, cinchonism (tinnitus)

Table 6–3. Vaughan-Williams Classification of Antiarrhythmics*

Class I (block sodium channels,slowing action potentials)	IA (block sodium channels and slow repolarization)	Procainamide, quinidine
	IB	Lidocaine, phenytoin
	IC (greatly prolongs QRS)	Flecainide
Class II		Beta-blockers
Class III	Block potassium channels (slowing repolarization and ↑ refractoriness) (↑ QT)	NAPA (metabolite of procainamide), amiodarone, sotalol, ibutilide
Class IV		Calcium blockers

*The sole purpose of this is to torture interns and students.
NAPA = *N*-acetyl procainamide.

Table 6–4. Indications for Antiarrhythmics

Arrhythmia	*Terminators*	*Preventives*
Atrial fibrillation/flutter (don't forget to rate control first)	Procainamide, ibutilide	Quinidine, sotalol, flecainide, amiodarone
Supraventricular tachycardia	Diltiazem, adenosine	Verapamil, propranolol
Ventricular tachycardia	Lidocaine, procainamide	Flecainide, sotalol, amiodarone

- Amiodarone: thyroid (usually hypo, sometimes hyper), pulmonary fibrosis
- Quinidine, amiodarone, verapamil, and diltiazem all increase digoxin toxicity

Pacemakers
Code:
First letter (chamber paced—A [atrial], V [ventricular], or D [dual])
Second letter (chamber sensed—A, V, or D)
Third letter (ppm response—I [inhibited by a beat], T [triggered by a beat], or D [dual])

- The most common pacemakers are VVI and DDD.
- VVI is used when the atria are expendable and should not be sensed (eg, atrial fibrillation).
- VVI and complete heart block patients can get jugular cannon a waves.
- DDD is used in everyone else, especially young patients and those dependent on atrial kick.
- Paced EKGs are generally unreadable (usually have LBBB pattern as pacing wire is in RV) (*EKG 19*); keep in mind that for several hours after the last paced beat, ST elevation is common on EKG and should not be considered infarction.

Valve Disease

General Principles

1. Remember endocarditis prophylaxis.
2. For stenotic valves, surgery is indicated when symptoms start.
3. For regurgitant valves, monitor EF and perform surgery at the first sign of trouble.

Aortic Stenosis

- Aortic senosis is due to degeneration (associated with HTN) or bicuspid valve.
- Symptoms include angina, syncope, and CHF (prognostically worse in that order).
- Signs include systolic murmur at the second right intercostal space, radiation to carotids, diminished S2 or paradoxically split S2, LVH, and diminished carotid upstroke (*parvus et tardus*).
- Catheterize prior to surgery so that CABG can be done simultaneously if need be.
- Replace the valve in patients with symptoms and in asymptomatic patients with severe AS and LV dysfunction and perhaps also those with severe LVH.
- Age per se is not a contraindication to surgery.

Aortic Regurgitation

- Differential diagnosis: aortic root dilation, endocarditis, syphilis, Marfan syndrome, ankylosing spondylitis

- Findings: (occur in chronic, not acute, AR) (see Table 6–5 for signs)
  - Wide pulse pressure
  - Dilated LV, diastolic murmur, pulsus bisferens (split in two), pistol-shot femoral pulse
  - Regurgitation against mitral valve leads to physiologic mitral stenosis and sometimes diminished S1 due to mitral preclosure.
  - Acute AR does not have wide pulse pressure. It is, however, a surgical urgency, and the valve should be replaced even in the presence of endocarditis.
  - Chronic AR requires valve replacement if there are symptoms, or LVEF is heading down toward 55%.
  - Medical therapy is the same as for CHF and also vasodilators.

Table 6–5. Eponymous Signs of Aortic Regurgitation

Sign	Findings
Austin Flint murmur	Diastolic rumble
Corrigan's (water-hammer) pulse	Rapid rise and fall or carotid/femoral pulse
Hill's sign	Popliteal BP > 60 mm Hg more than brachial BP
Duroziez's sign	Diastolic and systolic femoral bruits
de Musset's sign	Head bobbing
Müller's sign	Uvula bobbing
Quincke's pulse	Systolic blushing and diastolic blanching of nailbed during traction

Mitral Stenosis

1. Due to rheumatic heart disease.
2. Chronically leads to CHF (occasionally hemoptysis), LAE (chronically leads to atrial fibrillation + emboli and hoarseness due to recurrent laryngeal nerve impingement), pulmonary HTN (and signs of RV overload/failure).
3. Cannon a waves on Swan.
4. Signs: loud S1, opening snap, diastolic rumble, sternal lift if RV overload, Graham Steell's murmur if chronic pulmonary regurgitation.
5. Use balloon valvuloplasty or commissurotomy in those with moderate-severe mitral stenosis or bad symptoms.

Mitral Regurgitation

- Differential diagnosis is MVP, rheumatic disease, myxomatous degeneration, MI, and endocarditis.
- Mitral regurgitation causes volume overload (increases preload), eccentric dilation of LV, initial increase in LVEF (due to increased preload and lower afterload from having two open valves).
- It chronically leads to atrial fibrillation, CHF, and cannon v waves on Swan.
- Do surgery as soon as EF goes down to 60% or when LV starts to dilate. Repair (not replace) the valve if possible, as intact papillary muscle (especially chordal apparatus) is key to LV function. Surgery is bad in those with end-stage mitral regurgitation (LV is dead and replacing valve only increases afterload).
- Medical therapy is vasodilators and CHF medications.

Right-sided valve defects (TR, tricuspid stenosis [TS], pulmonic stenosis [PS], pulmonic regurgitation [PR]) are rare except for congenital heart disease. They are made worse by inspiration. TR and TS occur in carcinoid syndrome.

CARDIOMYOPATHIES

Dilated

- Differential diagnosis is ethanol, hemochromatosis, beriberi, Chagas' disease, coxsackievirus B, cocaine, and thyroid disease.
- Treat for CHF.
- ACE inhibitors and carvedilol may prolong survival; a transplant is needed.

Hypertrophic, Obstructive

Quick Points
- Old name is idiopathic hypertrophic subaortic stenosis; new name is hypertrophic obstructive cardiomyopathy (HOCM); autosomal dominant with reduced penetrance; bimodal age peak
- Asymmetric, disorganized septal hypertrophy with dynamic obstructive gradient to outflow from aortic valve ("symmetric anterior motion" [SAM] of mitral leaflet)
- Symptoms: sudden death, CHF (diastolic dysfunction), syncope, atrial fibrillation, VT

6

- Murmur: systolic, made worse by Valsalva, has components of AS and MR, but S2 is preserved (as opposed to AS)

Initial Management
- Interventions:
  - Beta-blockers (maximize metoprolol up to 100 mg PO bid as tolerated)
  - Calcium blockers (give cardioselective agents, eg, verapamil, diltiazem [maximize diltiazem up to 180 mg PO bid as tolerated])
  - Myomectomy
  - Dual-chamber pacemaker (improves contraction sequence, giving symptomatic relief)
  - Ethanol given into septal perforators in a catheter
- Need to make diagnosis as traditional CHF therapy (digoxin, nitrates, diuretics, afterload reduction) makes HOCM worse (digoxin increases inotropy, reduced preload increases SAM, and reduced afterload increases gradient)

Restrictive

1. Rare; due to myocardial infiltration (sarcoid, amyloid, hypereosinophilia); S3 and S4 are present
2. Can do biopsy; not much else to do, except steroids in some cases
3. Need to differentiate from constrictive pericarditis (which can be improved by pericardiotomy)

Pericardial Disease

- If you hear a rub, make sure you have others listen (they are rare and fleeting).
- Acute pericarditis: occurs post-MI, in Dressler's syndrome (autoimmune reaction weeks post-MI), rheumatic disease, TB, drugs (procainamide, hydralazine, isoniazid), lung and breast cancer, uremia, coxsackievirus B
- Tamponade: pulsus paradoxus (greater than a 20-point fall in systolic blood pressure with inspiration), JVD, narrow pulse pressure
- Constrictive pericarditis: right-sided heart failure, eggshell calcification on CXR, square-root sign and equalization of end-diastolic pressures on catheter, Kussmaul's sign (neck vein distension with inspiration)

Intra-aortic Balloon Pump

1. Balloon placed in aorta above infrarenal arteries and below great vessels
2. Contracts during systole (reducing afterload by creating vacuum in aorta) and expands in diastole (improving diastolic perfusion to heart, brain, and periphery)
3. Great for cardiogenic shock, severe MR (as a bridge to surgery)
4. Great for acute MI by reducing heart's workload and thus improving electrical stability
5. Contraindications: AR (expansion in diastole would be bad), aortic dissection, and DIC
6. Remember that augmented diastolic pressure should be higher than systolic; if not, use the following tips for troubleshooting:
   - Consider the volume status (the patient may be dehydrated)
   - Check the balloon's marker position on CXR
   - If the heart rate is too fast, the machine can't synchronize properly
   - The heart may not need the balloon's support anymore
   - The balloon may be clotted

MURMURS

See Table 6–6 for valve disease signs and Table 6–7 for maneuvers.

1. Describe when and how long (systolic vs. diastolic, early vs. mid vs. late vs. holo/pan) and sound (loud, harsh, soft, blowing, musical/cooing)
2. Austin Flint: diastolic, heard at apex. Due to AR causing mitral preclosure. Different from MS because there is no opening snap.
3. Innocent cardiopulmonary murmur: due to movement of heart; disappears on breath hold.
4. Diamond-shaped: crescendo-decrescendo murmur (eg, AS, PS)
5. Graham Steell: early diastolic murmur of pulmonic regurgitation due to MR-induced pulmonary HTN, best heard at Erb's point
6. MVP: MR + midsystolic click
7. Machinery: long, continuous rumble occurring in patent ductus arteriosus (occurs in both systole and diastole)
8. Pulmonary stenosis and ostium secundum atrial septal defect are the only defects not needing endocarditis prophylaxis
9. Still's murmur: innocent musical murmur resembling a string being twanged
10. Roger's murmur: loud pansystolic murmur at left sternal border, due to a small ventricular septal defect

Table 6–6. Valve Disease and Associated Signs

Valve Defect	Murmur/Sound	Pulse
Aortic stenosis	Diamond-shaped systolic ejection murmur at second right intercostal space, ejection click, loss of S2 and S4	Slowed carotid upstroke
Acute aortic regurgitation	Short diastolic murmur, S3	Thready pulse
Chronic aortic regurgitation	Holodiastolic murmur, Austin Flint	Cool signs
Mitral stenosis	Diastolic rumble, opening snap, loud S1	Cannon a waves and attenuated v descent on Swan
Mitral regurgitation	Apical pansystolic murmur, S3	Cannon v waves on Swan
Mitral valve prolapse with murmur	Pansystolic murmur, S3, midsystolic click	
Pulmonic stenosis	Ejection click, persistent, widely split S2	Cannon jugular a wave
Tricuspid stenosis	Diastolic murmur at LSB	Cannon jugular a wave
Tricuspid regurgitation	Systolic murmur at LSB	Cannon jugular v wave
Atrial septal defect	Systolic ejection murmur at LSB (increased flow across pulmonic valve), fixed split S2	
Ventricular septal defect	Holosystolic murmur at LSB	
Patent ductus arteriosus	Continuous machinery murmur, paradoxically split S2	
Hypertrophic obstructive cardiomyopathy	Harsh midsystolic murmur, preserved S2 and S4	See above
Aortic coarctation	Upper back midsystolic or continuous murmur	

Table 6–7. Maneuvers and Murmurs

Murmur Louder With	Signs	Defect
Squatting, expiration, after PVCs	Congestive heart failure/ angina/syncope, left ventricle hypertrophy	Aortic stenosis
Squatting, expiration	Left atrial enlargement hemoptysis, pulmonary hypertension, history of rheumatic fever	Mitral stenosis
	Left ventricle hypertrophy, history of endocarditis, Marfan syndrome, syphilis	Chronic aortic regurgitation
	Shock, pulmonary edema	Acute aortic regurgitation, aortic dissection
	Pulmonary edema, endocarditis, myocardial infarction	Acute mitral regurgitation
Valsalva, standing, handgrip, expiration	Left atrial enlargement	Mitral valve prolapse
Valsalva, standing, decreased murmur with handgrip		Hypertrophic obstructive cardiomyopathy
Inspiration	Right ventricle hypertrophy	Pulmonic stenosis
Squatting, inspiration	Right ventricle hypertrophy, carcinoid, endocarditis, rheumatic fever, jugular venous distension, liver pulsation	Tricuspid regurgitation
	Right atrial enlargement, carcinoid jugular vein distension	Tricuspid stenosis
Handgrip	Right ventricle hypertrophy + left ventricle hypertrophy; myocardial infarction; new systolic murmur	Ventricular septal defect
	Right ventricle hypertrophy, RBBB, LAFB (left axis deviation)	Ostium primum atrial septal defect

Continued on next page

Table 6–7. continued

Right ventricle hypertrophy, RBBB, LPFB (right axis deviation)	Ostium secundum atrial septal defect
Rib notching, loss of aortic notch	Aortic coarctation

BIBLIOGRAPHY

Reviews

Abernethy DR, Schwartz JB. Calcium-antagonist drugs. N Engl J Med 1999;341:1447–57.

Baker DW, et al. Management of heart failure. JAMA 1994;272:1528–34, 1614–8.

Braunwald E, et al. Unstable angina: diagnosis and management. AHCPR publication no. 94-0602. U.S. Department of Health and Human Services, March 1994.

Cigarroa JE, et al. Diagnostic imaging in the evaluation of suspected aortic dissection. N Engl J Med 1993;328:35–43.

Collins R, et al. Aspirin, heparin, and fibrinolytic therapy in suspected acute MI. N Engl J Med 1997;336:847–60.

Curabello BA. Valvular heart disease. N Engl J Med 1997;337:32–42.

Kennedy KD. Natural history of moderate aortic stenosis. J Am Coll Cardiol 1991;7:313–9.

Kushaba SS. Restrictive cardiomyopathy. N Engl J Med 1997;336:267–76.

LaRosa JC, Vupputuri S. Effect of statins on risk of coronary disease. JAMA 1999;282:2340–6.

Smith SC, et al. Preventing heart attack and death in patients with coronary disease. Circulation 1995;92:2–4.

Spirito P, et al. The management of hypertrophic cardiomyopathy. N Engl J Med 1997;336:775–85.

Wigle ED, et al. Hypertrophic cardiomyopathy. Circulation 1995;92:1680–92.

Guidelines

American College of Cardiology and American Heart Association. Guidelines for implantation of cardiac pacemakers and antiarrhythmia devices. J Am Coll Cardiol 1991;18:1–13.

American College of Cardiology and American Heart Association. Guidelines for clinical intracardiac electrophysiological and catheter ablation procedures. J Am Coll Cardiol 1995;26:555–73.

American College of Cardiology and American Heart Association. Guidelines for the evaluation and management of heart failure. J Am Coll Cardiol 1995; 26:1376–98.

American College of Cardiology and American Heart Association. Guidelines of perioperative cardiovascular evaluation for noncardiac surgery. Circulation 1996;93:1278–317.

26th Bethesda Conference. Recommendations for determining eligibility for competition in athletes with cardiovascular abnormalities. J Am Coll Cardiol 1994;24:845–9.

Hirsh J, Hoak J. Management of deep vein thrombosis and pulmonary embolism. Circulation 1996;93:2212–45.

Lee TH, Goldman L. Evaluation of the patient with acute chest pain. N Engl J Med 2000;342:1187–95.

Mangrum JM, Dimarco JP. Evaluation and management of bradycardia. N Engl J Med 2000;342:703–9.

Panju AA, et al. Is this patient having a myocardial infarction? JAMA 1998; 280:1256–63.

Studies and Trials

Arrhythmias

The Antiarrhythmics vs. Implantable Defibrillator Trial (AVID). A comparison of antiarrhythmic drugs vs. implantable defibrillators in patients resusciated from near-fatal ventricular arrhythmias. N Engl J Med 1997;337:1576–83. (*An RCT showing that defibrillators had 75.4% 3-year survival vs. 64.1% for amiodorane or sotalol when used in patients who had had VF or sustained VT.*)

Buxton AE, et al. A randomized study of the prevention of sudden death in patients with coronary artery disease. N Engl J Med 1999;341:1882–90. (*In patients with CAD, a LVEF < 40%, asymptomatic, unsustained but inducible ventricular tachycardia, implantable defibrillators reduced the risk of cardiac arrest or death by 76%, whereas antiarrhythmic drugs had no benefit.*)

Cardiac Arrhythmia Suppression Trial (CAST). Effect of encainide and flecainide on mortality in a randomized rial of arrhythmia suppression after myocardial infarction. N Engl J Med 1989;321:406–12. (*This landmark trial concluded that the class IC agents encainide and flecainide more than tripled the arrhythmic mortality of post-MI patients.*)

Coplen SE, et al. Efficacy and safety of quinidine therapy for maintenance of sinus rhythm after cardioversion. Circulation 1990;82:1106–16. (*This meta-analysis showed that qunidine nearly tripled mortality in this situation.*)

Manning WJ, et al. TEE facilitated early cardioversion from cardioversion from atrial fibrillation using short-term anticoagulation. J Am Coll Cardiol

1995;25:1354–61. (*TEE allowed for immediate conversion of atrial fibrillation if no thrombus was found.*)

Mason JW. A comparison of electrophysiologic testing with Holter monitoring to predict antiarrhythmic drug efficacy for ventricular tachyarrhythmias. N Engl J Med 1993;329:445–51. (*This CT showed no difference in arrhythmia recurrence between the two groups.*)

Multicenter Automatic Defibrillator Implantation Trial (MADIT). Improved survival with an implanted defibrillator in patients with coronary disease at high risk for ventricular arrhythmia. N Engl J Med 1996;335:1984–5. (*This seminal trial showed that implanted defibrillators prolonged survival compared to standard medical therapy in patients with a prior MI, an EF of < 35%, and inducible sustained VT.*)

Roy D, et al. Amiodarone to prevent recurrence of atrial fibrillation. N Engl J Med 2000;342:913–20. (*Amiodarone is more effective than sotalol or propafenone in preventing atrial fibrillation recurrences [35% risk of recurrence in amiodarone-treated patients vs. 63% for other group] over 16 months.*)

Singh SN, et al. Amiodarone in patients with CHF and asymptomatic ventricular arrhythmia. N Engl J Med 1995;333:77–82. (*Although amiodarone was effective in suppressing ventricular ectopy in this RCT, there was no reduction in incidence of sudden death or improvement in survival.*)

Teo KK. Effects of prophylactic antiarrhythmic drug therapy in acute myocardial infarction. JAMA 1993;270:1589–95. (*A meta-analysis concluding that beta-blockers reduced mortality by 16% and amiodarone by 24%, whereas class I agents increased mortality by 10%. Calcium blockers had no significant effect on mortality.*)

Coronary Artery Disease

Boden WE. Outcomes in patients with acute non-Q-wave MI randomly assigned to invasive vs. conservative management. N Engl J Med 1998;338:1785–91. (*Non–Q-wave MI patients who had early catheter [vs. conservative medical management] had worse outcomes in the first year and no mortality difference at 2 years.*)

Boushey CJ, et al. A quantitative assessment of plasma homocysteine as a risk factor for vascular disease. JAMA 1995;27:1049–57. (*A meta-analysis concluding that homocysteine is a risk factor for atherosclerotic disease that is likely reversible with folic acid.*)

Cannon RO, et al. Imipramine in patients with chest pain despite normal coronary angiograms. N Engl J Med 1994;330:1411–7. (*An RCT showing that imipramine 50 mg qhs reduced chest pain episodes in this population.*)

Cholesterol and Recurrent Events Trial. The effect of pravastatin on coronary events after myocardial infarction in patients with average cholesterol levels.

N Engl J Med 1996;335:1001–9. (*An RCT of 4,019 post-MI patients in which pravastatin produced a 24% reduction in incidence of fatal or nonfatal MI, as well as need for revascularization.*)

Craven TE, et al. Evaluation of the association between carotid artery atherosclerosis and coronary artery stenosis. Circulation 1990;8:1230–42. (*This case-control study found carotid ultrasound to be equivalent to other risk factors for identifying patients with coronary heart disease.*)

The Framingham Heart Study. Incidence of CHD and lipoprotein cholesterol levels. JAMA 1986;256:2835–8. (*This RCT found that total cholesterol was directly proportional to the rate of CHD and that HDL cholesterol was a protective factor against risk of CHD.*)

Global use of strategies to open occluded coronary arteries (GUSTO IIb Trial). A clinical trial comparing primary coronary angioplasty and tissue plasminogen activator for acute myocardial infarction. N Engl J Med 1997;336:1621–8. (*PTCA had a 9.6% incidence of negative endpoints [death, nonfatal reinfarction, and nonfatal CVA] versus 13.7% for TPA, a statistically significant difference, in this RCT of 1,138 patients with acute ST elevation.*)

Gottlieb S, et al. Effect of beta-blockade on mortality among high and low risk patients after MI. N Engl J Med 1998;339:489–97. (*Beta-blockers decreased mortality by 40% even in those with contraindications [CHF, COPD, old age] and also in subendocardial infarctions.*)

Graham IM. Plasma homocysteine as a risk factor for vascular disease. JAMA 1997;277:1775–81. (*This study showed that elevated homocysteine was a risk factor for vascular disease equal to smoking and hyperlipidemia.*)

Grines CL, et al. Coronary angioplasty with or without stent implantation for acute MI. N Engl J Med 1999;341:1949–56. (*This RCT found that routine implantation of a heparin-coated stent in acute MI patients undergoing angioplasty reduced negative outcomes [death, ischemia, reinfarction, or stroke] from 20.1% to 12.6%.*)

Gruppo Italiano per Lo Studio Della Soprovvivenza Nell'infarto Miocardio (GISSI-3 Trial). Effects of lisinopril and transdermal glyceryl trinitrate singly and together on 6 week mortality and ventricular function after acute MI. Lancet 1994;343:115–22. (*In this RCT of 19,394 patients, lisinopril begun within 24 hours of onset of MI produced a 12% reduction in mortality and 10% reduction in LV dysfunction. Nitrates had no effect on either outcome.*)

He J, et al. Passive smoking and the risk of coronary heart disease. N Engl J Med 1999;340:561–5. (*Passive smoking causes a 25% increase in the risk of CHD.*)

The Helsinki Heart Study. Primary prevention trial with gemfibrozil in middle-aged men with dyslipidemia. N Engl J Med 1987;317:1237–45. (*Gemfibrozil increased HDL, reduced LDL, and decreased coronary heart disease by 30% in a large RCT.*)

International Study of Infarct Survival (ISIS-2). Randomized trial of intravenous streptokinase, oral aspirin, both, or neither among 17,187 cases of suspected acute MI. Lancet 1988;2:349–60. (*Aspirin produced a 25% reduction in mortality, and streptokinase a 24% reduction. Combined use resulted in a 42% reduction in mortality.*)

ISIS-4. A randomized trial of oral captopril versus placebo, oral mononitrate versus placebo, and intravenous magnesium versus control among 58,043 patients with suspected acute MI. Lancet 1995;345:669–85. (*Captopril produced a 7% mortality reduction. Nitrates and magnesium had no significant effects.*)

The LIPID Group. Prevention of cardiovascular events and death with pravastatin in patients with coronary heart disease and a broad range of initial cholesterol levels. N Engl J Med 1998;339:1349–57. (*Pravastatin cut mortality by 24% in this RCT of 9,014 patients [more benefit in high cholesterol patients, but mortality was reduced by 19% even in those with normal cholesterol].*)

Mark DB, et al. Cost effectiveness of thrombolytic therapy with tPA as compared with streptokinase for acute MI. N Engl J Med 1995;332:1418–24. (*TPA was most cost effective in patients over 60 and in those with anterior infarctions.*)

The Multiple Risk Factor Intervention Trial (MRFIT). JAMA 1990;263:1795–801. (*In a large RCT primary prevention trial of multifactorial interventions [targeted at smoking, hypertension, and cholesterol], the special intervention group had 24% less mortality from acute MI, 10.6% less mortality from CAD, and 7.7% decreased all-cause mortality.*)

Ridker PM, et al. C-reactive protein in the prediction of cardiovascular disease in women. N Engl J Med 2000;342:836–43. (*Elevated levels of high-sensitivity C-reactive protein were a strong predictor of cardiovascular disease in women [relative risk = 4.4].*)

Scandinavian Simvastatin Survival Study Group (4S). Randomized trial of cholesterol lowering in 4,444 patiens with coronary heart disease. Lancet 1994;344:1383–9. (*In an RCT of patients with angina or previous MI, simvastatin produced a 25% reduction in total cholesterol, 35% decrease in LDL, 8% increase in HDL, 30% decrease in all-cause mortality, 42% decrease in cardiac mortality, and 30% decrease in need for revascularization procedures.*)

Shepherd J, et al. Prevention of coronary heart disease with pravastatin in men with hypercholesterolemia. West of Scotland Coronary Prevention Study Group (WOSCOP). N Engl J Med 1995;333:1301–7. (*An RCT of primary prevention of cardiac events in 6,595 men with a mean LDL of 192 using pravastatin, which produced a 31% reduction in coronary death, nonfatal MI, and need for revascularization.*)

Thrombolytics in Myocardial Ischemia (TIMI IIIb Trial). A randomized comparison of tPA vs. placebo and early invasive vs. early conservative strategies in unstable angina and non-Q-wave MI. J Am Coll Cardiol 1995;26:1643–50. (*In this RCT of 1,473 patients, TPA patients had a higher rate of fatal and nonfatal MI. There was no difference in outcome between early invasive and conservative strategies, except for the invasive group having a lower rate of rehospitalization.*)

Weaver WD, et al. Comparison of PTCA and IV thrombolytics for acute MI. JAMA 1997;278:2093–8. (*A meta-analysis showing that PTCA was slightly superior to thrombolytics with respect to rates of mortality, stroke, and reinfarction.*)

Zijlstra F, et al. Long-term benefit of primary angioplasty as compared with thrombolytic therapy for acute MI. N Engl J Med 1999;341:1413–9. (*Over 5 years, primary angioplasty patients had a mortality of 13% compared with 24% for streptokinase group. Angioplasty also reduced the rate of nonfatal reinfarction, heart failure, and recurrent ischemia.*)

Congestive Heart Failure

The CIBIS Trial. The Cardiac Insufficiency Bisoprolol Study. Lancet 1999;353:9–13. (*Bisoprolol reduces the mortality of CHF patients by 34%.*)

The Digitalis Investigation Group. The effect of digitalis on morbidity and mortality in patients with heart failure. N Engl J Med 1997;336:525–33. (*Digitalis did not decrease mortality, but it did decrease hospitalizations for CHF.*)

Hjalmarson A, et al. Metoprolol CR/XL Randomized Intervention Trial in CHF (MERIT). JAMA 2000;283:1295–1302. (*Extended-release metoprolol reduces mortality and hospitalizations by 31% and improves the quality of life in patients with CHF.*)

Pfeffer MA, et al. Effect of captopril on mortality and morbidity in patients with LV dysfunction after MI. N Engl J Med 1992;327:669–77. (*In this RCT with a median of 3.5 year follow-up, captopril produced a 19% reduction in all-cause mortality, 21% reduction in cardiovascular death, 25% decrease in reinfarction, and 37% decrease in progression to heart failure.*)

Hypertension

The ALLHAT Trial. Major cardiovascular events in hypertensives randomized to doxazosin vs. chlorthalidone. JAMA 2000;283:1967–74. (*Chlorthalidone and doxazosin offer equal risk reduction of mortality and nonfatal MI, whereas chlorthalidone reduces the risk of CHF, stroke, angina, and need for coronary revascularization more than doxazosin.*)

Appropriate Blood Pressure Control in Diabetes (ABCD) Trial. The effect of nisoldipine compared to enalopril on cardiovascular outcomes in patients with type 2 diabetes mellitus and hypertension. N Engl J Med 1998;338:645–52. (*Nisoldipine patients had 9.5 times the risk of MI as those on enalopril.*)

Kostis JB. Prevention of heart failure by antihypertensive drug therapy in older patients with isolated systolic hypertension. JAMA 1997;278:212–6. (*Chlorthalidone reduced heart failure by 49%; in those with prior MI, it reduced CHF by 80%.*)

Packer M, et al. The effect of carvedilol on morbidity and mortality in chronic heart failure. N Engl J Med 1996;334:1349–55. (*Carvedilol reduced all-cause mortality by 65%. However, there were few patients with advanced heart failure.*)

Pitt B, et al. Randomized trial of losartan versus captopril in patients over 65 with heart failure. Lancet 1997;349:747–52. (*Losartan was associated with a 32% risk reduction in all-cause mortality.*)

Valvular and Structural Heart Disease

Konstantinides S, et al. A comparison of surgical and medical therapy for atrial septal defect in adults. N Engl J Med 1995;333:469–73. (*Surgical closure of ASD reduced mortality and functional deterioration.*)

Lieberman EB, et al. Balloon aortic valvuloplasty in adults. J Am Coll Cardiol 1995;26:1522–8. (*Balloon valvuloplasty did not change the course of outcome of aortic stenosis.*)

Lin M, et al. Vasodilator therapy in chronic asymptomatic aortic regurgitation. J Am Coll Cardiol 1994;24:1046–53. (*Enalapril was superior to hydralazine in improving LV functional parameters.*)

Vascular Disease

Colucci WS, et al. IV Nesiritide for decompensated CHF. N Engl J Med 2000; 343:246–53. (*Nesiritide, a natriuretic peptide, improved hemodynamics and clinical status on a short-term basis for patients admitted with decompensated CHF.*)

Evans JM. Increased incidence of aortic aneurysm and dissection in giant cell (temporal) arteritis. Ann Intern Med 1995;122:502–7. (*Patients with temporal arteritis were 17.3 times more likely to develop thoracic aortic aneurysms and more than twice as likely to develop abdominal aortic aneurysms.*)

Ridker PM, et al. Factor V Leiden and risks of recurrent idiopathic venous thromboembolism. Circulation 1995;92:2800–2. (*In this segment of the Physicians' Health Study, Factor V Leiden increased the risk of recurrent DVT by 4 to 5 times.*)

Schomig A, et al. Coronary stenting + abciximab vs. tPA for acute MI. N Engl J Med 2000;343:385–91.(*Stenting plus abciximab is superior to TPA alone with respect to myocardial salvage and clinical outcomes over 6 months post-MI.*)

Schulman S, et al. A comparison of 6 weeks with 6 months of oral anticoagulant therapy after a first episode of venous thromboembolism. N Engl J Med 1995;332:1661–5. (*Six months of anticoagulation produced a 9.5% recurrence rate over 2 years vs. 18.1% for 6 weeks of therapy.*)

7

Pulmonary Medicine

Honor a physician with the honor due unto him for the uses which you may have of him: for the Lord hath created him. —Ecclesiastes 38:1

Our greatest glory is not in never falling but in rising every time we fall. —Confucius

INTRODUCTION

The pulmonary floor is not the ICU; therefore, some topics such as mechanical ventilation, acute respiratory distress syndrome (ARDS), and pneumothorax will be covered elsewhere. Overall, this is a busy service, as the diagnoses of asthma and COPD are common ones, especially in the fall and winter months. This chapter is intended to give you a general guide to the common types of pathology seen on this type of service, so some restrictive lung diseases like pneumoconiosis, byssinosis, and leiomyomatosis will be given short shrift. One of the most important things to remember on this floor is (as always) to WASH YOUR HANDS! Infective bronchitis and upper respiratory infections (URIs) are really communicable and you'll see a lot here, so be careful. Also, the patient with end-stage COPD in room 4 really doesn't need room 3's *Klebsiella* pneumonia, so wear gloves (see Chapter 5).

Lung Volumes

See Figure 7–1 for a graphic description.
- TLC = total lung capacity
- FRC = functional residual capacity, which is the volume of the lung at the end of normal expiration
- Inspiratory capacity (IC) = TLC – FRC
- Residual volume (RV) = volume of the lung at the end of full expiration
- Vital capacity (VC) = TLC – RV
- Tidal volume (TV) = volume of normal breath

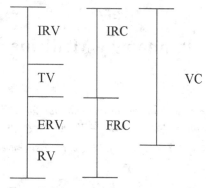

Figure 7-1. Lung volumes.

- Expiratory reserve (ERV) = FRC – RV
- Inspiratory reserve (IRV) = VC – TV – ERV

Flow Volume Loops

- A restrictive pattern causes a much smaller volume with a similar shape to normal breathing (ie, low VC). See Table 7-1 for obstructive patterns.

Table 7-1. Obstructive Patterns

	Causes	Pattern
Fixed upper airway obstruction	Tumors, tracheal stenosis	Flat curves both with inspiration and expiration
Extrathoracic obstruction	Tracheomalacia, vocal paralysis	Inspiratory obstruction with flat curve
Intrathoracic obstruction	Superior vena cava syndrome	Flat expiratory phase

FEV_1/FVC

FEV_1/FVC = ratio of expiratory volume in the first second of expiration to forced vital capacity; low in obstructive disease.

DLCO

DLCO = diffusion capacity for carbon monoxide, which is affected by anything blocking gas-blood oxygen exchange (especially interstitial lung disease).

ASTHMA

Quick Points
- Asthma is defined as reactive airway disease that shows a 12% or more response to bronchodilators by FEV_1 from a technical standpoint.
- A true asthmatic who smokes probably has psychological problems, as this behavior is not only self-destructive but also extremely unpleasant for the person involved.
- Asthma has two peaks, one in childhood and one in middle age; it is very rare to present with asthma for the first time at 65.
- Occupational asthma is related to workplace allergens and tends to be worse after return to work on Monday after an allergen-free weekend.
- Exercise-induced asthma is defined as a drop in FEV_1 by 15% on exposure to cold, dry air. It is seen a lot in young people and athletes.

Initial Management
- Peak flow meter, ABG, and pulse oximetry are all quite useful in evaluation of an acute attack.
- Asthmatics in an acute attack should have a low carbon dioxide partial pressure (PCO_2), as they are tachypneic; if he or she has a normal or elevated PCO_2, that is an ominous sign indicating that the person is tiring out and running out of respiratory reserve.
- Interventions:
  - Nebulized albuterol (can be given continuously or at any frequency indicated)
  - Albuterol via metered-dose inhaler (switch to this once the patient is more stable)
  - Steroids (for severe attacks, start methylprednisolone [Solu-Medrol] 60 mg IV q6h; give lower doses or even oral prednisone for less severe attacks)
  - Oxygen

- In severe cases, give theophylline (eg, Theo-Dur 100–300 mg PO bid) or aminophylline (6 mg/kg IV loading dose, followed by 1 g/250 cc D_5W at 0.7 mg/kg/hr). Be careful with this drug, as it has many contraindications and toxicities and is generally not routinely used.
- Intubation: this decision is primarily clinical and should not hinge on ABG or pulse oximetry.

Further Discussion

A. In reality, patients will call almost any episode of shortness of breath, wheeze, or cough asthma, and you need to make this determination by history (Table 7–2).

Table 7–2. Key Questions in Asthma History

When did it first start?

How many hospitalizations?

How many intubations?

What medications (inhalers)?

What is the pattern of inhaler/nebulizer use?

Any history of atopy (eczema)?

Any triggers (upper respiratory infection, animals, and smoking)?

B. *Asthma tests* include the peak flow meter, spirometry (useful in both diagnosis and following the disease course), and the methacholine challenge test (useful only in diagnosis). The latter is rarely used as history, for spirometry and physical findings will almost always yield a diagnosis.

1. *Peak flow.* This handy little device is simple to use (for most people) and is handy for determining how bad an attack is and how the patient is doing over time. A drop in peak flow to < one half of baseline is defined as an admittable asthma attack, and patients should be encouraged to use this device at home to monitor themselves.

2. *Spirometry.* We use spirometers all of the time in our clinic, and every patient with asthma gets an FEV_1/FVC done at each visit. Like the EKG, it is a change from baseline rather than any absolute

numbers that should worry you. Once again, this device is good for overall, over-time measurement of disease progression.

3. *Formal spirometry.* This is useful in diagnosis as the patient is evaluated both before and after bronchodilator use, and the percent change in FEV_1 is shown. Note that in asthma, which is basically obstructive, you will see a decrease in the FEV_1/FVC ratio (normal is 0.8, but it will be less in a patient having an acute attack).

4. *ABG.* This test shows hypoxia and usually normal or low PCO_2. If an asthmatic has a high PCO_2, this is a bad sign, as it shows that he or she is tiring out and has impending respiratory failure.

5. *Pulse oximetry.* This is another rough measure as to how the patient is doing, and the target should be at least 92% saturation for O_2 therapy.

C. Treatment (Inpatient)

1. *Beta agonists.* these drugs are wonderful in either acute or chronic asthma. Generally well tolerated, their major side effect is tachycardia and jumpiness from a proadrenergic effect. They act by opening up airways via smooth muscle contraction, simulating a fight or flight response in the lung only. Giving beta agonists by metered-dose inhaler (MDI) or nebulizer yields similar results, assuming that the patient has a proper technique with the MDI. All patients should be given beta-agent MDIs at the bedside for use once they feel up to it so that nebulizer treatments can be tapered.

2. *Steroids.* These are a powerful weapon against asthma but are often misunderstood. First, *there is no difference between IV and oral steroids.* This may shock you, but, if pressed, no one can cite a convincing study that shows any difference. Remember, steroids have very good bioavailability. Nevertheless, IV methylprednisolone (Solu-Medrol) is often given in the acute setting, usually 60 mg q6 hours for 24 hours in order to "break" an asthma attack. Steroids should actually take a few hours to have an effect as they act to decrease airway inflammation and mucus secretion and do not act instantly like beta agonists. Patients should be kept on a substantial dose of oral steroids until improvement shows (40-mg prednisone qd) and then be tapered off.

3. *Antibiotics.* Pneumonia or bronchitis commonly triggers asthma. If either is suspected, a course of antibiotics is warranted. Give IV

medicines in pneumonia and oral agents in bronchitis (eg, cefuroxime, clarithromycin [Biaxin]) with an eye toward covering common
respiratory invaders.

4. *Theophylline.* This phosphodiesterase inhibitor leads to bronchodilation. It is not commonly used due to drug interactions and
side effects.

D. Treatment (Outpatient)

1. *Beta agonists* are best used with a spacer and on an as-needed basis.
Use is usually two to four puffs every 4 to 6 hours, depending on
severity. Overuse is associated with an increase in mortality (pre-
sumably due to worse or worsening disease) and is an indicator that
the patient may require hospitalization and/or steroids. Albuterol
(Proventil) is a mainstay of acute bronchodilation, whereas salme-
terol (Serevent) has effects for 12 hours. *Never* let your patient run
out of this medicine. It is a ticket to the ER.

2. *All asthmatics need both influenza vaccine and Pneumovax.* "An
ounce of prevention is worth a pound of worry."

3. *Oral steroids* can be used on an outpatient basis in various ways.
For an acute attack, a short course of prednisone 40 mg for 4 to
5 days with no taper is allowable. In more brittle asthmatics or in
those who are more chronically steroid dependent, a more gradual
taper is indicated, usually starting at 40 and dropping by 10 every
3 to 4 days. Some patients are taught to keep their own bottles of
10-mg prednisone at home for just such an emergency and self-
administer and taper this drug.

4. *Inhaled steroids* are very useful in that they are essentially topical
(lung only) without side effects of adrenal axis suppression or bone
demineralization. They also work quite well in that they greatly
decrease the rate of attacks. Inhaled steroids (eg, Vanceril, Azma-
cort, Flovent) are used for chronic maintenance of asthma: use the
least dose needed to prevent attacks. Too often, patients just don't
get the idea that this is a preventive medicine! You *have* to drum it
into them that it is *not* for acute attacks and *not* to be used like a
beta agonist. Furthermore, to avoid giving your patients ricotta
cheese throat (candidiasis), they *must* use a spacer and rinse their
mouth after use.

5. *Cromolyn sodium (Intal)* is a useful, mast cell stabilizing drug with few to no side effects that reduces the frequency of attacks (not for use in an acute attack). It can be used as two puffs via MDI qid or 200 mg PO qid.

6. By blocking leukotrienes (specifically leukotriene D_4), *antileukotrienes* reduce bronchoconstriction. Clinically, they seem to be useful as out-patient medications to reduce the frequency of attacks (not for acute use). Zafirlukast (Accolate) is 20 mg PO bid and zileuton (Zyflo) is 600 mg PO qid. Montelukast (Singulair) is a newer agent.

CHRONIC OBSTRUCTIVE PULMONARY DISEASE

Quick Point
- Symptoms are very similar to asthma, although the pathogenesis involves the destruction of lung tissue from smoking.

Initial Management
- Nebulized albuterol
- Nebulized ipratropium (anticholinergics seem to have a better effect in COPD patients than asthma)
- Steroids can be used in COPD but are not great.
- Mucomyst (*N*-acetylcysteine) is useful to break up mucus secretions.
- Antibiotics (eg, cefuroxime 750 mg IV q8h) seem to reduce the duration of exacerbations of chronic bronchitis.
- Continuous long-term oxygen therapy is indicated for resting arterial oxygen < 55 mm Hg, oxygen saturation < 88%, or arterial oxgyen < 59 mm Hg with erythrocytosis or cor pulmonale. Noncontinuous therapy is indicated during exercise or sleep if those activities have arterial oxygen < 55.

Further Discussion

A. *Emphysema* is a destructive dilation of the alveoli due to loss of their septa and the formation of bullae with a lower surface area. This acts not to decrease O_2 absorption but to increase airway compliance, making for a hyperdistensible lung that never fully deflates. On spirometry, the residual volume takes up a proportionally greater portion of the triple-lumen catheter (TLC) (even though the baggy lung has a higher total lung capacity), so it's sort of like breathing at a higher baseline resting volume—not a pleasant feeling. Like in asthma, the FEV_1/FVC ratio is decreased and is usually below 0.8. There is little to no response to bronchodilators with this problem as it is not hyperreactivity of smooth muscle but actual destruction of lung architecture. Not surprisingly, there is no cure, although bullectomy has been tried with some success.

1. Centroacinar affects the area right near the terminal bronchiole; this is the type seen in smokers.
2. Panacinar affects all of the acini and is usually seen in α_1-antitrypsin disease.
3. Note that only 15% of smokers develop emphysema.
4. The air trapping in this disease, like in asthma, results in "auto-peep" (self-made increases in peak end expiratory pressure), which can make putting these patients on vents somewhat tricky as their ravaged lungs have a tendency to burst when too much pressure is applied.
5. Treatment is usually with atropine or ipratroprium bromide in addition to the normal antiasthma medications and oxygen. Note that steroids may not be of any use in emphysema unless there is also a component of mucus hyperproduction.

B. *Chronic bronchitis* is defined as 3 consecutive months of increased secretions (symptoms) for at least 2 consecutive years.

1. This is not always directly due to a bacterial infection, so antibiotics are not always needed; however, cefuroxime, clarithromycin, or TMP-SMX (Bactrim) is frequently given in acute exacerbations as prompt use may avert longer-term illness or complications. Antibiotics seem to frequently shorten the duration of exacerbation.
2. Treatment is once again similar to asthma but with the addition of atropine for further mucus control.
3. Mucomyst. This is used to dissolve and break up excess secretions in especially bad COPD or asthma and can be used for a day or two (any more leads to severe drying problems and thence ulceration).

C. *Bronchiectasis* is recurrent inflammatory damage to the small airways, resulting in pathologic dilation, bleeding, and mucus hypersecretion. It is usually found in those whose airways are immunocompromised (cystic fibrosis, Kartagener's syndrome, dysmotile cilia) and is almost always caused by infection, usually with *Staph.* or *Pseudomonas*.

D. General notes
   1. "Pink Puffer" = emphysema (normal to low O_2, high CO_2; thus, increased rate)
   2. "Blue Bloater" = bronchitis (low O_2; hence blue skin, but CO_2 not as high as above)

INTERSTITIAL LUNG DISEASE

A. Interstitial lung disease (ILD) reflects a group of problems presenting with a restrictive, not obstructive, picture with corresponding loss of FVC and normal FEV_1/FVC ratios and low DLCO. Damage is in the lung interstitium, causing fibrosis and thickening of the walls between the alveoli and vasculature. Interstitial diseases are rare and not overly treatable; they tend to be more in the domain of occupational medicine specialists (many occur from exposure to industrial materials). However, even though you will most likely never see this type of disease and, if you do, will be mostly unable to treat it, the Medical Boards love this stuff, so you still have to learn it. So much for pragmatism.

B. *Occupational Exposures*
   1. *Hypersensitivity pneumonitis* (bird fancier's lung, hay mold/thermophilic actinomyces, grain dust, air conditioning systems, and isocyanates).
      a. "Farmer's lung" is due to moldy hay.
      b. Poorly formed granulomas (unlike sharp ones in sarcoid).
      c. Suspect if the patient has recurrent pneumonia and occupational risk.
      d. Corticosteroids are useful in acute exacerbations.
      e. Similar to eosinophilic pneumonia but there are no peripheral eosinophils.
      f. Treatment is removal from work.
   2. *Organic dust (cotton dust)* causes byssinosis characterized by chest tightness regularly at the end of Monday (first day of the work week); treatment is removal from the work environment.
   3. *Inorganic dust* (the biggie) (see Table 7–3 for characteristics):
      a. *Asbestosis* occurs with > 10 years of exposure. Exposure can cause mid-thoracic pleural thickening and plaques but may not lead to impairment. Asbestosis results in pulmonary fibrosis (due

to repeated attacks on indigestible asbestos fibers by macrophages resulting in the full inflammatory cascade) at the lung bases, an increased risk of non–small cell lung cancer (NSCLC), and mesothelioma (the latter is not caused by smoking).

b. *Silicosis* takes years of exposure to develop; simple silicosis is characterized by upper lobe calcifications (eggshells), unlike asbestosis, which is lower lobe. Complicated nodular silicosis (progressive massive fibrosis) has large > 1-cm nodules and is due to massive exposure. It is similar to pulmonary alveolar proteinosis. Silicosis may or may not increase cancer risk, but it does increase the risk of TB (treat for TB in anyone with silicosis and a positive tuberculin skin test [PPD]).

c. *Coal workers' pneumoconiosis* looks a bit like silicosis on x-ray (upper lung field nodules) and has simple and progressive forms. The progressive form, like the complicated type of silicosis, has large nodules < 2 cm and is due to severe exposure; it leads to melanoptysis and is synergistic with smoking for loss of function.

d. *Berylliosis* also affects the upper lobes with hilar lymphadenopathy and granulomas that look identical to sarcoid. Because it is a cell-mediated response, even small exposures can cause this disease.

Table 7–3. Selected Interstitial Pulmonary Diseases

Condition	Exposure	Characteristics
Asbestosis	Pipe fitting, boilermaking, brake linings, navy yards, fire insulation	Pleural thickening, pulmonary fibrosis, increased risk for mesothelioma and non–small cell lung cancer
Silicosis	Mining, foundry, stonecutting	Eggshell hilar calcification, nodular pulmonary fibrosis, increased risk of TB
Berylliosis	Ceramics, electronics	Granulomas similar to sarcoid, hilar nodes
Coal miners' pneumoconiosis	Coal mining	Nodular opacities, rarely fibrosis
Byssinosis	Cotton handling	Monday afternoon asthma

4. A few things to remember are that (1) the Occupational Safety and Health Administration is working hard to make these diseases obsolete with the use of respirators and better safety conditions, and (2) once the damage is done, it is not really reversible; the only treatment is to take the person out of the job. So much for occupational interstitial disease.

C. *Nonoccupational Interstitial Lung Disease*
   1. *Collagen vascular disease* (CVD) (see Chapter 17 for full details). Remember, ILD is due to inflammatory processes at the vascular/alveolar level, so any CVD is a good candidate for causing this.
      a. You may be surprised to note that rheumatoid arthritis (RA) can cause pulmonary fibrosis in one-third of cases (Caplan's syndrome + RA + pulmonary fibrosis). It can also happen from the use of gold or methotrexate (MTX) to treat the disease. Necrobiotic nodules are occasionally seen on CXR in the upper lung zones. Pleurisy is present and sometimes effusion with a low glucose.
      b. SLE, of course, can cause idiopathic pulmonary fibrosis (IPF) (SLE can do anything it wants), affecting both lung and pleura (+ pleurisy, ± effusion, hemoptysis).
      c. Scleroderma also causes interstitial fibrosis and will also cause intimal proliferation leading to pulmonary HTN. This and RA increase your risk for bronchogenic cancer.
   2. *BOOP* (a funny name, but not a funny disease)
      a. Bronchiolitis obliterans with organizing pneumonia (BOOP) is insidious in onset and has fever, dyspnea, cough, malaise, and myalgia (looks like flu).
      b. X-ray shows bilateral patchy infiltrates.
      c. Penicillamine can sometimes cause this.
      d. Treatment is corticosteroids, and definitive diagnosis is by open lung biopsy. This problem is differentiated from IPF by the fact that IPF never has fever.
   3. *Sarcoidosis*
      a. This is a common disease that you will actually see.
      b. It is most common in African-American females but can occur in anyone.
      c. It forms noncaseating granulomas, usually with bilateral hilar adenopathy seen on x-ray.

    d. Pulmonary function tests (PFTs) are restrictive ± an obstructive component.

    e. You may see on labs increased calcium, increased gammaglobulin, and increased ACE (the latter is nondiagnostic, however).

    f. The best diagnosis is by transbronchial biopsy showing non-caseating granuloma.

    g. Erythema nodosum can also occur, and this designates a good prognosis.

    h. Seventy-five percent recover without treatment, but severe disease is treated with corticosteroids; however, these have not been shown to cause remission and are usually only used when other organs are involved.

    i. Remember, sarcoid can involve almost any tissue besides the lung, including the kidney, brain, skin, eye, and heart muscle conduction fibers.

4. Eosinophilic Granuloma

    a. Also known as Langerhans' cell granulomatosis

    b. Occurs in smokers, males more than females

    c. Can cause pneumothorax in 50% of affected people

    d. Smoking cessation is the best treatment; steroids don't do much.

    e. CXR positive for honeycomb lung characterized by interstitial change and small cystic spaces in the upper lung fields

    f. We don't know anyone who has ever seen this.

5. Lymphangioleiomyomatosis

    a. Occurs in premenopausal females

    b. Result of lymphatic and vasculature smooth muscle hyperprofusion

    c. Results in honeycombing on CXR, but this is diffuse (not upper lobe, only in eosinophilic granuloma)

    d. Pneumothorax is also common

    e. Chylous pleural effusions

    f. We had never even heard of this until we did a Board review.

6. Vasculitides (see Table 7–4 for characteristics)

    a. Wegener's: causes necrotizing granulomas, pulmonary vasculitis with cavitary nodules, associated with purulent nasal discharge, hematuria, or renal failure

    b. Churg-Strauss: look for in patients with preexisting asthma and eosinophilia

Table 7–4. Vasculitides Affecting the Lung

Condition	Characteristics
Wegener's	Necrotizing granulomas, cavitary nodules, nasal polyps, hematuria, renal failure
Churg-Strauss	Asthma, eosinophilia
Goodpasture's	Anti-basement membrane antibody causing hemoptysis + hematuria

    c. Goodpasture's syndrome: remember, hemoptysis precedes kidney failure from all of the attacks on the basement membrane. It resembles Wegener's without upper airway signs (like epistaxis).

    d. Idiopathic pulmonary hemosiderosis: like Goodpasture's but no kidney involvement

    e. As you can probably guess, treatment for all of this involves immunosuppressive therapy, which is best left to the rheumatology people.

D. A Few Last Notes

    1. Diagnosing the type of ILD is a headache as you can see from the above, and the rarity of these disorders makes it tougher still. Bear in mind that if you have a dyspneic patient who hasn't responded to inhalers, send them for PFTs and make sure to check the DLCO. If an abnormality is seen, then further work-up can commence. This usually involves CT and bronchoscopy, as well as tests for vasculitis, autoimmune disorders, and the like. If all of these tests bear no fruit, and all one sees is an interstitial fibrosis of the lung, then you have IPF.

    2. IPF is a diagnosis of exclusion.

      • It is slow, progressive, and ultimately fatal, and probably autoimmune in nature.

      • It sort of looks like BOOP in presentation, but there is never any fever, and the patient doesn't become acutely ill with it.

      • Onset of SOB is around 6 months, and x-ray shows diffuse infiltrates, not patchy like in BOOP.

      • Only 20% show improvement on (you guessed it) corticosteroids, with improvement being followed with lung volumes, DLCO, and ABG to track progression.

PULMONARY EMBOLISM

Quick Points

- Signs and symptoms include dyspnea (78%), tachypnea (73%), pleuritic pain (59%), rales on auscultation (55%), cough (43%), tachycardia (30%), and low-grade fever (rarer).
- Risk factors are Virchow's triad (venous damage, stasis, and hypercoagulability), which occurs in or due to cancer, oral contraceptives, smoking, postoperative patients (especially hip replacement), invalids, and protein C/S deficiency.
- ABG shows a high alveolar-arterial gradient (see below).
- X-rays will show atelectasis or density (69%), pleural effusions (47%), or an elevated hemidiaphragm (28%) in PE, but it is usually going to be a biggie if you see this. The classic sign is Westermark's sign (triangular area of peripheral lung opacity due to infarction).

Initial Management

- There is an old proverb, "Patients die from their second PE, not their first." Rapid intervention does make a difference.
- Recommended diagnostic approach to a stable patient with a possible PE (see Chapter 2, Figure 2–1):
  - Perform a leg Doppler (if positive, anticoagulate).
  - Check serum D-dimer (if negative, it is almost impossible for the patient to have a PE, which almost always gives fibrin degradation products, which are picked up on D-dimer).
  - If the leg Doppler is negative and the D-dimer is positive, go to spiral CT or MRI.
  - Pulmonary angiogram remains the gold standard for any questionable or unstable cases.
- Anticoagulate with heparin (check guaiac concurrently and make sure the patient has no bleeding problems elsewhere).
- Once the patient is stable, think about coumadinization versus placement of an inferior vena cava (Greenfield) filter to prevent future emboli (see discussion below).

Further Discussion

A. PE is a frustrating disease condition for a multitude of reasons. First, it is often not even thought of. Second, it tends to mimic other problems, like MI, pneumonia, or costochondritis. The best advice we can give is to be on the lookout for it in the susceptible and to never forget that every tachycardic, tachypneic individual you see may, in fact, be suffering from this common and serious disorder.

B. General Notes
   1. If properly treated, the mortality rate of acute PE is 5 to 8%.
   2. If not properly treated, the mortality rate is 25 to 30% (yikes!).
   3. Two-thirds of deaths occur within 1 to 2 hours of the event.
   4. Recurrent emboli kill most people, developing in 70% of patients with prior PE.
   5. The symptoms mimic other disorders.

C. Arterial Blood Gases
   1. Contrary to what you may expect, you will not have a high PCO_2 and you may or may not have a low PO_2. It really depends on how big a PE it is. Don't use pulse oximetry alone; if you suspect PE, do a room air ABG and calculate the alveolar-arterial gradient.
   2. Alveolar – arterial gradient = $150 - ([PCO_2/0.8] + PO_2)$ on room air. Nasal cannula will mess up your fraction of inspired oxygen (FIO_2) as you can't know how much the person is really getting (the rule of thumb is that each liter by nasal cannula increases the oxygen amount by 3%, so 2 L of nasal cannula = room air (21%) + 6% = 27% (approximately).
   3. The gradient is normally 10 to 20, or age $\times$ 0.4 if over 40 years.

D. The V/Q Scan
   1. This test results, all by itself, in much of the irritation factor in dealing with PEs.
   2. The test is nonspecific, reader dependent, and probably overused, especially in light of newer diagnostic developments.
   3. This test is rarely read as either normal or as high probability. Usually, you get something noncommittal like "intermediate or low probability." Even if read as low probability, if the clinical picture fits, there is still a 40% chance of PE. In short, this test does much to rule in but little to rule out the disease.

E. The Spiral CT of Pulmonary Circulation
   1. A CT/angiogram is of great help in diagnosis. Although not useful in finding small peripheral emboli, it is good (95%) at finding large central

ones. Overall, it is the latter that are actually worrisome and liable to kill a patient, so this test is pragmatically the best one. (In renal failure patients, MRI may be an alternative [less contrast load]).

2. It is also useful in patients who cannot tolerate or cooperate with V/Q or have underlying lung disease, making V/Q unreliable (emphysema, lung cancer, pneumonia).

F. Pulmonary Angiogram
   1. This is the gold standard, but it is not done much as it is more invasive. Furthermore, with spiral CT, it is less difficult to make the diagnosis.
   2. Basically, only do this if the clinical picture is in contradistinction to all of your diagnostic tests and you have to be sure it's not a PE.

G. Ultrasound
   1. Most PEs come from DVT of the leg (deep and superficial femoral veins, popliteal, etc, but not varicose veins).
   2. In the face of a negative ultrasound, PE is highly unlikely unless V/Q or CT strongly opposes this.

H. Treatment
   1. In our hospital, we use a weight-based algorithm for heparinization, namely, 80 U/kg load, and then 18 U/kg IV starting drip.
   2. Before rushing in to do this, you must check for bleeding problems and guaiac the patient. We have all seen the horrors of heparin.
   3. *Oxygen, oxygen, oxygen* (give them a nice O_2 saturation of 92% or so).
   4. Once the patient is stabilized, you must decide what to do next.
      a. Greenfield filters should be placed in those who have failed previous warfarin (Coumadin). (This is a nasty umbrella-like thing that is permanently inserted in a femoral or inferior vena cava [IVC]. It stops big clots but if left in long enough forms clots of its own and severe leg swelling. Avoid them in young patients.)
      b. A Greenfield, however, is not an anticoagulant, so in the infirm, unsteady, alcoholic, or very aged, it may be a safer alternative.
      c. Warfarin, as you know, is rat poison, and you should treat it as such. It is a difficult drug to dose and control and can be fatal if either too much or too little is taken.

    d. Usually, this is begun about 24 hours after a stable PTT is reached (a feat in itself) and then fiddled with to attain an INR of 2 to 3, usually throughout the entire course of treatment as this medicine has a funny way of being completely unpredictable.

    e. Patients normally start at around 10 mg of loading dose for 1 to 2 days, and then this is adjusted. Remember that the INR you see today actually reflects the warfarin dose taken yesterday.

5. Note that low molecular weight heparin is approved for treatment of DVT and negates all of this cumbersome INR testing; its place is really in the treatment of uncomplicated DVTs in patients who can be treated at home (ie, young, otherwise healthy).

6. Treatment is usually around 6 months for the DVT to resorb, but it can also be chronic depending on the patient's reason for hypercoagulability.

TUBERCULOSIS

Quick Points

- Infection is generally via inhalation. Disease may never ensue (90% are disease free), but a person's risk of conversion (positive PPD) is 5% in the first 5 years and then 10% thereafter. AIDS patients have a 40% risk of conversion within the first several months (not years).
- TB likes oxygen, so it has a proclivity for the upper lobes and lung apices.
- Signs and symptoms include cough, night sweats, frequent fevers, weight loss, hemoptysis, and weakness, with CXR changes showing upper lobe infiltrates or hilar adenopathy.

Further Discussion

A. This nasty mycobacterial disease is on the rise as it has found its niche ecologically as a mutualist with HIV. As such, its prevalence has increased in urban areas and areas of low socioeconomic status as this problem grows. Fortunately, in New York City at least, the enforcement of directly observed therapy and rigorous screening has actually lowered the TB prevalence from what it was 5 to 10 years ago.

B. Infection begins when an aerosolized droplet of sputum from an infected person is inhaled. The drop goes right down into the lung by gravity and the tubercle bacteria set up shop in an alveolus.

C. Even those who convert may not get active disease, but if they do, the common symptoms are as above.

D. Note that 15% of TB is extrapulmonary, sometimes causing meningitis, vertebral disease (Pott's disease), or arthritis. Almost any other organ in the body is susceptible. Pathology shows caseating granulomas.

E. Screening (see Table 7–5 for screening interpretation)
1. Those who need to be screened are HIV patients, close contacts of those with TB or recent conversion, IDUs, low-income populations, the homeless, and immigrants from endemic areas.
2. Tests are the PPD or serial, once-a-year, CXRs.
3. The PPD is only contraindicated in those with prior necrosing reactions; however, if a patient is known to be PPD+, there is little indication for retesting.
    a. False negatives occur in cases of anergy or too recent exposure. You can fix this by doing concomitant mumps/*Candida* inoculation and by retesting in 1 month, respectively.
4. So what does one do with a positive PPD?
    a. In the high-risk group, give prophylactic therapy regardless of age.
    b. In the moderate-risk group, use prophylaxis for the IDUs, HIV patients (non-AIDS), diabetics, patients with renal failure or hema-

Table 7–5. Guidelines for Interpreting Tuberculin Skin Test Induration

> 15 mm	Positive in all patients
10–15 mm	Positive in moderate-risk groups:
	Homeless
	Injection drug users
	Health care workers
	Diabetics
	Those on steroids
	Children
5–10 mm	Positive for high-risk groups:
	HIV-positive patients
	Patients with a positive chest x-ray
	Close contacts of documented case

tologic malignancy, those on prednisone use, or otherwise debilitated people. In those who are from endemic areas, migrant workers, homeless, or inmates, do not treat unless under 35 years old.

c. Everybody else is treated only if under 35 years (if over 35, treatment hepatotoxicity is worse than not treating).

d. Note that if you are negative but had a high-risk contact (eg, a full-blown TB case coughs into your open mouth as you inhale), you need treatment until a repeat PPD is negative 10 to 12 weeks later.

5. What is this booster effect, anyway?

a. This is a phenomenon seen in the elderly and infirm.

b. Basically, it means that a person can have a negative PPD if the initial exposure was long enough ago.

c. To test, just repeat the PPD in 1 to 3 weeks after the initial negative.

F. Treatment

1. Treatment is with four agents for the first 2 months and then two drugs for the last 4 months.

2. Yes, it's a 6-month ordeal.

3. The "big two" are isoniazid (300 mg PO qd) and rifampin (300 mg PO bid): these are the drugs that go the whole 6-month period.

4. The other two are pyrazinimide (1,000 mg PO bid) and ethambutol (800 mg PO bid) or streptomycin (weight based).

5. In patients with a very low risk of having multidrug-resistant TB, a three-drug regimen may be used, dropping the fourth drug (ethambutol or streptomycin).

6. Toxicities of TB drugs:

- Isoniazid and rifampin both cause hepatotoxicity (monitor LFTs and look for right upper quadrant pain and hepatomegaly).
- Isoniazid causes peripheral neuropathy (give vitamin B_6 to pre-empt this).
- Ethambutol causes retrobulbar optic neuritis (if there are any visual problems, call Ophthalmology immediately).

7. Exceptions: if the patient can't use pyrazinamide, then isoniazid and rifampin are given for 9 months; if the TB is resistant to isoniazid, then give the other three drugs for 6 months.

8. Multidrug-resistant TB is dangerous and hard to treat; antibiotics are based on sensitivities.

LUNG CANCER

Quick Points
- Risk factors include smoking (10×), asbestos (6×), and uranium and nickel mining.
- Stopping smoking decreases the risk over time until year 15, when it is again at baseline.
- The symptoms are oddly similar to those of TB; hemoptysis, weight loss, malaise/low energy, and fevers occur in both conditions.
- Lung cancer is the leading cause of death among both men and women (it recently beat breast cancer in females), and 85% of these deaths are smoking related. So much for Phillip-Morris's research.

Further Discussion

A. *Cancers*
  1. Adenocarcinoma: peripheral, most common, early metastases (CNS, adrenals, bone), usually a solitary nodule. Subtype is bronchoalveolar carcinoma (which is associated with scars).
  2. Squamous carcinoma: central, doesn't metastasize early, causes obstructive picture, cavitates.
  3. Small cell lung cancer (SCLC): central, aggressive, doesn't cavitate, 80% positive metastases at diagnosis.
  4. Large cell lung cancer: peripheral, CNS, and mediastinal metastases; superior vena cava syndrome.

B. *Solitary Pulmonary Nodule*
  1. Middle to lateral one-third of lung with normal surrounding parenchyma.
  2. Thirty-five percent are malignant.
  3. Calcifications usually imply benignity.
  4. Follow it every 3 months with x-rays.
  5. Biopsy if a high-risk person (ie, a smoking asbestos worker).

C. *Paraneoplastic Clues*
  1. Elevated calcium occurs in squamous cell cancer (which secretes parathyroid hormone [PTH]-related peptide.

2. SIADH, Cushing's syndrome, and Eaton-Lambert myasthenic syndrome (see Chapter 8) occur in SCLC (which can produce endocrine hormones).
3. Gynecomastia occurs in large cell cancer.
4. Hypertrophic osteoarthropathy occurs in all three types of NSCLC.

D. *Diagnosis* is made by a variety of techniques, starting with basic labs, followed by imaging, and then to either bronchoscopy (if the lesion is less peripheral) or mediastinoscopy, or mediastinotomy/open thoracotomy.

E. *Treatment*
   1. NSCLC. The type doesn't matter much with regard to survival.
   2. Stage I (in situ) NSCLC is treated with surgery and stage II (local nodes) with radical surgery.
   3. Stage II NSCLC is resected if the node involvement is ipsilateral.
   4. Stage IIIb NSCLC is generally nonsurgical due to lymph node or local extension. Thoracotomy is the only way to cure this, and if there are metastases, palliative treatment with radiation is all that can be done.
   5. SCLC is a rapid divider and therefore not all that amenable to surgery as it is usually metastatic at discovery. SCLC is classified by limited (no known metastases) or disseminated disease. Treatment is with chemotherapy and radiation and is usually palliative.

MISCELLANEOUS

A. *Sleep Apnea*
   • Associated with obesity, HTN, cor pulmonale, daytime hypersomnolence, car accidents
   • Treat with weight loss, avoidance of alcohol or sedatives, proper sleep hygiene, and nasal continuous positive airway pressure (CPAP) or BIPAP

B. *Cystic Fibrosis*
   • This once pediatric disease now goes into adulthood as treatment prolongs survival.

- Chloride channel defect (cystic fibrosis transmembrane conductance regulator) impairs cilia function, causing recurrent pneumonias, pancreatic insufficiency, and sterility.
- Treatment includes antibiotics, chest physiotherapy, and DNase.

BIBLIOGRAPHY

Reviews

Arcasoy SM, Kotloff RM. Lung transplantation. N Engl J Med 1999;340:1081–91.

Barnes PJ. Chronic obstructive pulmonary disease. N Engl J Med 2000;343:269–80.

Bassetti C, Aldrich MS. Narcolepsy. Neurol Clin 1996;14:545–72.

Beckett WS. Occupational respiratory diseases. N Engl J Med 2000;342:406–13.

Crapo RO. Pulmonary-function testing. N Engl J Med 1994;331:24–30.

Davis PB, et al. Cystic fibrosis. Am J Respir Crit Care Med 1996;154:1229–56.

Drazen JM, et al. Treatment of asthma with drugs modulating the leukotriene pathway. N Engl J Med 1999;340:197–206.

Goldhaber SZ. Pulmonary embolism. N Engl J Med 1998;339:93–104.

Heffner JE, et al. Diagnostic value of tests that discriminate between exudative and transudative pleural effusions. Chest 1997;111:970–80.

Hillberg RE, Johnson DC. Noninvasive ventilation. N Engl J Med 1997;337:1746–52.

Joseph J, Sahn SA. Connective tissue diseases and the pleura. Chest 1993;104:262–70.

Kollef MH, Schuster DP. Acute respiratory distress syndrome. N Engl J Med 1995;332:27–37.

Light RW. Management of spontaneous pneumothorax. Am Rev Respir Dis 1993;148:245–8.

Newman LS, et al. Sarcoidosis. N Engl J Med 1997;336:1224–34.

Raghu G. Interstitial lung disease. Am J Respir Crit Care Med 1995;151:909–14.

Rubin LJ. Primary pulmonary hypertension. N Engl J Med 1997;336:111–7.

Sahn SA. The pleura. Am Rev Respir Dis 1988;138:184–234.

Slutsky AS. Mechanical ventilation. Chest 1993;104:1833–59.

Smetani GW. Preoperative pulmonary evaluation. N Engl J Med 1999;340:937–44.

Strollo PJ, Rogers RM. Obstructive sleep apnea. N Engl J Med 1996;334:99–104.

Ware LB, Matthay MA. Acute respiratory distress syndrome. N Engl J Med 2000;342:1334–9.

Guidelines

American Sleep Disorders Association. Practice paramenters for the treatment of obstructive sleep apnea. Sleep 1996;19:152–5.

American Thoracic Society. Guidelines for the initial management of community-acquired pneumonia. Am Rev Respir Dis 1993;148:1418–26.

American Thoracic Society. Hospital-acquired pneumonia. Am J Respir Crit Care Med 1996;153:1711–25.

American Thoracic Society. Standards for the diagnosis and care of patients with COPD. Am J Respir Crit Care Med 1995;152:S77–120.

American Thoracic Society. Treatment of TB. Am J Respir Crit Care Med 1994;149:1359–74.

Cahil BC, Ingbar DH. Massive hemoptysis. Clin Chest Med 1994;15:147–68.

Studies and Trials

Critical Care

Connors AF, et al. The effectiveness of right heart catherization in initial care of critically ill patients. JAMA 1996;276:889–97. (*This controversial study found that Swan-Ganz catheterization did not reduce mortality but increased the cost and length of stay.*)

Prod'hom G, et al. Nosocomial pneumonia in mechanically ventilated patients receiving antacid, ranitidine, or sucralfate. Ann Intern Med 1994;120:653–62. (*An RCT showing that patients on sucralfate had much less late-onset pneumonia than those on ranitidine or other antacids, with similar rates of GI bleeding.*)

Rouby JJ, et al. Risk factors and clinical relevance of nosocomial maxillary sinusitis. Am J Respir Crit Care Med. 1994;150:776–83. (*Nasal tubes [intubation or gastric tubes] increased the risk of maxillary sinusitis [from 22.5 to 95.%];67% of sinusitis patients developed nosocomial pneumonia.*)

Valles J, et al. Continuous aspiration of subglottic secretions in preventing ventilator-associated pneumonia. Ann Intern Med 1995;122:179–86. (*An RCT showing that continuous aspiration of subglottic secretions reduced the risk of ventilator-associated pneumonia.*)

Pulmonary Embolism

Prospective investigation of PE diagnosis (PIOPED). JAMA 1990;263:2753–9. (*Specificity of V/Q scans was only 10% for PE. Sensitivity of high-probability scans was only 41%. Thus, V/Q scans are generally not clinically useful.*)

Interstitial Lung Disease

Abenhaim L, et al. Appetite-suppressant drugs and the risk of primary pulmonary hypertension (PPH). N Engl J Med 1996;335:609–16. (*Use of appetite suppressants for more than 3 months increased the risk of primary pulmonary HTN by 23.*)

Barst RJ, et al. A comparison of continuous IV prostacyclin with conventional therapy for primary pulmonary hypertension. N Engl J Med 1996;334:296–302. (*An

RCT showing that IV prostacyclin continuously improved survival and function in primary pulmonary HTN patients.)

Gibson GJ, et al. Effects of long-term corticosteroid treatment in sarcoidosis. Thorax 1996;51:238–47. (*Steroids improved long-term outcomes in sarcoid patients.*)

Ziesche R, et al. Long-term treatment with IFN gamma-1b and low-dose prednisolone in patients with IPF. N Engl J Med 1999;341:1264–69. (*One year of treatment with IFN-γ-1b + prednisolone improved lung capacity and resting oxygenation.*)

Cystic Fibrosis

Fuchs HJ, et al. Effect of DNase on exacerbations of respiratory symptoms and on pulmonary functions in cystic fibrosis. N Engl J Med 1994;331:637–42. (*An RCT showing that qd or bid inhalation of DNase reduced respiratory exacerbations by one-third and slightly improved pulmonary function.*)

Chronic Obstructive Pulmonary Disease/Asthma

Anthonisen NR, et al. Effect of smoking intervention on rate of decline of FEV1. JAMA 1994;272:1497–505. (*An RCT showing that quitting halved the rate of decline of FEV1 [from 63 mL/yr to 34 mL/yr].*)

Geddes D, et al. Effect of lung-volume reduction in emphysema. N Engl J Med 2000;343:239–45. (*Lung-volume reduction increased FEV, walking distance, and quality of life.*)

Saint S, et al. Antibiotics in COPD exacerbations. JAMA 1995;273:957–60. (*A meta-analysis showing that antibiotics are of some benefit, especially in severe cases of COPD and in those needing hospitalization.*)

Suissa S, et al. Low dose inhaled steroids and prevention of death from asthma. N Engl J Med 2000;343:332–6. (*Regular use of low-dose beclomethasone decreased asthma mortality by 21%.*)

Thompson WH, et al. Controlled trial of oral prednisone in outpatients with acute COPD exacerbation. Am J Respir Crit Care Med 1996;154:407–12. (*An RCT showing that prednisone helped hasten recovery and reduced treatment failure.*)

8

Neurology

Diagnose, then Adios! We don't treat disease, we admire it. — Simmons Lessell, on neurology

Knowledge and experience are like a pair of shoes: you can go farther with both than one alone. — Anonymous

HISTORY AND PHYSICAL

- Time course:
  - Acute events suggest strokes or seizures.
  - Subacute (hours to days) course suggests infectious or demyelinating etiologies.
  - Chronic disease is likely to be degenerative or neoplastic in origin.
  - Progressive focal deficits suggest mass lesion.
- Somatization is often unmasked by inconsistencies in gait, sensation, and muscle strength that do not correlate with one another or with basic anatomy.
- Sensory examination: see Clinical Neuroanatomy below
- See Table 8–1 for upper versus lower motor neuron signs.
- Cerebellar function is assessed by checking gait, finger-to-nose touching, heel-shin sliding test, and rapid alternating movements. Signs of dysfunction are
  - Ataxia and broad-based gait
  - Dysmetria: past pointing on finger-to-nose testing
  - Dysdiadochokinesia (inability to rapidly alternate movements, eg, to hit one hand alternately with the palm and back of the other hand)
  - Poor ability to slide heel down one's shin
- Pupils (see Table 8–2 and Chapter 18)

Table 8–1. Upper versus Lower Motor Neuron Signs of Pathology

	Upper Motor Neuron	*Lower Motor Neuron*
Reflexes	Hyperreflexia	Hyporeflexia
Tone	Spastic	Flaccid
Other	Positive Babinski's sign (upgoing toe)	Fasciculations

Table 8–2. Selected Pupil Syndromes

Syndrome	*Characteristics*
Horner's	Loss of sympathetics causing anhidrosis, ptosis, and miosis
Adie's	Denervation of parasympathetics causing tonic dilation of pupil that reacts poorly to light but constricts with accommodation
Argyll Robertson	Often due to syphilitic midbrain damage, these are small pupils that accommodate but don't react ("prostitute's pupil")
Marcus Gunn's	Afferent pupillary defect (detected on swinging flashlight test)

DIAGNOSTICS

- MRI is superior for posterior fossa lesions, spine, and small lesions.
- CT is superior to rule out hemorrhage.
- EEG is useful in seizures, but normal EEG does not rule out epilepsy. It is useful in coma, herpetic encephalitis (temporal discharges), hepatic encephalopathy (triphasic waves), and Creutzfeldt-Jakob disease (bilateral synchronous repetitive sharp waves).
- Electromyogram/nerve conduction velocity (EMG/NCV) is useful for peripheral neuropathies, myopathies, and determining the origin of muscle weakness. Demyelinating disorders cause slow NCV.
- Myelography is useful in patients with disk disease and tumor and also allows sampling of CSF.
- Muscle biopsy is done for multiorgan conditions and for myopathies.
- Nerve biopsy is good for asymmetric, multifocal neuropathy (do the sural nerve).
- Evoked potentials are useful for multiple sclerosis (where they can find a second lesion in patients with only one known lesion) and detecting subclinical lesions in spinal cord or cranial nerve [CN] III.

Clinical Neuroanatomy

See Table 8–3 for dermatome distribution.

1. Cranial nerves: remember the "Oh, Oh, Oh, To Touch And Feel" and "Some Say Marry Money But My Brother Says..." mnemonics for CN names and sensorimotor function. In brief:

   - I = olfactory nerve. Supplies the sense of smell. Lost in the anterior cerebral artery (ACA) infarct.
   - II = optic nerve. Runs from the eye, decussates at the chiasm (where nasal axons [carrying temporal visual field] cross to the other side). Optic tracts originating from the chiasm then go to the lateral geniculate body in the thalamus, which sends axons along optic radiations (geniculocalcarine tract) to the occipital lobe (near calcarine fissure). Some fibers from the optic tract divert away to the brachium of the superior colliculus as part of the pupillary reflex pathway. Some inferior optic radiation fibers course into the temporal lobe (Meyer's loop) en route to the occipital lobe.

Table 8–3. Selected Spinal Levels and Dermatomes

Level	Distribution		
C3–5	Phrenic nerve (needed for breathing)		
C5 to T1 (brachial plexus)	Sensory	C5	Lateral arm
		C6	Lateral forearm, thumb, and index finger
		C7	Middle finger
		C8	Medial forearm
		T1	Medial arm
	Motor	C5–6	Biceps
		C7	Triceps
T4	Nipple		
T10	Umbilicus		
L4	Knee		
L5	Great toe and its extensor (motor loss causes foot drop when standing on heel)		
S1	Lateral foot; motor loss results in difficulty standing on toes		
S2–4	Anal sphincter (S2, 3, and 4 "help keep it off the floor")		

- Lesions anterior to the chiasm will cause visual defects in only one eye; posterior lesions generally cause defects in both eyes (contralateral homonymous hemianopsia).
- Pituitary tumors affect the chiasm and cause "pie in the sky" visual field defects (superior temporal defects), progressing to bitemporal field defects.
- Internal carotid aneurysms affect the lateral chiasm, causing monocular nasal field defect.
- Meyer's loop lesions cause homonymous superior quadrantanopia.
- Occipital lobe lesions usually spare the macula.
- III = oculomotor nerve. Arises from the superior colliculus in the tectum of the midbrain and runs underneath the uncus (which is why it is susceptible to uncal herniation. Supplies all of the extraocular muscles except the superior oblique and lateral rectus.
- IV = trochlear nerve. Arises from the midbrain as well and is the longest CN, as it is the only CN to arise from the dorsum of the brain. Thus, it is the most vulnerable to closed head trauma.
- V = trigeminal nerve. Arises from the pons and goes to the trigeminal ganglion in Meckel's cave in the skull base. Divides into ophthalmic (V1), maxillary (V2), and mandibular (V3) branches.
  - V1 supplies sensation to the eye and forehead. See Chapter 18 for further detail.
  - V2 supplies sensation to the cheek and maxilla. In blunt facial trauma, damage to V2 causes numbness.
  - V3 is the only part of the trigeminal nerve that has both a sensory (mandibular area) and a motor (muscle of mastication) component.
- VI = abducens nerve. From the lower pons, this supplies the lateral rectus.
- VII = facial nerve. Arises from the cerebellopontine angle. The part of its nucleus that supplies the forehead is innervated by both hemispheres; hence, only peripheral facial nerve injury can cause loss of wrinkling of the forehead (unlike central lesions). The geniculate branch supplies the anterior two-thirds of the tongue.
  - Surgery or damage to parotid glands can cause facial nerve injury.
  - Bell's palsy = idiopathic peripheral nerve injury, which can cause corneal exposure (inability to fully blink), loss of smile on

the affected side, loss of taste, loss of lacrimation, and hyper-acusis. Treat with prednisone + acyclovir.

- VIII = vestibular nerve. Arises from the cerebellopontine angle (hence, acoustic neuromas and cerebellopontine angle tumors affect both VII and VIII). See Chapter 18 for more information.
- IX = glossopharyngeal nerve. Arises from the medulla and supplies the tongue and pharynx.
- X = vagus nerve. Arises from the medulla and supplies much of the autonomic system. The recurrent laryngeal nerve supplies the vocal cords.
- XI = spinal accessory nerve. The cranial component joins the vagus, whereas the spinal component supplies the sternocleido-mastoid and trapezius (so loss of XI causes you to "drop your shoulder and look at it").
- XII = hypoglossal nerve. Arises from the medulla and passes through the foramen magnum. Loss causes tongue deviation toward the affected side.

2. Spinal Cord:
- Posterior columns carry deep touch, vibration, and proprioception and are affected in syphilis (lues) and vitamin B_{12} deficiency (sub-acute combined degeneration). Their destruction causes Romberg's sign (on closing the eyes, patients lose balance).
- The lateral corticospinal tract carries the primary motor tract, which synapses on anterior horn cells at appropriate levels. Lateral corti-cospinal tracts are affected in B_{12} deficiency, whereas anterior horn cells are killed in polio and Lou Gehrig's disease (amyotrophic lateral sclerosis [ALS]).
- The lateral spinothalamic tract carries pain and temperature. These fibers decussate in the spinal cord about two levels above entry, which accounts for why syringomyelia (dilation of canal of spinal cord) affects pain and temperature primarily.
- Arnold-Chiari malformation is associated with syringomyelia and cerebellar herniation through the foramen magnum, causing severe weakness.

3. Stuff Inside the Head (see also Stroke Syndromes, below):
- Superior sagittal sinus mass lesions can cause increased intracranial pressure (ICP) and headache without other focal signs

- Cavernous sinus lesions affect the VI nerve first (as it passes inside the sinus), but also III, IV, V1, and V2 (which pass in the wall of the sinus). Sympathetics traveling with the carotid artery can also be affected, causing Horner's syndrome.
- Basilar artery disease causes bilateral motor weakness and nerve VI palsy.
- Posterior inferior cerebellar artery infarcts cause Wallenberg's syndrome (see Stroke Syndromes) and cerebellar findings. Posterior interior communicating artery aneurysms can cause painful nerve III palsy with efferent pupillary defect.

ALTERED MENTAL STATUS

Coma

Commonly Confused Terms

- Abulia = severe apathy and delay in response due to frontal lobe lesions.
- Brain death = unresponsiveness, no pupillary function (midbrain), no doll's eyes (pontine), and apnea (off ventilator, no response to PCO_2 > 60). EEG is helpful but not necessary to establish this diagnosis.
- Locked-in syndrome = pontine infarction causing loss of all motor function except eye motions (remember CN V is at the pons, so that and everything below are gone).
- Persistent vegetative state: absent cognition after brain damage.

Initial Management
- Approach to coma:
  - Ensure airway.
  - Give coma cocktail: thiamine, glucose, naloxone. Consider flumazenil.
  - Assess consciousness, pupils, ocular motility, posturing.
  - Check pupils (see Table 8–4)
- Check posturing:
  - Decerebrate (extensor) posturing = extension of lower extremities and elbows.
  - Decorticate (flexor) posturing = flexion of elbows with extension of legs.
  - Decorticate is better to have (the brain stem is probably okay).

Table 8–4. Pupil Syndromes in Coma

Pupillary Characteristics	Probable Cause(s)
One dilated unreactive pupil	Parasympathetic denervation (CN III compression from uncal herniation, subarachnoid hemorrhage, etc)
One pinpoint pupil	Horner's (eg, hypothalamic or lateral medullary stroke)
Two pinpoint pupils	Pontine infarct or opiate overdose
Two midpoint nonreactive pupils	Midbrain injury (anoxia, hypothermia, barbiturates)
Two dilated nonreactive pupils	Encephalopathy (anoxia, barbiturates)

- Check ocular motility:
  - Horizontal disconjugate gaze at rest indicates cranial neuropathy.
  - Skew deviation (disconjugate vertical gaze) implies brainstem lesion.
  - Horizontal conjugate gaze implies ipsilateral hemispheric or pontine lesion or contralateral thalamic lesion.
  - Nystagmus during coma may mean there is status epilepticus.
  - Calorics:
    - Normally, cold water in the ear canal will cause slow motion of the eyes to the same side, and warm water will cause slow motion to the other side.
    - If the brain stem is injured, then COWS will happen (cold, opposite, warm, same).
  - Doll's eyes: if the brain stem is intact, the eyes will move opposite to head motion in an attempt to stay fixed.
- Tests include CBC, SMA, toxicology screen, CT, LP (if meningitis is suspected and only after CT rules out mass lesion), and EEG (if seizures or brain death is an issue).
- See Chapter 15 for management of ↑ ICP and Chapter 16 for the Mini-Mental State Examination (MMSE).
- Ninety-six percent of patients with nontraumatic coma who had abnormal brainstem responses or absent motor responses at 72 hours die or

have severe disability. If there is no improvement within 1 month, a persistent vegetative state is common.

Delirium

Quick Points
- Delirium is an acute change in mental status with altered alertness, disturbed attention, disorganized thinking, sleep problems, abnormal behavior, altered psychomotor activity, and perceptual dysfunction. It is often worse in the evening ("sundowning").
- Risk factors are age, prior CNS disease, history of dependence on sedatives/alcohol/opiates, and recent surgery.
- Causes include medications (anticholinergics, opiates, sedatives), metabolic causes (hypoxia, cirrhosis, renal failure, CHF, hypoglycemia/hyperglycemia), hip fractures, bypass surgery, strokes, seizures, and subdural hematomas.
- On examination, multifocal myoclonus indicates anoxia, anticholinergics, narcotics, or uremia. Asterixis indicates hepatic or renal failure.
- Triphasic waves on EEG imply hepatic encephalopathy.

Initial Management
- Check medications and history.
- Treat the underlying cause. Support with environmental orientation (clocks, windows, calendars). Lorazepam (Ativan) or haloperidol (Haldol) should be used sparingly for severe agitation.

Dementia

Dementia is progressive and persistent impaired congitive function. Memory, language, executive function, orientation, and abstract thinking can all be affected. Consciousness is normal.

- *Alzheimer's disease* causes insidious cognitive dysfunction progressing to incontinence and psychosis. Risk factors are age, prior head trauma, Down syndrome, low education level, and family history. Apolipoprotein E4 (on chromosome 19) is also a risk factor. On pathology, neurofibrillary tangles and plaques are present. Pick's disease is clinically identical but different on histology. Treatment includes tacrine and donepezil (CNS anticholinesterases), which slow progression. Tacrine causes a lot of liver toxicity, whereas donepezil is safer. Antidepressants with minimal anticholinergic effect (eg, trazodone) may be needed.

- *Multi-infarct dementia.* Multiple strokes cause a stepladder increase in dysfunction. Focal neurologic deficits are commonly present.
- *Normal pressure hydrocephalus.* This is a triad of dementia, ataxia, and incontinence. There is no specific treatment.
- *Creutzfeldt-Jakob disease* is due to a slow virus (onset 20 years after exposure), causing rapid progression (myoclonus, dementia, and death within 1 year).
- Other causes include vitamin B_{12} deficiency, hyper- and hypothyroidism, and HIV (for which zidovudine [AZT] prevents and partially reverses dementia).

STROKE AND CEREBROVASCULAR DISEASE

Quick Points
- Cerebrovascular disease can be thrombotic, embolic, or hemorrhagic.
- TIA = neurologic deficits reversing within 24 hours (usually 5–20 minutes).
- Thrombotic strokes are usually preceded by a TIA (embolic strokes are not). Emboli go to the middle cerebral artery (MCA) most commonly, followed by the posterior cerebral artery (PCA), and then the ACA. Thrombosis frequency is the internal carotid artery and then the middle cerebral, vertebral, and basilar artery.

Initial Management
- CT without contrast to rule out hemorrhage (blood appears white).
- Neurologists prefer NS to D_5NS.
- If the patient has mild-to-moderate HTN, do not normalize it (you want to maintain cerebral perfusion pressure). If the BP is > 200/120, consider decreasing it; otherwise, it is okay to have a patient with systolic BP in the 160 to 190 range. If BP control is required, use labetalol instead of nitroprusside (the latter decreases cerebral perfusion).
- If the stroke is *not* hemorrhagic, decide whether the patient is a candidate for thrombolysis:
  - Inclusion criterion for TPA is presentation within 3 hours of onset.

- Exclusion criteria are previous stroke or head trauma in the last 3 months, any history of intracranial hemorrhage, BP > 185/110, history of bleeding disorder or current anticoagulation, or recent invasive surgical procedure.
- New research shows that intra-arterial prourokinase may be effective if given within 6 hours of onset into the specific artery that is thrombosed.
- Do EKG, echocardiography, and carotid Doppler to rule out embolic sources (looking for atrial fibrillation, patent foramen ovale, other structural heart disease, cardiac thrombi, carotid stenosis, and/or anomalies). Transcranial Doppler and magnetic resonance angiography (MRA) are useful to detect intracranial occlusive disease. Angiography is the gold standard.
- Do a hypercoagulability work-up for patients who have stroke and are < 50 years old, or if they have a personal or family history of thromboses.
- Heparin anticoagulation to 1.5 to 2× PTT is often used (depending on the hospital) for ischemic stroke for the initial course (make sure there is NO hemorrhage, and keep PTT < 2× normal). However, there is no conclusive proof that this is effective, and considerable controversy remains about heparin in stroke.
- North American Symptomatic Carotid Endarterectomy Trial (NASCET). The risk of recurrent ipsilateral stroke was reduced in patients with CVA/TIA and > 50% carotid stenosis in institutions with experienced surgeons and low operative mortality. For 100% stenosis lesions, endarterectomy should not be done.
- Asymptomatic Carotid Artery Stenosis Trial (ACAS). In patients with asymptomatic carotid artery stenosis (detected by bruit or Doppler), the rate of ipsilateral stroke in those with > 60% carotid stenosis decreased by 53% by endarterectomy.
- Long-term medical management includes antiplatelet agents (ticlopidine, ASA, or clopidogrel), which should be given to patients with nonsurgical stenoses. Coumadinize if the patient has hypercoagulability, has atrial fibrillation, or fails antiplatelet agents.

Hemorrhagic Strokes

Any intracranial hemorrhage can cause increased ICP, brainstem compression, or coma. Hemorrhagic strokes are most common in the putamen (sign is stroke in the internal capsule, which is damaged as it is adjacent to the putamen). Other hemorrhagic areas are listed in Table 8–5.

- For subarachnoid hemorrhage, work-up includes both CT and LP (CT is only 90% sensitive). LP may show frank blood or xanthochromia if the hemorrhage is old. Treatment includes nimodipine (reduces spasm), adequate hydration, management of BP, stool softeners to reduce straining, and surgery. Transcranial Doppler is useful to diagnose spasm.
- Intracerebral hemorrhage is associated with cocaine and arteriovenous malformations (AVMs).
- Cerebellar hematomas are surgical emergencies (they can rapidly cause brainstem compression; conversely, they are rapidly decompressible).
- Epidural hematomas (usually due to laceration of the middle meningial artery in the foramen spinosum) often occur after trauma (classic presentation is injury, a brief unconsciousness, a few hours of normal function, and then a sudden decline).
- Subdural hematomas present with a chronic course (may mimic dementia) and are usually venous in origin.
- On imaging, epidural hematomas have a biconvex shape, whereas subdural hematomas are concave toward the brain.
- In general, for intracranial hemorrhage, get Neurosurgery involved as soon as possible.

Table 8–5. Hemorrhagic Stroke Areas

Affected Area	Manifestations
Internal capsule	Contralateral hemiparesis, sensory loss, hemianopsia, and deviation of eye away from lesion
Thalamus	Sensory loss, possible hemiplegia, eyes turn down and in, unequal pupils
Pons	Locked-in syndrome, coma, miosis
Cerebellum	Ataxia, vomiting, ocular bobbing

Stroke Syndromes

- Middle cerebral artery (MCA): contralateral weakness, sensory loss, homonymous hemianopsia.
- Left MCA stroke causes aphasia (impaired language function).
- Right MCA causes impaired spatial function.
- Right brain lesions cause neglect of the left side.
- Frontal lobe lesions cause the eyes to turn toward the lesion.
- Parietal lesions cause loss of two-point discrimination, graphesthesia, and stereognosia: patients can't touch or direct gaze at objects that they see.
- Gerstmann's and Balint's syndromes (Table 8–6) are due to MCA disease.
- Posterior cerebral artery: contralateral homonymous hemianopsia.
- Anterior cerebral artery: weakness of distal contralateral leg.
- Vertebrobasilar artery: bilateral extremity sensorimotor findings (crossed findings, ie, left face, right arm), loss of consciousness, and CN dysfunction. Wallenberg's, Weber's, and Benedikt's syndromes (see Table 8–6) are due to vertebrobasilar disease.

Table 8–6. Selected Eponymous Stroke Syndromes

Syndrome Name	Affected Area	Manifestations
Gerstmann's	Left parietal lobe	Acalculia, dysgraphia, left-right confusion, and right hemiparesis
Balint's	Biparietal lobes	Optic and ocular ataxia (inability to visually guide limb or eye motions); inability to avoid objects in one's path
Weber's	Ventral midbrain	Ipsilateral nerve III palsy and contralateral hemiparesis
Wallenberg's	Lateral medulla	Nausea and vomiting, nystagmus, ipsilateral Horner's syndrome, ipsilateral palate weakness, crossed sensory loss
Benedikt's	Dorsal midbrain and red nucleus	Ipsilateral nerve III palsy + contralateral ataxia

Further Discussion
- Cocaine, migraine, and oral contraceptives in smokers are also associated with stroke.
- Neck trauma causing stroke is likely due to carotid dissection, which requires heparin and possibly surgery.
- Lacunar infarcts occur in the thalamus (pure sensory), internal capsule (pure motor), or pons (dysarthria, ataxia, clumsy hand) and are due to small artery disease from HTN or DM. Treat the disease and use antiplatelet agents.
- Syncope occurs from stroke only with hemorrhagic, large MCA, or brainstem strokes.

Epilepsy

Quick Points
- Syncope, psychogenic causes, TIAs, and migraine can simulate seizures. Psychogenic seizures show bizarre motor activity (pelvic thrusting) and no lip biting, incontinence, or postictal confusion.
- Epilepsy classification:
  - Simple partial: consciousness unimpaired, focal convulsions
  - Jacksonian march: simple partial seizure with secondary generalization
  - Complex partial: impaired consciousness, aura of visceral sensation, stereotypes (lip smacking, chewing, automatisms)
  - Generalized: (loss of consciousness)
    - Absence (petit mal): brief lapses of consciousness with 3-Hz spike-wave complexes on EEG
    - Myoclonic: 4- to 6-Hz spike-wave discharges, family history, chromosome 6
    - Tonic-clonic (grand mal): generalized convulsions

Initial Management
- Status epilepticus = two or more seizures without full recovery of function in between or continuous seizure activity for > 30 minutes
  - Secure airway; give thiamine + glucose.
  - Lorazepam (0.1 mg/kg) is effective. Then give phenytoin (Dilantin) (20 mg/kg) IV at a rate < 50 mg/min (lest there be hypotension).
  - If there is still no response, pentobarbitol coma with intubation is a last resort.

∞

- H&P, EEG, and MRI are needed for new-onset seizures. Anticonvulsant blood levels should be drawn on those not adequately controlled on present medications.
- The recurrence rate after the first seizure in the presence of a normal examination, EEG, and MRI is only 5%, so not all patients need medication, especially if precipitants are preventable (alcohol, hypoglycemia, fever).
- Use monotherapy when possible (see Table 8–7).
- Key toxicities of drugs are listed in Table 8–8.

Table 8–7. Recommended Agents for Epilepsy Subtypes

Type	Recommended Drugs
Primary generalized epilepsy	Valproate (Depakote); alternatives are phenytoin or carbamazepine
Secondary generalized epilepsy (eg, post-trauma or mass lesion)	Phenytoin (Dilantin); alternatives are valproate or carbamazepine
Partial	Carbamazepine; alternative is valproate
Absence	Ethosuximide or valproate
Myoclonic	Clonazepam or valproate

Table 8–8. Key Toxicities of Drugs

Drug	Toxicity
Carbamazepine	Agranulocytosis, hepatotoxicity (check WBC, LFTs regularly)
Phenytoin	Slurred speech, ataxia, confusion, gingival hyperplasia; fast IV infusion can cause ventricular fibrillation and severe hypotension
Valproate	Nausea/vomiting; rarely thrombocytopenia
Felbamate	Aplastic anemia, hepatotoxicity

- *Approach to pharmacotherapy:*
  - Increase the dose of medications until seizures are controlled or until toxicity occurs.
    - Antiepileptics show a linear relationship between dose and serum level, except phenytoin, where even small increases in dose can cause large elevations in serum levels.
  - If one drug fails, try a different drug before using combinations (combinations have more risk of interactions and toxicity).
  - In pregnancy, antiepileptic drugs cause a 5% risk of congenital malformations (cleft lip, heart lesions, neural tube defects [last with valproate or carbamazepine]).
    - Monitor levels closely; discontinue drugs if possible.
    - Folate reduces the risk of neural tube defects.
  - Check drug levels routinely if control is difficult; many patients will need doses giving levels above the therapeutic range for adequate control. Once seizures are controlled without toxicity, you can check drug levels less frequently.
  - Attempt to discontinue medication if the patient is seizure free for > 2 years, has a normal EEG, has no organic brain disease, and/or has a known preventable precipitant. Taper over a few weeks; patients should not drive while on taper.
- Epilepsy surgery can be done for recurrent partial seizures that are refractory.
- New agents:
  - Felbamate is useful for Lennox-Gastaut syndrome (found in children, this has a 3-Hz frequency with multiple seizure forms).
  - Gabapentin (Neurontin) is useful as an adjunct to carbamazepine (Tegretol) or phenytoin (Dilantin) and has almost no toxicity.
  - Lamotrigine (Lamictal) is as effective as carbamazepine but is much more expensive and also has more drug interactions (increases carbamazepine and decreases divalproex)

HEADACHE

See Table 8–9 for treatment.
  1. Migraine headaches are unilateral, throbbing headaches with sensitivity to light and sound. Aura is classically present.

Table 8–9. Treatment of Headache

Type	Prophylactic Treatment	Abortive Treatment
Migraine	Propranolol, verapamil	NSAIDs, ergotamine, sumatriptan
Cluster	Verapamil	Oxygen, steroids
Trigeminal neuralgia		Carbamazepine, surgery
Pseudotumor cerebri	Weight loss, avoidance of medications	Acetazolomide, prednisone, lumbar puncture, surgery
Tension		NSAIDs, antidepressants
Hemicrania	Indomethacin	Indomethacin

2. Cluster headaches occur daily for several weeks at the same time every day. Very severe in intensity, these can also cause tearing and Horner's syndrome. Patients are usually male and smoke.
3. Trigeminal neuralgia (tic douloureux) causes lancing pain across the face and is often due to vascular compression of the trigeminal nerve.
4. Pseudotumor cerebri occurs in obese, premenopausal women. Associated drugs are tetracycline and vitamin A. Withdrawal of chronic steroids may precipitate it. Symptoms include headache, diplopia, and visual field loss. Optic disc edema and/or hemorrhages are usually present. CT/MRI show small ventricles but otherwise a normal brain; LP shows high opening pressure.
5. Tension headache is the common headache that everyone gets.
6. Hemicrania is more frequent than cluster headaches (several times a day), is briefer, and occurs in women.

NYSTAGMUS

- Congenital nystagmus is horizontal.
- Downbeat vertical nystagmus is due to multiple sclerosis, basilar infarct, cervical lesions, seizure medications, and cerebellar atrophy.
- Upbeat nystagmus is due to lesions in the rostral medulla or caudal pons.

NEUROMUSCULAR DISORDERS

1. *Amyotrophic lateral sclerosis* (Lou Gehrig's disease): death of anterior horn cells in the spinal cord (possibly due to excitotoxicity or

superoxide dismutase dysfunction on chromosome 19) leading to progressive weakness (with death from aspiration/asphyxiation once respiratory muscles are involved), upper and lower motor neuron signs on examination (weakness, spasticity, fasciculations). Do MRI to rule out structural C-spine disease. Postpolio syndromes are nonprogressive but have similar deficits (polio destroys the anterior horn). Riluzole (antiglutamate agent) slows progression in patients with bulbar-onset disease. Baclofen reduces spasm.

2. *Peripheral neuropathies*:
   - Work-up includes glucose, creatinine, CXR, CBC, ESR, and T4. In patients over 40, do serum and immune protein electrophoreses (SPEP and IPEP).
   - Guillain-Barré: autoimmune reaction to peripheral myelin.
     - Occurs after virus (CMV, EBV, HIV), or *Campylobacter* infection.
     - Weakness ascends from the legs.
     - Treat with support (intubate if needed) + plasmapheresis + IV gamma globulin.
     - Negative inspiratory force (NIF) is useful in the decision to intubate.
   - Charcot-Marie-Tooth disease: autosomal-dominant sensorimotor neuropathy causing atrophic calves (champagne bottle legs), high arched feet, hammer toes, and enlarged nerves. Type 1 (chromosome 17) is demyelinating (slow NCV); type 2 (chromosome 1) is axonal (almost normal NCV).
   - Vasculitides: Wegener's syndrome, polyarteritis nodosa, lupus, and rheumatoid arthritis can cause mononeuropathy multiplex (multiple peripheral nerves). It is usually asymmetric.
   - Diabetes is a major cause of distal peripheral neuropathies.
   - Compressive neuropathies include:
     - Carpal tunnel syndrome from median nerve entrapment (due to repetitive stress) causing weakness, atrophy, and pain, especially in the thumb, index finger, and middle finger.
     - Wrist drop is produced by radial nerve compression (can happen with nephrosis and in alcoholics who pass out with their arms underneath—"Saturday night palsy").

- Peroneal nerve compression (at proximal head of fibula) causes foot drop, as can L5 radiculopathy. Peroneal nerve injury patients can invert the foot, whereas L5 radiculopathy patients cannot.
- Sciatic nerve compression (sciatica) causes difficulty standing on the tips of the toes but no decrease in ankle jerk (S1 radiculopathy patients have both).
- Other: didanosine, zalcitabine, vincristine, paclitaxel, and cisplatin cause peripheral neuropathy. Gammopathies (myeloma, amyloidosis, Waldenstrom's) also cause neuropathies. These are usually symmetric.
- The pain of peripheral neuropathy can be treated with low-dose tricyclics (amitriptyline or nortriptyline 20 mg PO qd), phenytoin, carbamazepine, mexiletine, and capsaicin cream.

3. *Neuromuscular junction diseases*:
   - Myasthenia gravis. Diagnose with pathologic fatigability in voluntary muscles (especially eye muscles).
     - Weakness gets worse with exercise, over the course of the day, and with hot environments.
     - Confirm with EMG, serum acetylcholine-receptor antibody, and edrophonium (Tensilon) test (edrophonium, an acetylcholinesterase inhibitor, will briefly improve muscle function).
     - Treat with thymectomy in anyone with generalized myasthenia gravis, steroids, plasmapheresis, and cholinesterase inhibitors (eg, pyridostigmine [Mestinon]).
   - Eaton-Lambert syndrome. Autoimmune antibody to the presynaptic nerve terminal causes weakness that improves with effort and exercise. Commonly seen in SCLC. Treat with plasmapheresis, IV gammaglobulin, and 3, 4 diaminopyridine (increases available acetylcholine).

4. *Myopathies*:
   - Thyroid: hypo- and hyperthyroidism cause weakness. Hypothyroidism elevates CPK as well (mimicking polymyositis).
   - Kearns-Sayre syndrome: mitochondrial disorder with heart block, chronic progressive external ophthalmoplegia, high CSF protein, and retinitis pigmentosa. Diagnose on muscle biopsy.
   - Inclusion body myositis: slowly progressive weakness in elderly. Pain is rare. Diagnose on biopsy. CPK is slightly high. No treatment is available.

- Dermatomyositis/polymyositis: proximal weakness and high CPK. On biopsy, dermatomyositis has perifascicular atrophy due to perivascular antibodies; polymyositis has inflammatory infiltrates due to cytotoxic T cells. See Chapter 17 for more information.
- Drug induced: zidovudine, steroids, aminoglycosides, and paralytics cause myopathy.

5. *Muscular dystrophies*: hereditary progressive wasting and weakness.
   - Duchenne's disease: X-linked (only males get the disease) absence of dystrophin causing infantile weakness, elevated CPK, abnormal EKG, and early death.
   - Myotonic dystrophy: autosomal-dominant trinucleotide repeat expansion (which gets worse with every generation, increasing severity) on chromosome 19. Symptoms include myotonia (patients can't release grip, eg, aren't able to change facial expressions or let go of a handshake), Christmas tree cataracts, frontal baldness, testicular atrophy, and weakness in the 20s. CPK is normal, but EKG is not.

MOVEMENT DISORDERS

Parkinson's Disease

Quick Points
- This is an idiopathic condition with degeneration of substantia nigra causing loss of striatal dopamine (with associated signs and symptoms), response to levodopa, and Lewy bodies in substantia nigra. See Table 8–10 for differential.
- Triad = rigidity, tremor, and bradykinesia. Mask facies, resting tremor ("pill-rolling tremor"), and decreased arm swing are frequent. Depression or dementia can occur.
- Patients < 40 years of age should be ruled out for other conditions (eg, Wilson's disease) and should undergo work-up, including CT and MRI of the head.

Initial Management
- Sinemet (levodopa + carbidopa; the latter slows the metabolism of levodopa) is used when symptoms interfere with a patient's function.
   - Start 1 tablet (25/250: 25-mg carbidopa + 250-mg levodopa) PO tid and then raise the dose as needed.

- Toxicity includes nausea, psychosis, and chorea, especially at high doses or after prolonged treatment. Reducing the dosage or taking holidays from the medication may be needed. With time, the duration of the Sinemet effect becomes shorter, resulting in an on-off effect (you may need to go to Sinemet-CR [controlled release] or more frequent Sinemet).
- Anticholinergics (eg, benztropine [Cogentin] 1–2 mg PO bid) and amantadine (Symmetrel) 100 mg PO bid are used for mild disease.
- Selegiline, a monoamine oxidase (MAO)-B inhibitor (5 mg PO bid), is an effective alternative to Sinemet.
- Bromocriptine (Parlodel) 1.25 mg PO bid (raise to 20 mg PO bid) and pergolide (Permax) 0.05 mg PO qd (raise to 1 mg PO tid) are other alternatives.
- Recently, an implanted subthalamic nucleus pacemaker has been shown to be of benefit.

Table 8–10. Differential of Parkinson's Disease

MPTP (contaminant in street meperidine)

Medications (neuroleptics)

Tumors

Progressive supranuclear palsy (parkinsonism + vertical gaze palsy)

Shy-Drager syndrome (parkinsonism + dysautonomia, causing orthostatic hypotension treatable with saline, fludrocortisone, and midodrine)

Gilles de la Tourette's Syndrome

Idiopathic motor and vocal tics (including occasionally coprolalia). Treat with haloperidol, clonidine, or clonazepam.

Huntington's Chorea

Autosomal-dominant disorder with chorea, dementia, and psychosis beginning in the 40s. The gene is on chromosome 4 (genetic testing is available). Caudate nucleus and Meynert's nucleus become atrophic. Treatment includes clozapine for psychosis. It is eventually fatal.

Miscellaneous

1. Benign essential tremor. This is an intention tremor, relieved by alcohol and beta-blockers. Frequency is 7 Hz (physiologic tremor has a 9-Hz frequency). It is made worse by hyperthyroidism, stress, and caffeine.
2. Ballism. Wild, flailing motions due to destruction of the subthalamic nucleus.
3. Tardive dyskinesia. A consequence of neuroleptics, this disorder with bradykinesia, and occasional chorea may be irreversible. Clozapine and risperidone (nondopaminergic antipsychotics) don't cause this.
4. Neuroleptic malignant syndrome. Triad is rigidity, fever, and mental status changes due to neuroleptics. It can be fatal. CPK is very high (rhabdomyolysis can occur). Treat with discontinuing neuroleptics, hydration, support, dantrolene, and/or bromocriptine.

MULTIPLE SCLEROSIS

Quick Points
- Idiopathic chronic entity with demyelination of the CNS (optic nerves, cerebellum, brain stem, and spinal cord are favorite targets).
- Multiple sclerosis is more prevalent in northern latitudes, areas of cleaner sanitation, and the children of affected parents. Some think it to be an autoimmune reaction to a virus that, if exposed to as a child, there is no adverse effect, but if exposed to later in life, multiple sclerosis occurs (this tries to explain why it is almost unheard of in the Third World, where children are exposed to everything growing up).
- Patterns include relapsing-remitting, primary progressive, secondary progressive, and progressive relapsing disease. Relapsing-remitting and secondary progressive patterns are 80% of patients.

Key Clinical Syndromes

1. *Optic neuritis.* This often serves as a prelude to multiple sclerosis. Signs and symptoms include pain on eye motion, blurred vision, afferent pupillary defect (APD) (also known as Marcus Gunn's pupil), and decreased color vision. The Optic Neuritis Treatment Trial (ONTT) showed that methylprednisolone 250 IV q6h × 3 days, followed by prednisone taper, reduced recurrences, sped visual recovery, and reduced progression to multiple sclerosis at 2 years, benefits seen

mostly when there were white-matter signal abnormalities in the brain on MRI. However, starting off with oral prednisone was bad, as it increased recurrences and slowed recovery. In any case, final visual acuity and the rate of multiple sclerosis at 5 years was the same in all groups, including placebo.

2. *Transverse myelitis.* Inflammation in the spinal cord produces weakness and sensory loss (dermatomal levels). Bowel and bladder function may be compromised.

3. *Internuclear ophthalmoplegia.* Demyelination in medial longitudinal fasciculus compromises communication between CN III and contralateral CN VI (eg, on right gaze, the left eye cannot turn inward, whereas the right eye turns out).

Work-up

ANA, ESR, vitamin B_{12}, CT/MRI should be done. LP is useful in questionable cases, showing slight mononuclear pleocytosis (< 50 cells) and elevation of immunoglobulins.

Symptomatic Therapy

1. Spasticity, depression, pain, and bladder dysfunction can all be disabling.

2. Baclofen (γ-aminobutyric acid [GABA] agonist) is first-line treatment for spasticity.

3. Oxybutynin (Ditropan) can alleviate urinary urgency or incontinence.

4. Pain can be treated with tricyclics or carbamazepine.

5. Remember to support the families' and the patients' psychologic well-being.

6. Multiple sclerosis activity is reduced during pregnancy, but relapse occurs 2 months postpartum.

Disease Therapy

1. Steroids (methylprednisolone 250 mg IV q6h × 3–5 days, followed by prednisone taper) are the mainstay for relapses. Chronic steroids are not effective for slowing progression.

2. IFN-β is useful for relapsing-remitting multiple sclerosis. It decreases the frequency of relapse and new lesions. IFN-β-1a (Avonex) and IFN-β-1b (Betaseron) are two preparations. IFN-β-1a also slows the progression of disability. Toxicity includes flu-like symptoms.

3. Glutiramer (Copaxone) is an alternative to IFN, as it also reduces the relapse rate in the relapsing-remitting multiple sclerosis.
4. Low-dose MTX (7.5 mg every week) slows disability in patients with progressive multiple sclerosis.

PHAKOMATOSES

Phakomatoses are rare conditions that you will likely never see anywhere but on an examination. They are generally autosomal dominant, except Wyburn-Mason's syndrome. What you need to know is outlined in Table 8–11.

Table 8–11. Phakomatoses and Clinical Features

von Hippel-Lindau disease	Cerebellar hemangioblastomas, renal cell carcinoma, pheochromocytoma, retinal hemangiomas
Neurofibromatosis type I (von Recklinghausen's)	Café-au-lait spots, axillary freckles, plexiform neurofibromas, optic gliomas, glioblastomas, gastrointestinal hamartomas, pheochromocytomas (Type 3 MEN syndrome)
Neurofibromatosis type II	Little skin involvement, bilateral acoustic neuromas, pheochromocytomas
Wyburn-Mason's syndrome	Arteriovenous malformation in retina and midbrain; only phakomatosis that is not autosomal dominant
Tuberous sclerosis	Adenoma sebaceum, shagreen patches, astrocytic hamartomas in brain and retina, seizures, mental retardation
Sturge-Weber syndrome (encephalotrigeminal hemangiomas)	Facial angioma (nevus flammeus), leptomeningeal hemangiomas, mental retardation, seizures, choroidal cavernous hemangioma in eye

BRAIN TUMORS

Glioblastomas comprise half of all primary brain tumors. Other tumors include low-grade astrocytomas, oligodendrogliomas, and ependymomas. Meningiomas and schwannomas are rarer still. Primary CNS lymphomas occur most often in HIV patients. Metastases from the lung, breast, melanoma, kidney, and colon occur. Dural metastases are usually from the breast or prostate. See Chapter 10 for a discussion of epidural metastases and cord compression. Treatment includes surgery and radiation. Recurrence is high; survival for glioblastomas is only 8 to 12 months. Chemotherapy is experimental. Factoid: Cerebellar degeneration is a paraneoplastic syndrome occurring with breast cancer, ovarian cancer, SCLC, and Hodgkin's disease, due to antibodies against Purkinje's cells of the cerebellum.

BIBLIOGRAPHY

Reviews

Brodie MJ, Dichter MA. Antiepileptic drugs. N Engl J Med 1996;334:168–75.

Cummings JL. Dementia. Lancet. 1995;45:211–8.

Dalakas MC. Polymyositis, dermatomyositis, and inclusion-body myositis. N Engl J Med 1991;325:1487–98.

Drachman DB. Myasthenia gravis. N Engl J Med 1994;330:1797–810.

Furman JM, Cass SP. Benign positional vertigo. N Engl J Med 1999;341:1590–6.

Hotson JR, Balon RW. Acute vestibular syndrome. N Engl J Med 1998;339:680–6.

Lang A, Lozano A. Parkinson's disease. Part II. N Engl J Med 1998;339:1130–43.

Lowenstein DH, Alldredge BK. Status epilepticus. N Engl J Med 1998;338:970–7.

Posner JB. Brain metastases. J Neurooncol 1996;27:287–93.

Rodick RA, et al. Management of multiple sclerosis. N Engl J Med 1997;337:1604–11.

Ropper AD. The Guillain-Barré syndrome. N Engl J Med 1992;326:1130–6.

Guidelines

Adams HP, et al. Guidelines for the management of patients with acute ischemic stroke. Stroke 1994;25:1901–14.

American College of Medical Genetics. Use of apolipoprotein E testing for Alzheimer's. JAMA 1995;274:1627–9.

American College of Physicians. Guidelines for medical treatment for stroke prevention. Ann Intern Med 1994;121:54–5.

Bates D. The management of medical coma. J Neurol Neurosurg Psychiatry 1993;56:589–98.

Feinberg WM, et al. Guidelines for the management of TIAs. Circulation 1994;25:1320–35.

Mayberg MR, et al. Guidelines for the management of aneursymal subarachnoid hemorrhage. Stroke 1994;25:2315–8.

Rummans TA, et al. Delirium in elderly patients. Mayo Clin Proc 1995;70:989–98.

Studies and Trials

Stroke

Bracken MB, et al. Administration of methylprednisolone in the treatment of acute spinal cord injury. JAMA 1997;277:1597–604. (*If given in the first 3 hours, give methylprednisolone for 24 hours; if given within 3 to 8 hours, give it for 48 hours.*)

Cannagieter SC, et al. Optimal oral anticoagulant therapy in patients with mechanical heart valves. N Engl J Med 1995;333:11–7. (*INR in these patients should be targeted for 3.0 to 4.0.*)

Endarterectomy for Asymptomatic Carotid Artery Stenosis (ACAS Trial). JAMA 1995;273:1421–8. (*Carotid endarterectomy reduces the risk of stroke in patients with asymptomatic carotid artery stenosis > 60%.*)

The French Study of Aortic Plaques in Stroke. N Engl J Med 1996;334:1216–21. (Aortic plaques thicker than 4 mm increase the risk of stroke recurrence by 5.2.)

Furlan A, et al. Intra-arterial prourokinase for acute ischemic stroke. JAMA 1999;282:2003–11. (*Treatment with intra-arterial prourokinase within 6 hours of onset of ischemic stroke decreases mortality and neurologic disability.*)

Joshipura KJ, et al. Fruits and vegetables and risk of ischemic stroke. JAMA 1999;282:1233–9. (*Each serving of fruits and vegetables reduced the risk of ischemic stroke by 6%.*)

The National Institute of Neurological Disorders. TPA for acute ischemic stroke. N Engl J Med 1995;333:1581–7. (*An RCT showing that giving TPA within 3 hours of acute ischemic stroke improved outcomes at 3 months.*)

The North American Stroke and Carotid Endarterectomy Trial (NASCET). N Engl J Med 1998;339:1415–25. (*Carotid endarterectomy reduced the risk of stroke in symptomatic patients if carotid stenosis was greater than 50% and surgical mortality was low [ie, in places with experienced surgeons] [earlier result indicated benefit only if stenosis was >70%].*)

Perry HM, et al. Effect of treating isolated systolic hypertension on risk of stroke. JAMA 2000;284:464–71. (*Treatment of systolic HTN reduced the risk of ischemic stroke by 37% over 2 years and hemorrhagic stroke by 63%.*)

White HD. Pravastatin and risk of stroke. N Engl J Med 2000;343:317–26. (*Pravastatin reduced risk of ischemic stroke by 19% in patients with prior MI or unstable angina.*)

Yin D, Carpenter JP. Cost-effectiveness of screening for asymptomatic carotid stenosis. J Vasc Surg 1998;27:245–55. (*One-time screening with carotid ultrasound for asymptomatic carotid stenosis is cost effective when its prevalence is > 4.5% [generally in the over-60 population].*)

8

Multiple Sclerosis

Jacobs LD, et al. Intramuscular interferon beta-1a for disease progression in relapsing multiple sclerosis. Ann Neurol 1996;39:285–94. (*An RCT showing that weekly IFN-β slowed progression of disability in relapsing patients with multiple sclerosis.*)

The Optic Neuritis Treatment Trial (ONTT). N Engl J Med 1993;329:1764–9. (*An RCT showing that IV methylprednisolone followed by oral prednisone decreased the 2-year risk of multiple sclerosis in patients with optic neuritis from 16.7 to 7.5%. Oral prednisone alone did not decrease risk. The benefit of IV therapy was most when patients had three or more MRI lesions at study entry [which was also a strong risk factor for later development of multiple sclerosis].*)

Degenerative Disorders

Bensimon G, et al. A controlled trial of riluzole in ALS. N Engl J Med 1994;330:585–91. (*Riluzole improved 1 year survival in ALS from 58 to 74%.*)

Knapp MJ, et al. The Tacrine Study. JAMA 1994;271:985–91. (*Tacrine 160 mg/d improved cognitive parameters and family assessments for mild-moderate Alzheimer's cases. Toxicities included high LFTs and cholinergic effects.*)

Seizure Disorders

Treiman DM, et al. A comparison of four treatments for generalized convulsive status epilepticus. N Engl J Med 1998;339:792–8. (*Lorazepam was superior to phenobarbitol, phenytoin, and diazepam for initial IV treatment of status.*)

Brain Tumors

Patchell RA, et al. A randomized trial of surgery in the treatment of single brain metastases to the brain. N Engl J Med 1990;322:494–500. (*Surgery is superior to radiation for solitary brain metastasis.*)

9

Nephrology

Don't be nervous, Ma. — Alan Dubrow, MD

Remember how much you do not know. Do not pour strange medicines into your patients. — Sir William Osler

BASICS OF NEPHROPHYSIOLOGY

Nephrology is a bête noire that has plagued many a physician since Physiology in first year of medical school, inscrutable yet still invaluable. We will attempt to clarify and connect the fundamentals of what you need to know with respect to how the kidney works, what happens when it does not, and how various pharmacologic agents do their job.

To start, the kidney has a cortex, where the glomeruli are located, and a medulla, where the loops of Henle and collecting ducts are located. Bear in mind throughout the ensuing discussion that the medulla is a hypertonic environment, due to the actions of the thick ascending loop of Henle. See Figure 9–1 for a graphic description.

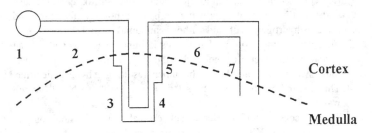

Figure 9–1. Schematic of the nephron. See text on the following page for descriptions of numbered parts of the nephron.

1. Glomerulus. This is a tuft of capillaries where ultrafiltration of a protein-free solute occurs into Bowman's space. Afferent and efferent arterioles carry blood in and out. Prostaglandins keep the afferent arteriole open (so ASA, a prostaglandin blocker, constricts the afferent arterioles and reduces inflow to glomeruli), whereas angiotensin II causes efferent arteriolar constriction, maintaining glomerular perfusion. Renin is secreted by the juxtaglomerular apparatus in response to hypoperfusion of the kidney (eg, CHF, renal artery stenosis, dehydration), which converts angiotensinogen to angiotensin I, which is converted by angiotensin-converting enzyme (ACE; located in the lung) to angiotensin II. Thus, ACE inhibitors cause efferent arteriolar dilation, reducing glomerular filtration. So, ASA + ACE inhibitors or renal artery stenosis + ACE inhibitors precipitate acute renal failure (ARF). The glomerular filtration rate (GFR) is determined by plasma flow, capillary permeability, and the hydrostatic and oncotic pressures in the capillaries and Bowman's space. Thus, GFR decreases with hypotension, urinary tract obstruction, CHF, hemoconcentration, and glomerulonephritis, among other reasons. Proteinuria reflects glomerular injury.

2. Proximal collecting tubule (PCT). This area carries out isomotic resorption of the glomerular ultrafiltrate, resorbing about two-thirds of the sodium and water filtered by the glomerulus. It also reabsorbs amino acids, glucose, phosphate, and lactate. Glucose is completely reabsorbed up to a serum level of about 180 (so uncontrolled diabetics get glucosuria, whereas patients with type I renal tubular acidosis [RTA] [see below] get aminoaciduria and glucosuria). The PCT also reabsorbs bicarbonate (with the help of carbonic anhydrase) and secretes hydrogen (with and without ammonia).

3. Thin descending loop of Henle. This is impermeable to sodium but permeable to water. Remember that the loop of Henle is in the hypertonic medulla, so water leaves the lumen, resulting in hypertonic urine.

4. Thin ascending loop of Henle. This is permeable to NaCl but not water.

5. Thick ascending loop of Henle. This critical part of the nephron features the Na-K-2Cl active cotransporter, which pumps out those ions in that proportion into the medullary interstitium, resulting in the hypertonic medulla and a dilute tubular fluid. This transporter is blocked by the loop diuretics (eg, furosemide [Lasix]).

6. Distal convoluted tubule (DCT). The dilute urine entering the DCT stays dilute or is diluted further as the DCT is impermeable to water while NaCl is actively resorbed. Antidiuretic hormone (ADH) increases water permeability, concentrating the urine. Aldosterone increases sodium resorption (followed by water), which is compensated by secretion of potassium and hydrogen (which is why hyperaldosteronism causes hypokalemic metabolic alkalosis). This is why ADH controls plasma osmolarity, whereas aldosterone controls plasma volume. The more sodium seen by the DCT, the more is resorbed and the more potassium and hydrogen are excreted: loop diuretics and thiazides cause hypokalemia and alkalosis. Thiazides and metolazone block NaCl resorption in the DCT, and water follows the unresorbed salt, leading to diuresis. Angiotensin II increases aldosterone secretion (so CHF, cirrhosis, and dehydration lead to volume retention by the kidney, which is blocked by ACE inhibitors).

7. Collecting duct. Na continues to be actively resorbed here. ADH and aldosterone work here as well with similar actions as in the DCT to concentrate the urine and resorb sodium, respectively. Atrial natriuretic peptide (ANP) (released in response to hypervolemia stretching the atria) blocks sodium resorption here, causing natriuresis. Spironolactone blocks the aldosterone receptor, whereas triamterene and amiloride block sodium resorption directly; both thus reduce potassium and hydrogen secretion, causing an acidosis and hyperkalemia (these are called potassium-sparing diuretics).

Notes on Diuretics and Clinical Situations

See Table 9–1 for an overview of diuretics.

1. Carbonic anhydrase inhibitors cause metabolic acidosis.

2. Furosemide and thiazides cause hypokalemic alkalosis as noted above, whereas potassium-sparing diuretics cause hyperkalemic acidosis as noted above.

3. Furosemide increases excretion of free water (as it blocks both urine concentration and dilution by interfering with the function of the thick ascending loop of Henle) and calcium, causing hypocalcemia, whereas thiazides reduce free water clearance (by blocking only urinary dilution through affecting only the DCT) and calcium clearance, causing hypercalcemia.

Table 9–1. Diuretics

Class	Common Drugs	Site of Action	Mechanism
Carbonic anhydrase inhibitors	Acetazolamide (Diamox), methazolamide (Neptazane)	Proximal collecting tubule	Block $NaHCO_3$ resorption
Loop diuretics	Furosemide (Lasix), bumetanide (Bumex)	Thick ascending loop of Henle	Blocks active Na-K-2Cl transport
Thiazides	Hydrochlorothiazide	Distal convoluting tubule	Blocks NaCl resorption
K-sparing diuretics	Spironolactone (Aldactone), triamterene, amiloride	Collecting duct	Block Na resorption and K secretion

4. In nephrogenic diabetes insipidus (DI) (see Chapter 14), the kidney is unresponsive to ADH, leading to loss of free water. Thiazides are helpful here: they cause volume contraction and sodium depletion, decreasing GFR and increasing PCT resorption; hence, less sodium comes to the thick ascending loop of Henle, and the urine is less diluted. Furosemide is not indicated as it increases free water clearance.

5. In sickle cell patients, the hypertonic medulla is great for sickling, so much of the medulla is infarcted, and the urinary concentration mechanism is wrecked. These patients are consequently prone to dehydration, making the situation worse.

6. Patients with cirrhosis and ascites frequently have hyperaldosteronism, so spironolactone is a good diuretic in these cases.

7. Osmotic diuretics (eg, mannitol) get into the renal tubules and draw water into them, blocking sodium and water resorption throughout the nephron.

PATIENT WITH SUSPECTED RENAL DISEASE

See Table 9–2 for nephropathy previews.

Taking a detailed history is extremely important. The diagnosis of uremia seems simple on the surface; however, uremia can present as many other

Table 9–2. Preview of Nephropathies

Problem	Signs and Symptoms
Urinary tract infection	Bacteriuria, pyuria, WBC casts
Rapidly progressive renal failure	Anuria, oliguria, low glomerular filtration rate
Chronic renal failure	Azotemia > 3 mo, small kidneys, broad casts, signs of uremia or renal osteodystrophy
Nephrotic syndrome	Proteinuria > 3.5 g/d, hypoalbuminemia, hyperlipidemia, edema, lipiduria
Nephritis	Proteinuria, edema, hypertension, hematuria, RBC casts, oliguria
Obstruction	Azotemia, hydronephrosis, oliguria or polyuria, urinary retention
Renal tubule defects	Electrolyte or acid-base disturbances, polyuria

diseases. It is important to realize this and, in turn, understand that under-dialysis is common. If a patient is undergoing dialysis, an assessment of dialysis adequacy should be made.

The history should include a review of the patient's recent complaints, past medical history, and prescription and nonprescription medications. It is important to know the patient's BP, pulse, weight, and input and output (always know the input and output). The physical examination should be thorough and should include a careful evaluation of the patient's volume status, localizing signs and symptoms (eg, suprapubic tenderness, CVA tenderness), and any other signs of systemic disease (eg, palpable purpura, suggesting vasculitis).

The H&P can help in classifying the type of renal compromise into the following groups: prerenal, intrarenal, or postrenal (see the section below on Acute Renal Failure). The next step is the examination of the urine. This should include a baseline U/A and examination of the sediment. A crude assessment of the patient's GFR can be made using the creatinine clearance.

Urinalysis

Analysis of the urine was the beginning of laboratory medicine. Early physicians examined the urine color, turbidity, volume, viscosity, odor, and sweetness (don't ask how they checked the last one). U/A gives us information about pH, specific gravity, glucose, protein, ketones, and cells.

Normal urine pH is 4.6 to 8.0 (average 6), depending on the patient's diet. Urea splitting organisms (eg, *Proteus*) can increase urine pH.

Normal specific gravity is 1.003 to 1.030. Specific gravity compares the mass of a solution to an equal volume of water. See Table 9–3 for causes of abnormal urine specific gravity.

Proteinuria is a clinical marker indicating underlying renal disease. The urine dipstick is the method used to identify proteinuria (Table 9–4).

A positive dipstick should always be followed by a sulfosalicylic acid test (sensitive to 5–10 mg/dL). If a sulfosalicylic acid test shows a significantly higher concentration than the dipstick, rule out Bence Jones proteinuria. Significant proteinuria is > 300 mg/d. Classify proteinuria: postural versus transient versus persistent. Persistent proteinuria can be further classified by source: glomerular, decreased tubular reabsorption, or increased plasma levels of normal or abnormal proteins.

Ketonuria is used for screening for ketoacidosis. It occurs in DM, starvation, high-fat diets, hyperthyroidism, fever, and pregnancy.

Table 9–3. Abnormal Urine Specific Gravity

Low	High
Polydipsia	Proteinuria
Sickle cell anemia	Glucosuria
Papillary necrosis	Antibiotics
Diabetes insipidus	After use of contrast media
Phenacetin/acetaminophen abuse	After use of mannitol or dextran
	Diuretics

Table 9–4. Approximate Urine Dipstick Values for Proteinuria

1+	100 mg/dL
2+	300 mg/dL
3+	500 mg/dL
4+	1,000 mg/dL

Urine urobilinogen is rarely useful instead of direct and indirect bilirubin. It is usually increased in hemolysis, tissue hemorrhage, hepatic cell damage, ands cholangitis. Porphobilinogenuria is in porphyria, lead poisoning, cirrhosis, and infectious hepatitis.

Bilirubinuria implies conjugated hyperbilirubinemia.

Cells in the urine can make the diagnosis. Zero to two RBCs per high-power field (hpf) are normal. They look like colorless discs in the urine. Dysmorphic forms are consistent with glomerular bleeding. See Table 9–5 for discussion of cells in the urine.

Table 9–5. Significance of Cells and Components in Urine

RBCs (> 2 RBCs/high-power field)	Glomerulonephritis Nephrolithiasis Neoplasms Menstrual contamination
Hemoglobin	Intravascular hemolysis
Myoglobin	Rhabdomyolysis
Pyuria (> 5 WBCs/high-power field)	Infection (pyelonephritis, cystitis, prostatitis, urethritis) Glomerulonephritis (eg, lupus) Neoplasms
Renal tubular cells	Tubular damage
Oval fat bodies	Lipid nephrosis
Eosinophils (detected with Hansel's stain)	Acute interstitial nephritis Vasculitis or glomerulonephritis Prostatitis or pyelonephritis IgA nephropathy Cholesterol emboli
Transitional cells	Neoplasms

Casts and Crystals

Casts are formed in the lumen of the distal convoluted tubule and collecting duct. The width of a cast reflects where it's formed. Casts are made of Tamm-Horsfall (TH) protein. Cellular casts are cells enmeshed in the TH protein matrix. See Tables 9–6 and 9–7 for causes of casts and crystals.

Table 9–6. Urinary Casts

Type	Predisposing Conditions
Hyaline	Most common; seen with exercise, dehydration, heat exposure, and stress
RBC	Glomerulonephritis
WBC	Pyelonephritis or glomerulonephritis (need culture)
Broad	From collecting duct; due to decreased perfusion from distal collecting tubule to collecting duct (often seen in chronic renal failure)
Coarse granular	Nonspecific; occur in acute tubular necrosis
Pigmented granular	Ischemic or toxic acute renal failure
Waxy (oval fat bodies)	Nonspecific; occur in nephrosis

Table 9–7. Urinary Crystals

Type	Description	Predisposing Conditions
Urates	Rhombic rosettes, negatively birefringent	Leukemia, gout
Calcium oxalate	Colorless octahedrals resembling envelopes (can be dumbbell or oval, too)	High oxalic acid diets, antifreeze poisoning, vitamin C toxicity
Cystine	Colorless hexagonal plates	Inherited metabolic defect
Other		Sulfonamides, ampicillin, acyclovir, contrast dye

ACUTE RENAL FAILURE

Quick Points
- Acute renal failure (ARF) is a deterioration in renal function over a period of hours to days. Subsequently, the kidneys can't maintain fluid/electrolyte balance and excrete nitrogenous wastes.
- Commonly used definitions of ARF:
  - Increase in serum creatinine of 50% over baseline
  - Reduction in creatinine clearance of 50%
  - Decreased renal function resulting in the need for dialysis

- Risk factors:
  - Prerenal azotemia
  - Those with preexisting renal insufficiency are predisposed to ARF due to contrast, aminoglycosides, atheroembolism, and cardiovascular surgery
  - Renal insufficiency and DM—high risk with radiocontrast
- ARF can be oliguric (< 400 cc/d) or nonoliguric. Nonoliguric renal failure carries a better prognosis.

Initial Management
- Careful fluid management, correction of electrolyte abnormalities, and trying to reverse the underlying cause.
- Make sure you rule out obstruction relatively early on. All you have to do is insert a Foley catheter and get a renal ultrasound to look for hydronephrosis and kidney size (small kidneys = chronic renal failure [CRF]).
- Try to prevent further renal injury. Avoid nephrotoxic drugs.
- Adjust medications based on creatinine clearance.
- If metabolic acidosis is due to renal dysfunction, sodium bicarbonate may be necessary.
- Anemia is often a problem due to phlebotomy, decreased erythropoietin, and uremia. Platelet dysfunction may also be caused by uremia. Treatment includes packed red blood cells (PRBCs), vasopressin, and dialysis.
- For severe ARF, dialysis is the mainstay of therapy:
  - Indications for emergency dialysis (this is when you wake up the renal fellow at 2 AM). (*Make sure you know the indications listed in Table 9–8.*)
- Note that there is no absolute cutoff number for BUN or creatinine (Cr) that requires immediate dialysis.

Table 9–8. Indications for Emergency Dialysis

Metabolic Disturbances	Organ Dysfunction
Fluid overload unresponsive to diuretics	Pericarditis
Severe refractory acidosis (pH < 7.2)	Seizures, encephalopathy
Refractory hyperkalemia	Bleeding diathesis

Making the Diagnosis of Acute Renal Failure

- Take a careful H&P examination. Make sure to elicit a history of exposure to nephrotoxic agents (medications and contrast).
- Often volume status is difficult to assess on physical examination. Look for JVD at 30 degrees, cardiac gallop, and peripheral edema. A rash may accompany allergic interstitial nephritis. Livedo reticularis can accompany cholesterol emboli.
- The next step is to obtain a U/A and urine indices (see above for a discussion of U/A). Urine indices include osmolality, urinary sodium, and fractional excretion of sodium. FENa = ([urine sodium/plasma sodium] × [plasma creatinine/urine creatinine]). See Table 9–9 for evaluation of urine indices.
- Useful blood tests are SMA-7 (look at BUN/Cr), calcium, uric acid, CPK, and eosinophil count (almost always elevated with allergic interstitial nephritis).
- The presence of an osmolal gap suggests the presence of a low molecular weight nephrotoxin (ie, ethylene glycol).

Table 9–9. Urine Indices in Renal Failure

Prerenal	*Tubular Damage*
Urine osmolality > 500 mOsm/kg	Urine osmolality < 350 (loss of ability to concentrate urine)
Urine Na < 20 mmol/L	Urine Na > 40 mmol/L
BUN:Cr ratio > 20	
FENa < 1%	FENa > 1%

Further Discussion

Causes of ARF. (see Table 9–10 for an overview).

- *Prerenal:* Rapidly reversible if the underlying cause is discovered.
- *Intrinsic/renal:* Think of the site of injury: tubule, interstitium, vessels, or glomerulus. Prerenal azotemia and ischemic necrosis of the tubules are on a continuum. Glomerulonephritis needs to be diagnosed quickly, as patients may need immunosuppression or plasma exchange.

Table 9–10. Common Causes of Acute Renal Failure

| Prerenal (Volume Depletion) | Renal | | | Postrenal (Urinary Tract Obstruction) |
	Tubular	Interstitial	Glomerular	
Dehydration	Ischemia	Drug allergy	See glomerulo-nephritis section below	Prostate cancer
Congestive heart failure	Aminoglyco-sides	Autoimmune infiltration		Cervical cancer
Fever	NSAIDs			Retroperitoneal fibrosis
Diuretics	Contrast			Renal stones
Vomiting	Myoglobinuria			Benign prostatic hyperplasia
Diarrhea	Cisplatin			
	Myeloma			

- *Postrenal:* Urinary outflow obstruction—remember that both outflow tracts must be obstructed, or single-tract obstruction if the patient has only one working kidney.

Special Specific Causes.
1. HIV nephropathy causes large kidneys, rapid course, and heavy proteinuria, usually in African Americans. ACE inhibitors improve renal function.
2. Contrast nephropathy occurs in one-quarter of high-risk patients. Half-normal saline is protective. Nonionic contrast is protective in the high-risk pool (prior renal disease, diabetics, etc).
3. Papillary necrosis is caused by acetaminophen, phenacetin, ASA, diabetes, sickle cell anemia, obstruction, or multiple previous pyelonephritis episodes.
4. Lead nephropathy causes Fanconi's syndrome, aminoaciduria, glucosuria, hypokalemia, and gout (saturnine gout).

END-STAGE RENAL DISEASE/CHRONIC RENAL FAILURE

Quick Points
- CRF is characterized by progressive azotemia over weeks to months, isosthenuria, and HTN (in most patients).
- The diagnosis is made by bilateral small kidneys on ultrasound. Confirmation is obtained by radiologic evidence of renal osteodystrophy.

* CRF often progresses to end-stage renal disease (ESRD).

Initial Management
See Table 9–11 for common management issues.

Table 9–11. Common Management Issues in Chronic Renal Failure

Diet	Individualize; good base point is 2 g Na, 80 g protein, 80 mEq K
Anemia	Erythropoietin 50 U/kg 3×/wk
Calcium management	Calcitriol (Rocaltrol) 0.5–2.0 μg PO qd (for renal osteodystrophy)
	Calcium carbonate 500 mg PO tid
	Phoslo (for hyperphosphatemia; avoid aluminum-containing agents, as aluminum can cause neurologic disease in these patients)
Gastritis	Famotidine (Pepcid) 20 mg PO qd (½ dose due to renal failure)
Hypertension + proteinuria	ACE inhibitors

Further Discussion

There are several goals in caring for patients undergoing hemodialysis: sufficient dialysis, good nutrition, good vascular access, avoiding hospitalizations, and maintaining a good quality of life.

* *Vascular access.* This is necessary for adequate dialysis. Remember that no BP or blood draws in that arm. Thrombosis and infection of vascular access account for 20 to 40% of hospitalizations. Native atrioventricular fistulas are superior to grafts. They have a lower incidence of thrombosis and infection. Note that fistulas and grafts are good ways to teach interns and students what thrills are. A thrombosed access can be treated with urokinase. If that is not successful, perform angioplasty or surgery. In terms of infection, the most common organism is *S. aureus.* Treatment with broad-spectrum antibiotics should be started without delay (vancomycin and gentamicin).

Patients should be treated for 3 to 4 weeks, and, if there is no response, then the access should be removed or ligated.

- *Nutrition.* Protein intake should be 1.5 g/kg/d. Salt intake has to be adjusted individually. If a patient is adequately dialyzed, then there is no reason to restrict potassium. Water-soluble vitamins are dialyzed out, and patients need replacement.

- *Cardiac status.* Half of the deaths of dialysis patients are secondary to cardiovascular disease. There is an increased incidence of MIs. The indications for CABG and PTCA are the same as in any other patients. In dialysis patients, there is an elevated baseline CPK (for unknown reasons), but the CPK-MB is still of clinical value. Pericarditis with pericardial effusions can occur in patients with inadequate dialysis. The treatment is intensive heparin-free dialysis.

- *Anemia.* This is caused by erythropoietin deficiency Once a target hematocrit of 36 to 40 is reached, the dose should be reduced (not discontinued). Make sure patients have adequate iron stores. Toxicity of erythropoietin is HTN. Most patients receive parenteral iron at dialysis. Patients also have an increased bleeding tendency, caused by altered platelet function (which can be improved with desmopressin, cryoprecipitate, and erythropoietin).

- *Infections.* Dialysis patients are immunosuppressed. TB is also common among dialysis patients. All dialysis patients should have immunizations: hepatitis B, flu shot, Pneumovax.

- *Renal osteodystrophy.* This is usually a consequence of secondary hyperparathyroidism. Serum parathyroid should be measured. Patients may have metastatic calcifications in the skin and joints, bone and joint pain, and lytic lesions. There is usually hypocalcemia and hyperphosphatemia. The treatment includes calcitriol (IV administration is more effective than oral, given at dialysis), calcium acetate (Phoslo) or carbonate with meals to maximize phosphate binding, and parathyroidectomy (if symptoms progress or there is a very high parathyroid level).

- *Sexual dysfunction.* Commonly, patients are impotent and infertile. Patients often have dysfunctional uterine bleeding. They should be referred for a gynecologic evaluation.

- *Gastroenterology.* Gastritis and duodenitis are common. AVMs are also common and may cause bleeding.

- *Neurology.* Uremic patients often have a mixed sensory and motor peripheral neuropathy. Altered mental status is seen with inadequate dialysis, hypercalcemia, infection, aluminum toxicity, and dialysis dysequilibrium.
- Some special issues. Patients should receive adequate dialysis prior to surgery. Urgent dialysis is not indicated after radiocontrast dye studies in patients who are receiving regular or adequate dialysis. Avoid demerol (its metabolites accumulate and can cause seizures).
- *Polycystic kidney disease.* Linked to chromosome 16, this disease can cause CRF. The adult form is autosomal dominant; the infantile form is autosomal recessive. It is associated with berry aneurysms, mitral valve prolapse, and diverticulosis.
- Shohl's solution (calcium citrate) increases aluminum absorption, decreasing bone turnover, making bone disease worse.

NEPHROTIC SYNDROME

Quick Points
See Table 9–12 for signs of nephrotic syndrome.
- The definition is urinary protein > 3.5 g per 1.73 m^2 of body surface area daily.
- Hypercoagulability occurs due to loss of proteins C and S, and antithrombin III, with liver overproduction of clotting factors to try to compensate for proteinuria.
- Patients are more susceptible to infections due to loss of immunoglobulins.

Initial Management
See Table 9–13 for intervention.

Table 9–12. Manifestations of Nephrotic Syndrome

Hypoalbuminemia

Hypernatremia

Hypercoagulability

Hyperlipidemia

Table 9–13. Interventions in Nephrotic Syndrome

Intervention	Purpose
ACE inhibitors	Reduce proteinuria; improves survival
Low-protein and low-sodium diet	Slow disease progression; reduce edema
NSAIDs	Reduce proteinuria
Loop diuretics	Reduce edema
Statins	Treat hypercholesterolemia
Anticoagulation	Treat deep vein thrombosis, pulmonary embolus, arterial thrombosis

Further Discussion

The most common cause of nephrotic proteinuria is diabetic nephropathy. Other causes of the nephrotic syndrome are the following:

- *Minimal change disease.* This is most common in children. Its pathogenesis is unknown. Glomeruli appear normal under light microscopy, but under electron microscopy (EM), there is fusion of the epithelial foot processes. You can see oval fat bodies on U/A. It usually does not progress to renal failure. Disorder responds to prednisone (1 mg/kg/d) for 4 to 6 weeks. There is a frequent rate of relapse, and some individuals require cyclophosphamide and chlorambucil.

- *Focal glomerular sclerosis.* Eighty percent of patients have microscopic hematuria at presentation. It is associated with heroin abuse, AIDS, reflux nephropathy, NSAIDs, and massive obesity. Individuals are usually hypertensive and have decreased renal function. Immunofluorescence reveals deposits of IgM and C3 on the sclerotic segments. Therapy is prednisone. Approximately 40% of patients respond. In spite of therapy, most patients progress to ESRD in 5 to 10 years.

- *Membranous glomerulonephritis.* This is the most common cause of primary nephrotic syndrome in adults, usually in the fifth and sixth decades. Approximately 50% of individuals have a slowly progressive loss of renal function over 3 to 10 years. It may be idiopathic or associated with hepatitis B, autoimmune diseases, lupus, diabetes, thyroiditis, mixed connective tissue disease, and cancer (membranous nephropathy is paraneoplastic syndrome). On immunofluorescence,

there are deposits of IgG and C3 along capillary loops. The natural history is variable. A 3-month course of prednisone may induce remission.
- *Membranoproliferative glomerulonephritis.* This is responsible for 10% of cases of idiopathic nephrotic syndrome. There are two subgroups. Type I is associated with granular subendothelial immune complex deposits, low levels of serum complement, and the presence of cryoglobulins and circulating immune complexes. One-third of patients have a history of a recent URI. Type II is rare and is characterized by circulating IgG and a C3 nephritic factor. There is no consensus that any form of therapy is of benefit. The majority of patients progress to ESRD in months to years. Other rarer causes of the nephrotic syndrome are amyloid, light chain deposition, preeclampsia, and infectious disease (viral, bacterial).

Clinical complications are as follows:
- *Sodium retention and edema formation.* There is primary retention of sodium by the kidney. Edema can be reversed only if there is a negative sodium balance (dietary restriction of sodium and diuretics).
- *Thromboembolic complications are a major complication.* Renal vein thrombosis is frequent in membranous glomerulonephritis. DVT is also common, and there is an increased risk of coronary events. Predictors of risk are low serum albumin, high rates of protein excretion, high fibrinogen levels, low antithrombin III, and hypovolemia. Hyperlipidemia is secondary to overproduction and impaired catabolism of apoprotein B containing lipoproteins.

URINARY TRACT INFECTION

Quick Points
- Acute uncomplicated UTIs are common in women. Approximately 25 to 35% of 20 to 40 year olds have had at least one episode. There is a far lower incidence in men (approximately 5 per 10,000 university men). The cost is approximately one billion dollars annually in the U.S. See Table 9–14 for pathogens.
- Common presenting complaints are increased urinary frequency, nocturia, urgency, suprapubic or flank pain, and dysuria.

- Diagnosis is usually made by urinalysis and urine culture. Usually, pyuria, hematuria, and bacteriuria are present (usually defined as > 100,000 cfu per mL).

Table 9–14. Common Organisms in Urinary Tract Infection

Acute Urethritis	Vaginitis	Acute Cystitis	Catheter-Associated UTI
C. trachomatis	Candida	E. coli	E. coli
Gonococcus	Trichomonas	S. saprophyticus	Pseudomonas
Herpes simplex virus		Proteus	Klebsiella
		Klebsiella	Proteus
		Enterococcus	S. aureus
			S. epidermidis
			Yeast

Initial Management
- Most lower UTIs resolve spontaneously (50–70%)
- Patients can be treated with 1-, 3-, or 7-day therapy. The shorter therapy has an increased rate of compliance, is more cost effective, and is probably just as effective.
- Recommendations are a 3-day regimen of oral TMP-SMX 1 tablet PO bid or ciprofloxacin 500 mg PO bid. Cranberry juice is also reported to reduce recurrences.
- For catheter-induced UTIs, the goal of treatment is prevention: remove the catheter as soon as possible. Alternatives are a condom catheter, intermittent catheterization, and suprapubic and intraurethral catheters.

Further Discussion

The differential includes acute cystitis, acute urethritis, and vaginitis.
- Acute urethritis. Patients have pyuria, without bacteriuria. Commonly, there will be a history of a new sexual partner or a history of STDs. There is a gradual onset of symptoms including vaginal discharge or bleeding.

- Vaginitis. Commonly, patients have vaginal symptoms of discharge, odor, pruritus, dyspareunia, and dysuria. Usually, there is no frequency or urgency.
- In the inpatient setting, we commonly see catheter-associated UTIs. Approximately 15 to 25% of patients have a catheter inserted. The incidence of bacteriuria is 3 to 10% per day. The greatest risk for bacteriuria is the duration of catheterization. Most patients will be bacteriuric by the end of 30 days. Short-term complications include fevers, pyelonephritis, bacteremia, and death. Long-term complications include stones, obstruction, chronic renal inflammation, renal failure, and bladder cancer.

NEPHROLITHIASIS

Quick Points
- The prevalence of nephrolithiasis is 7% in men and 3% in women. Peak incidence is age 20 for men, decreasing with age.
- Symptoms include severe colicky pain in the abdomen and flank and nausea and vomiting; patients are writhing and can't stay still, in contrast to peritonitis and appendicitis, where they try to stay still.
- A plain film of the abdomen and renal ultrasonography will diagnose most stones. Stones containing calcium are radiopaque, whereas those containing uric acid are radiolucent.

Initial Management
- Aggressive hydration and analgesia (ketorolac and/or narcotics) are essential.
- Extracorporeal shock wave lithotripsy and ureteroscopy are used in complicated cases where the stone does not pass.
- Urinalysis usually reveals microscopic or gross hematuria. Urinary pH is valuable. Persistent urinary pH less than 5.0 is suggestive of uric acid or cystine stones.
- Evaluation should include metabolic evaluation, especially for recurrent stones. At a minimum, patients should have urinalysis, SMA, 24-hour urinary calcium, uric acid, oxalate, and citrate.

Further Discussion

The most common stone produced is calcium (oxalate, then phosphate) and then struvite (magnesium ammonium phosphate), uric acid, and cystine. The pathogenesis of stones includes supersaturation of urine, conditions for crystallization, and absence of a crystal inhibitor. Normal urine contains inhibitors of stone formation. Citrate, magnesium, and pyrophosphate are inorganic inhibitors. The most common cause of kidney stones is hypercalciuria (60% of patients):

- Absorptive type I—hypercalciuria on a calcium-restricted diet, normal fasting urinary calcium, and exaggerated calciuric response to calcium loading
- Absorptive type II—urine calcium is normal on a restricted diet
- Renal—hypercalciuria on a restricted diet, elevated fasting urinary calcium, and elevated serum PTH with normal serum calcium

Hyperuricosuria is the next most common and then hypocitraturia. Both of these result in calcium nephrolithiasis.

Uric acid calculi commonly occur at a low urine pH. Struvite calculi are commonly seen in women with recurrent UTIs. Frequently, they are discovered as large staghorn calculi, which form a cast of the renal collecting system. These stones are radiodense and commonly form with a high urinary pH (7–7.5). They are formed secondary to urease-producing organisms (*Proteus, Pseudomonas, Providencia, Klebsiella, Staphylococcus,* and *Mycoplasma*). Cystine stones are a result of abnormal excretion of cystine, ornithine, lysine, and arginine.

If the diagnosis remains uncertain, then IV urography is indicated. Stone analysis should be performed on recovered stones. Medullary sponge kidney causes stones but not hypercalcemia.

Medications may be used to treat metabolic disorders:

- Potassium citrate for hyocitraturic calcium nephrolithiasis
- Allopurinol for hyperuricemic patients
- Thiazide diuretics for hypercalciuria (50 mg/d).
- Diet restriction for type II. Dietary treatment should include protein (60 g/d) and sodium (3–4 g/d) restriction and increased fluids.

RENAL TUBULAR ACIDOSIS

The rule of thumb classification is the higher the number, the higher the potassium. Types are as follows:

1. Distal—autosomal dominant; occurs in nephrocalcinosis and kidney stones; has low serum potassium; often associated with osteomalacia or rickets

2. Proximal—often occurs with Fanconi's syndrome; potassium is still low but closer to normal; needs lots of bicarbonate replacement. There is glucosuria, aminoaciduria, and mild proteinuria. Symptoms include thiazides and a low-salt diet.

3. Rare form in children; mix of distal and proximal; not discussed in medicine.

4. Distal—acquired; has high potassium; usually has low levels of renin and aldosterone (eg, DM, HTN, nephropathies). Can be treated with furosemide (Lasix) or fludrocortisone (Florinef).

RENAL NEOPLASMS

Quick Points
- Associations:
  - Male
  - von Hippel-Lindau disease (spinal and cerebellar hemangioblastomas, retinal angiomas, pheochromocytomas, renal and pancreatic cysts, cystadenomas of the epididymis, and renal cell carcinomas)
  - ESRD
- Symptoms:
  - Flank pain
  - Palpable mass
  - Hematuria

Initial Management
- Work-up
  - As an initial radiologic test, ultrasonography is useful. Ultrasonography can distinguish between cystic, solid, and complex renal masses.
  - Any mass that does not meet criteria for a simple cyst should be evaluated by CT.
- The only successful treatment for patients with localized renal cell carcinoma is surgical excision. The preferred surgical approach is radical nephrectomy (removal of the kidney with its surrounding fascia and the ipsilateral adrenal gland).
- Radiation therapy and chemotherapy are of limited value.
- Treatment of metastatic disease is interleukin-2. Stem cell or BMT is being attempted.

TUBULOINTERSTITIAL DISEASES

Allergic Tubulointerstitial Nephritis

Quick Points
- Acute tubulointerstitial nephritis makes up approximately 15% of cases of ARF. Most cases are drug related. The presentation is usually a sudden decrease in renal function in a patient who has been taking a new medication. See Table 9–15 for causes.
- Other common signs and symptoms are fever (85–100%) and transient maculopapular rash (25–50%). Less than 30% of patients have the classic triad of fever, rash, and eosinophilia.
- Common laboratory findings include gross or microscopic hematuria and peripheral eosinophilia. Greater than 1% eosinophils in the urine is 95% specific and 65% sensitive. Kidneys are normal sized or enlarged on ultrasonography.

Table 9–15. Common Causes of Allergic Interstitial Nephritis

Drugs	*Infections*
Beta-lactam antibiotics	Legionnaires' disease
NSAIDs	Epstein-Barr virus
Thiazides	Leptospirosis
Sulfonamides	Mycoplasma
Furosemide	Rocky Mountain spotted fever
Cimetidine	
ACE inhibitors	
Rifampin	

Initial Management
- Discontinue the offending drug.
- Acute dialysis may be necessary in up to 30% of patients.
- High-dose steroids are often used if renal function does not return to baseline after discontinuing the drug (there is no evidence for this).

Chronic Tubulointerstitial Nephritis

Quick Points
- Causes:
  - Prolonged obstruction of the urinary tract (eg, renal stones, prostate disease, cervical cancer, tumor involvement, or fibrosis of the retroperitoneum)
  - Reflux nephropathy (usually in children)
  - Analgesic abuse (generally acetaminopen, especially in combination with ASA and caffeine)
  - Heavy metal exposure (lead, cadmium—usually secondary to occupational exposure)
- Symptoms are due to the inability to concentrate the urine (ie, polyuria and nocturia out of proportion to the degree of renal impairment).
- Some patients also experience significant salt wasting.

Initial Management
- The urinalysis is usually nonspecific.
- Usually, there is an inability to acidify the urine in association with hyperchloremic metabolic acidosis.
- The diagnostic modality of choice is renal ultrasonography, with or without IVP.
- Treatment depends on identification of the underlying cause (eg, treat obstruction if there is hydronephrosis).
- Recovery of renal function depends on the degree of interstitial fibrosis.
- If there is evidence of parenchymal loss (small shrunken kidneys), ESRD is often inevitable.

MULTISYSTEM DISEASE WITH KIDNEY INVOLVEMENT

Wegener's Granulomatosis

Antineutrophil cytoplasmic autoantibodies have been seen in some patients with necrotizing glomerulonephritis (with or without pulmonary hemorrhage) and with patients with active Wegener's, which is a rare disorder (3/100,000). It is characterized by vasculitis and necrotizing granulomatous lesions of both the upper and lower respiratory tract and glomerulonephritis. Without treatment, the disease is fatal. It most commonly occurs in the fourth and fifth decades. The disorder usually develops over 4 to 12 months, with 90% of patients presenting with upper or lower respiratory tract symptoms. Renal involvement develops in 75% of cases. Most patients are slightly anemic, have mild leukocytosis, and have increased ESR. Chest CT is more sensitive than CXR, but lesions can range from infiltrates, nodules, and masses to cavities. Over 90% of patients with active Wegener's are positive for antineutrophil cystoplasmic antibody (ANCA). cANCA is more common and specific for this disorder than pANCA. Diagnosis must be made early. Early diagnosis can prevent renal failure and save lives. Remission can be induced in up to 75% of patients with cyclophosphamide and prednisone. Patients who do not have immediately life-threatening disease can be treated with methotrexate. TMP-SMX is useful in maintaining remission.

Polyarteritis Nodosa

Polyarteritis nodosa (PAN) is characterized by focal or segmental lesions of arteries of small to medium size. The hallmark of the disease is acute necrotizing inflammation of the arterial media, with fibrinoid necrosis and extensive inflammatory cell infiltration of all coats of the vessel and surrounding tissue. The cause is unknown, but hepatitis B and C have been strongly implicated. The clinical presentation is usually insidious. Extremity pain is often a prominent early feature. The combination of mononeuritis multiplex and systemic symptoms is an early clue to PAN. There is a wide variety of cutaneous manifestations. Kidney involvement occurs in up to 80% of cases. HTN presents in 50% of cases (it's rare in Wegener's syndrome). The renal lesion is segmental necrotizing glomerulonephritis with extracapillary proliferation. Abdominal "angina" is also common.

Laboratory findings include proteinuria, hematuria, and red cell casts. Most patients are anemic and have leukocytosis. Eosinophilia is more common with pulmonary manifestations. pANCA is found in 30% of patients with PAN but can also be found in other situations. However, diagnosis requires positive histology or angiography (aneurysms). High-dose steroids control symptoms. Cyclophosphamide improves survival.

Systemic Lupus Erythematosus

Lupus nephritis is an extremely serious complication of SLE. Patients can present with a nephritic or nephrotic picture. Renal biopsy is often done in order to document the type and severity of the kidney disease. The five types are as follows:

- Type I—normal
- Type II—minimal or mesangial proliferative
- Type III—focal and segmental proliferative
- Type IV—diffuse proliferative
- Type V—membranous

Types I and II require no therapy. Types III and IV should be treated with aggressive immunosupression. It is unclear as to how to treat Type V disease (steroids are often given). Serologic evidence includes increased levels of ANA, anti–double-stranded DNA, and reduced levels of C3, C4, and CH50.

Diabetic Nephropathy

In the U.S., diabetes is the major cause of ESRD (we're sure you've heard this before). High-risk groups include African Americans, males, and Native Americans. The earliest changes are an increase in kidney size secondary to cellular hypertrophy, proliferation, and an increased GFR. The rate of progression of kidney disease can be slowed down with ACE inhibitors (check for microalbuminuria), normalization of BP, and strict glycemic control. Patients with diabetic nephropathy are more prone to have papillary necrosis, type IV RTA, and an increased risk of ARF secondary to contrast (remember to hydrate).

Multiple Myeloma

MM is discussed in more detail in Chapter 4. Remember that Bence Jones proteinuria (light-chain immunoglobins) is a major contributor to renal failure. They can be directly nephrotoxic or can cause tubular obstruction. Patients usually present with the nephrotic syndrome. Patients are often hypercalcemic and hyperuricemic.

HEMATURIA/NEPHRITIS

Hematuria

Quick Points
- Hematuria is termed gross or macroscopic when the urine is red in color due to the presence of blood. When the urine appears visually

normal, the term microscopic is used. Hematuria can be persistent or intermittent.
- Unexplained hematuria in men or nonmenstruating women should be worked up with IVP, cystoscopy, and urine cytology.
- Try to assess the pattern of hematuria. Initial hematuria indicates a urethral lesion, whereas terminal hematuria indicates bladder disease.
- The presence of RBC casts in the urine is the essential component of the nephritic syndrome. It usually suggests a proliferative glomerular disease. Proteinuria with hematuria usually indicates that hematuria is renal in origin (blood may increase the level of protein in the urine, but if protein is > 500 mg/24 hours, it's safe to say that there is renal disease).
- Important labs also include CBC, SMA, and PT/PTT. In an African-American patient with hematuria, assess for sickle cell disease. If glomerular disease is suspected, early renal biopsy is important.

Further Discussion

Nephritic syndrome is characterized by the presence of RBC casts in the urinary sediment, modest proteinuria (usually < 1 g/d), azotemia, HTN, and edema. It is almost always associated with glomerular causes of hematuria.

The dipstick method is used to screen for hematuria (can detect as little as 3 RBC/hpf). False positives may be caused by hemoglobinuria, myoglobinuria, and povidone-iodine (Betadine).

Hematuria is divided into
1. Extrarenal (65% of patients): calculi, neoplasm, infection, drug, trauma
2. Glomerular
3. Nonglomerular

Glomerular disease is most common in children and young adults:
- Proliferative disease. These are the most common causes of glomerular hematuria. They usually present with the nephritic syndrome. Proliferative diseases are divided into primary and secondary.
- Primary proliferative disease:
  - IgA nephropathy (Berger's) disease. This is the most common cause of acute glomerulonephritis in the U.S. and is more common in Asia. The cause is unknown. It tends to present as an episode of macroscopic hematuria, frequently right after exercise or URI.

Gross hematuria usually lasts 2 to 6 days. In contrast to poststreptococcal glomerulonephritis, there is no latent period. Half of the patients develop progressive loss of renal function. There are mesangial deposits on EM. The same renal lesion is seen with Henoch-Schönlein purpura.

- Poststreptococcal glomerulonephritis. This is secondary to infection with beta-hemolytic *Streptococcus*. Most commonly present with pharyngitis or impetigo. The latent period between infection and onset of urinary symptoms is 6 to 21 days. It is characterized by abrupt onset of tea-colored urine, oliguria, edema, HTN, and mild to moderate proteinuria. Urinary sodium is low, with FENa < 0.5. Usually, there are decreased complements (CH50, C3). The disease is immune complex mediated. There are subepithelial deposits/ "humps" on EM. Disorder is usually self-limiting, with 95% of patients recovering renal function within 2 months of onset. There is no specific treatment, except antihypertensives, salt restriction, and diuretics.

- Rapidly progressive glomerulonephritis (RPGN). This is any glomerular disease associated with rapid loss of renal function. RPGN should be considered if renal biopsy reveals the presence of crescents in > 50% or more glomeruli. The causes of RPGN can be categorized according to immunofluorescence patterns on renal biopsy.

  - Immune complex disease. Granular deposits of immunoglobin (IgG and IgA) and complement along capillary walls. Glomerulonephritis is usually a manifestation of systemic disease (SLE, cryoglobulinemia, poststreptococcal). Treatment is high-dose methylprednisolone for 3 days, followed by oral prednisone (2 mg/kg/d) tapered over several months. In addition, cytotoxic drugs (cyclophosphamide) are added.

  - Idiopathic (Pauci-immune) crescentic glomerulonephritis. This may involve the kidney or may be part of a systemic disorder (Wegener's, PAN). It is associated with increased ANCA and normal serum complement levels. Men are affected twice as much as women. Flu-like symptoms with fevers, myalgias, and polyarthralgias are common. Therapy is the same as for immune complex disease.

  - Goodpasture's syndrome. This affects 5% of patients. Hemoptysis and hematuria are due to anti-glomerular basement membrane

(GBM) antibody deposits in the kidneys and lungs (Wegener's disease can also cause these symptoms). Disease occurs in young Caucasian males. Microscopic hematuria and proteinuria develop within 2 weeks of onset of pulmonary disease. Immunofluorescence shows linear deposition of IgG on the basement membrane, often with C3 in the same pattern. Treatment is combined plasma exchange therapy (to remove circulating antibodies) and immunosuppression (prednisone and cyclophosphamide).

- Familial
  - Alport's syndrome usually occurs in males (X-linked). Hematuria is associated with subsequent proteinuria and hearing loss.
- Nonglomerular renal causes
  - Renal cell carcinoma
  - Sickle cell disease (papillary necrosis)
  - Hypercalciuria and hyperuricosuria (thiazides, allopurinol)

CONTINUOUS AMBULATORY PERITONEAL DIALYSIS

A common form of renal replacement is peritoneal dialysis (PD). These patients are infrequently hospitalized. The key advantage of PD is that it can be done at home. Patients can lead normal lives. Other advantages include less hypotension (better for CHF) and improved glucose control in diabetics (you can add insulin to the PD fluid).

Depending on the country, 5 to 95% of ESRD patients entering maintenance therapy select PD. The major hazard and the most frequent cause of termination is peritonitis. On average, patients get peritonitis 0.5 times per year. The definition of peritonitis is a cell count $> 100/mm^3$ and $>$ 50% neutrophils. The working definition of peritonitis is the presence of at least two of the following:

- Positive Gram's stain or culture
- Cloudy fluid (cell count $> 100/mm^3$ with $> 50\%$ PMNs)
- Symptoms of peritoneal inflammation: abdominal pain, rebound, nausea, and fever

In order to establish an accurate microbiologic diagnosis of peritonitis,
- Take cultures early. The first cloudy bag is the best specimen. Remember that a delay in several hours from the time of collection to the time of culture does not decrease the accuracy of diagnosis.
- Culture large volumes.

- Do culture and sensitivity as soon as possible. The majority of cultures become positive in the first 24 hours. In more than 75% of patients, the diagnosis is established within 72 hours.

Gram's stain establishes the presence of microorganisms in about 20 to 30% of cases. It may be useful in diagnosing fungal peritonitis. Blood cultures are usually consistently negative but may indicate a source. Remember to send a daily cell count. PD cultures should be done every 3 days. The incidence of culture-negative peritonitis varies from 2 to 20%. Causes include

- Low-sensitivity culture methods
- Culture volumes that are too small
- A causative organism that requires special media (ie, *Mycobacterium*)
- Cultures taken from patients already on antibiotic therapy
- Symptoms and signs that are not due to the infectious agent

The most common cause of peritonitis is bacteria. Approximately 4 to 8% may be fungal, most commonly *Candida*. In most cases of peritonitis, symptoms decrease rapidly after starting therapy and disappear within 2 to 3 days. Other considerations include an exit site infection, in which the site is inflamed and has serous or purulent discharge. Also of concern is a tunnel infection (the tunnel under the skin, where the PD catheter is), which is more difficult to treat. An ultrasound may be useful in this situation to look for a fluid collection.

Recurrence is defined as the reappearance of symptoms, positive cultures (after they have been negative), or increased PMNs. This may indicate inadequate therapy or the appearance of an abscess that was previously inaccessible. Recurrence is defined as the reappearance of symptoms after therapy has been stopped, but within a 4-week period. This usually indicates inadequate treatment of a tunnel or exit site infection.

The major consequence of peritonitis is adhesions. This is frequently seen with *S. aureus* or fungal peritonitis. Remember that patients with peritonitis will have to go on hemodialysis for several weeks.

BIBLIOGRAPHY

Reviews and Guidelines

Adrogue HJ, Madias NE. Hyponatremia and hypernatremia. N Engl J Med 2000; 342:1493–9, 1581–9.

Badalamenti S, et al. Hepatorenal syndrome. New perspectives in pathogenesis and treatment. Arch Intern Med 1993;153:1957–67.

Bennett PH, et al. Screening and management of microalbuminuria in patients with diabetes mellitus. Am J Kidney Dis 1995;25:107–12.

Bidani A, et al. Permissive hypercapnia in acute respiratory failure. JAMA 1994; 274:957–62.

Brater DC. Diuretic therapy. N Engl J Med 1998;339:387–96.

Coe FL, et al. The pathogenesis and treatment of kidney stones. N Engl J Med 1992;327:1141–52.

Debroe M, Elseviers M. Analgesic nephropathy. N Engl J Med 1998;339: 446–452.

Ferris TF. Preeclampsia and postpartum renal failure. Am J Med 1995;99:343–7.

Gennari FG. Hypokalemia. N Engl J Med 1998;39:451–8.

Hricik DG, et al. Glomerulonephritis. N Engl J Med 1998;339:888–99.

Hruska KA, et al. Renal osteodystrophy. N Engl J Med 1995;333:166–74.

Klahr, S. The progression of renal disease. N Engl J Med 1988;318:1657–66.

Klahr S, Miller SB. Acute oliguria. N Engl J Med 1998;338:671–6.

Muirhead N, et al. Evidence-based recommendations for the clinical use of recombinant human erythropoietin. Am J Kidney Dis 1995;26:S1–24.

Orth SR, Ritz E. The nephrotic syndrome. N Engl J Med 1998;338:1202–11.

Ritz E, Orth SR. Nephropathy in patients with type 2 diabetes mellitus. N Engl J Med 1999;341:1127–33.

Thadhani R, et al. Acute renal failure. N Engl J Med 1996;334:1448–60.

Studies and Trials

Cattran DC, et al. Long-term benefits of ACE inhibitor therapy in patients with severe IgA nephropathy. Am J Kidney Dis 1994;23:247–54. (*A retrospective review of 115 patients revealing that ACE I reduced proteinuria and progression of renal failure more than other antihypertensives.*)

Diabetes Control and Complication Trial Research Group. The effect of intensive treatment of diabetes on the development and progression of long-term complications in insulin-dependent diabetes mellitus. N Engl J Med 1993;329:977–86. (*A seminal RCT showing the benefits of glucose control in type I diabetics with respect to preventing nephropathy, retinopathy, and neuropathy.*)

Donadio JV, et al. A controlled trial of fish oils in IgA nephropathy. N Engl J Med 1995;331:1194–9. (*An RCT showing that fish oil slowed progression of renal disease in IgA nephropathy.*)

Hoffman GS, et al. Wegener's granulomatosis: an analysis of 158 patients. Ann Intern Med 1992;116:488–98. (*National Institutes of Health long-term series showing improved survival in Wegener's with use of cytotoxic agents.*)

Hogan SL, et al. A review of therapeutic studies of idiopathic membranous glomerulopathy. Am J Kidney Dis 1995;25:862–75. (*A meta-analysis showing improved remission of nephrotic syndrome in membranous nephropathy with use of alkylating agents but not glucocorticoids.*)

Levine RJ, et al. Trial of calcium to prevent preeclampsia. N Engl J Med 1997; 337:69–76. (*An RCT showing that calcium supplementation did not affect the incidence, severity, or time of onset of preeclampsia and did not affect rate or severity of pregnancy-associated hypertension.*)

Lewis EJ, et al. The effects of ACE inhibition on diabetic nephropathy. N Engl J Med 1993;329:1456–62. (*An RCT showing that ACE inhibitors reduce proteinuria and progression of renal disease in diabetics.*)

Lucas MJ. A comparision of magnesium sulfate with phenytoin for the prevention of eclampsia. N Engl J Med 1995;333:201–5. (*An RCT showing that magnesium during labor in hypertensive nulliparous women reduced the rate of eclampsia [seizures] but slightly increased the rate of cesarean-section; there were no adverse effects on fetal outcome.*)

Maschio G, et al. Effect of the ACE inhibitor benazepril on progression of chronic renal insufficiency. N Engl J Med 1996;334:939–45. (*An RCT showing that benazepril slowed progression of chronic renal insufficiency, especially in men, diabetics, patients with glomerulopathies, and those with proteinuria greater than 1 g/24 hr, but not in patients with polcystic kidney disease.*)

Pedrini MT, et al. The effect of dietary protein restriction on the progression of diabetic and nondiabetic renal diseases. Ann Intern Med 1996;124:627–32. (*A meta-analysis showing that protein restriction slows but doesn't stop progression of renal failure.*)

Ponticelli C, et al. A 10 year follow-up of a randomized study with methylprednisolone and chlorambucil in idiopathic membranous nephropathy. Kidney Int 1995;48:1600–4. (*An RCT showing benefit with immunosuppression in membranous nephropathy.*)

Port FK, et al. Comparison of survival probabilities for dialysis patients vs. cadaveric renal transplant recipients. JAMA 1993;270:1339–43. (*Transplant patients had a better survival rate than dialysis patients [Michigan database of ESRD patients].*)

Sibai BM, et al. Risk factors for preeclampsia and adverse neonatal outcomes among women with chronic hypertension. N Engl J Med 1998;339:667–71. (*Proteinuria early in pregnancy increases the risk of adverse neonatal outcomes regardless of development of preeclampsia in women with chronic HTN.*)

10

Oncology

God grant me the serenity to accept the things I cannot change, the courage to change the things I can, and the wisdom to know the difference. — Anonymous

Concern for man himself and his fate must always be the chief interest of all technical endeavors...in order that the creations of our mind shall be a blessing and not a curse to mankind. — Albert Einstein

GENERAL ISSUES

Cancer is the second most common cause of death in the U.S. Prostate cancer is the most common cancer detected in American men. Breast cancer remains the most common cancer in women. In terms of cancer death, lung cancer is at the forefront for both men and women (you've come a long way, baby).

The key points of treatment are as follows:
1. Be compassionate. Many of these patients are at the end stages of their terminal disease and require some extra kindness.
2. Always assess pain. There is no reason for a patient to be in pain.
3. A discussion of advanced care directives is essential as soon as possible after diagnosis or admission. At a minimum, each patient should have a health care proxy.
4. A careful physical examination is necessary daily. Look for skin breakdown, oral lesions (ie, thrush), and the size of lymph nodes (use a ruler to measure).
5. Constipation is a relatively common problem. Often, these patients are immobile and on morphine products. Prevention is the key. Once pain medications are started, a bowel regimen should be started at the same time.

Oncologic Emergencies

Hypercalcemia

Quick Points
- Hypercalcemia occurs in 10 to 20% of patients with cancer, most commonly in patients with breast, lung, kidney, head and neck cancers, and MM.
- Hypercalcemia is caused by activation of osteoclasts by tumor-derived factors. Newly recognized is the PTH-related protein. Other tumor-derived factors are tumor necrosis factor (TNF), prostaglandins, IFN, interleukins, colony-stimulating factors, and transforming growth factor (TGF)-α.
- Signs and symptoms:
  - Nausea, vomiting, constipation, polyuria
  - Muscular weakness, hyporeflexia
  - Confusion, psychosis, tumor, and lethargy
  - Short QT on EKG

Initial Management
- Vigorous hydration with diuresis (*most important*). Give NS (4–6 L/d), followed by furosemide (Lasix) (increases urinary calcium loss). Make sure that the patient is well hydrated prior to starting furosemide. Watch out for fluid overload (strict input and output).
- Bisphosphonates (pamidronate is the main IV medication) — the mainstay of treatment. They inhibit osteoclast bone resorption and are nontoxic. Give 60 to 90 mg over 24 hours, with adequate hydration. Calcium usually normalizes in 7 days. Takes 2 to 3 days to achieve the maximum effect.
- Calcitonin — works immediately to inhibit bone resorption. Usual dose is 4 U/kg IM/SQ q12 hours. This can be increased to 8 U/kg q12 hours after 1 to 2 days. Be sure to skin test first to rule out hypersensitivity. Tachyphylaxis usually occurs after 1 to 3 days of treatment. Also good as adjuvant analgesic.
- Gallium nitrate — superior to calcitonin. Given by continuous infusion at a dose of 100 to 200 mg/m^2/d for 5 days.
- Mithramycin — rarely used. Inhibits osteoclast activity.

- *Treat the underlying malignancy.*
- *Mobilize the patient.*

Spinal Cord Compression

Quick Points
- Spinal cord compression is usually secondary to bone metastases to the vertebral column or due to a paraspinal or epidural mass. This is an emergency because delay can result in paraplegia.
- It is most commonly seen with prostate, breast, and lung cancer or MM.
- The most common signs and symptoms are back pain, progressive weakness, and sensory loss (usually in the lower extremities). Urinary retention and bladder/bowel incontinence are usually late findings. Neurologic deficits found at the time of diagnosis are usually irreversible. Early diagnosis is the key.
- MRI makes the diagnosis.

Initial Management
- The treatment of choice is radiation therapy to the area of the spinal cord and two adjacent vertebrae (above and below).
- Dexamethasone IV should also be started (10 mg IV immediately, then 4–6 mg IV q6 hours).
- Surgery is indicated in the following settings:
  - Spinal cord compression without the diagnosis of malignancy.
  - Radioresistant tumor or patients who have already received maximal radiation to that area.
  - Patients who develop progressive neurologic deficits during radiation and who have a favorable overall prognosis.
  - Vertebral collapse with mechanical cord compression.

Tumor Lysis Syndrome

Quick Points
- Tumor lysis syndrome is due to rapid release of cellular contents. This usually occurs after treatment of lymphoid malignancies with a

10

large tumor burden. This may also occur with rapidly proliferating malignancies.

- *The key players are uric acid, phosphate, calcium, and potassium.* LDH is also very high (especially in lymphomas and testicular cancer).
- Neoplasms with high nucleic acid turnover release large amounts of uric acid. Massive tumor cell necrosis releases phosphate.
- A serum urate concentration > 15 mg/dL is associated with a high risk for uric acid nephropathy.
- Phosphate may precipitate with calcium in nonskeletal tissues (ie, kidney), causing nephrocalcinosis and renal failure.
- Hyperkalemia, with consequent hypocalcemia, puts patients at risk for ventricular arrhythmias.
- Tumor lysis syndrome is most commonly associated with the following malignancies: high-grade lymphomas, Burkitt's lymphoma, acute lymphoblastic leukemia, Hodgkin's disease, chronic lymphocytic leukemia, and some solid tumors (breast, small cell, testicular).
- Initially, patients present with weakness, anorexia, and vomiting. Consequently, they develop muscle weakness, cramps, seizures, and then altered mental status.

Initial Management
- The mainstay of treatment is prevention.
- Make sure patients are well hydrated.
- Start allopurinol 12 to 24 hours prior to starting therapy (initial dose is 600 mg, then 300 mg qd) and continue for 1 week after initial chemotherapy.
- The next step is urinary alkalization.
- Volume status, renal function, uric acid levels, and urine pH should be monitored.
- Provide emergency hemodialysis and respiratory support if necessary.

Increased Intracranial Pressure

Quick Points
- May be secondary to primary brain tumors or metastases.
- Signs and symptoms are headache, decreasing mentation, and papilledema.

Initial Management

- Give dexamethasone (4–20 mg IV qid) to reduce cerebral edema from metastases.
- Phenobarbital may reduce cerebral metabolism and improve cerebral compliance.
- If herniation is a major concern, IV mannitol may reduce pressure.
- If the patient herniates, he or she needs to be intubated, and mechanical hyperventilation may reduce intracranial pressure temporarily.
- If the patient is a candidate, definitive therapy may include radiation, craniotomy, or burr holes (time to call Neurosurgery).

Malignant Effusions

Quick Points

- Malignant effusions can occur in any body cavity, most commonly the pleura, peritoneum, or pericardium.
- Signs and symptoms are based on location: SOB can occur with effusions of pleural, peritoneal, or pericardial spaces; evidence of tamponade (hypotension, right-sided heart failure) occurs with pericardial effusions.

Initial Management

- Obtaining a sample of the effusion is essential to confirming diagnosis; fix the fluid in formalin or ethanol as soon as it is obtained.
- Treating the cause is essential, of course.
- Repeated taps can be used for symptomatic relief.
- *For pleural effusions,*
  - Injection of talc via a chest tube or mechanical pleural stripping (either through video-assisted thoracoscopy or open thoracotomy) can be used to end malignant effusions.
  - Avoid taking more than 1 L off in a thoracentesis to reduce the risk of post–re-expansion pulmonary edema.
- *For peritoneal effusions,*
  - Surgical debulking of peritoneal metastases is generally necessary.
  - Avoid taking more than 2 L off in a single paracentesis to reduce the risk of hypotension.

10

- *For pericardial effusions,*
  - An opening of a pericardial window and pericardiectomy are the options to relieve tamponade.

Neutropenia

- G-CSF is good for prophylaxis in patients receiving chemotherapy regimens with a > 40% risk of developing neutropenic fever.
- Most clinicians use G-CSF in almost all patients who do develop neutropenic fever.
- Standard broad-spectrum coverage for neutropenic fever is ticarcillin-clavulanate (Timentin)/piperacillin plus aminoglycoside.

If fever persists for > 1 week, start empiric amphotericin.

Tumor Markers

Usually, tumor markers are used to trend the efficacy of treatment and screen for recurrence in those in whom it had been elevated before. The

Table 10–1. Cancers and Tumor Markers

Hairy cell leukemia	Tartrate-resistant acid phosphatase
Prostate	Prostate-specific antigen, prostate acid phosphatase
Gastrointestinal (colorectal, pancreas, stomach)	Carcinoembryonic antigen, CA 19-9
Hepatocellular	Alpha-fetoprotein, CA125
Ovary	CA 125
Germ cell tumors	Alpha-fetoprotein
Choriocarcinomas	Beta-human chorionic gonadotropin
Thyroid	Thyroglobin, calcitonin (for medullary cancer)
Myeloma	Immunoglobins (Bence Jones)
Bone	Alkaline phosphatase
Melanoma	S-100
Sarcoma	Vimentin
Breast cancer	Cytokeratin

only screening markers are prostate-specific antigen (PSA), alpha-feto-protein (AFP), and calcitonin. See Table 10–1.

Pain Management

When you are taking care of an oncology patient, never forget to address the issue of pain. Unfortunately, pain associated with cancer is frequently undertreated. As always, the initial assessment should include a detailed history, physical examination, psychosocial assessment, and appropriate diagnostic tests. Remember to ask the basic questions about pain: location, intensity/severity, aggravating/relieving factors, how the patient responds to pain, and pain control goals. Most clinicians use the standard numeric pain intensity scale (0–10, with 0 being no pain and 10 being the worst possible pain). See Table 10–2 for a pain management approach.

Remember (especially in the opiate naive patient) to start off with short-acting opiates for at least 24 hours. Once analgesics are begun, it is necessary to determine the efficacy and duration of relief. When large amounts of short-acting analgesics are needed, calculate the 24-hour dose and convert to intermediate-acting drugs (eg, morphine [MS Contin]) and, later, long-acting agents (fentanyl patch q72 hr). Keep short-acting agents available for rescue doses of breakthrough pain.

There are significant side effects to opiates:

1. Constipation: treat constipation prophylactically.
2. Nausea/vomiting: treat with antiemetics.
3. Sedation: reduce the dose and increase the frequency. You may need to use CNS stimulants.
4. Respiratory depression: usually doesn't occur in patients on long-term opiates. Give naloxone in small doses to improve respiratory function without reversing analgesia.

Table 10–2. World Health Organization Three-Step Analgesic Ladder

Step I	Mild to moderate pain	ASA, acetaminophen, or NSAIDs
Step II	Persistent mild to moderate pain	Add an opioid
Step III	Moderate to severe pain	Increase opioid potency or dose

Sometimes adjuvant drugs and modalities are useful in treating cancer pain: steroids, anticonvulsants, antidepressants, neuroleptics, pamidronate, radiation (especially for bone pain), nerve blocks, and, lastly, palliative surgery.

Chemotherapeutic Agents

Here are some commonly used chemotheraputic agents and their toxicities. Keep these in mind for your patients being treated on the floor.

- Aldesleukin (interleukin-2)
  - Acute toxicity: fever, hypotension, capillary leak syndrome
  - Delayed toxicity: nephrotic syndrome
- Anastrozole (Arimidex)
  - Acute toxicity: nausea, diarrhea, hot flashes, headache
- Bleomycin
  - Acute toxicity: nausea and vomiting, fever, anaphylaxis, phlebitis at injection site
  - Delayed toxicity: pneumonitis and pulmonary fibrosis
- Busulfan (alkylator of DNA)
  - Delayed toxicity: bone marrow depression, pulmonary infiltrates, and fibrosis
- Carboplatin
  - Acute: nausea and vomiting
  - Delayed: bone marrow depression, peripheral neuropathy
- Chlorambucil (alkylator)
  - Delayed: bone marrow depression
- Cisplatin (cross-link DNA)
  - Acute: nausea and vomiting, diarrhea
  - Delayed: renal damage, ototoxicity, bone marrow depression, hypomagnesemia, peripheral neuropathy, hypocalcemia, hypokalemia, hypophosphatemia, hyperuricemia
- Cyclophosphamide (alkylator)
  - Acute: nausea and vomiting, type I hypersensitivity (anaphylaxis)
  - Delayed: bone marrow depression, alopecia, hemorrhagic cystitis
- Daunorubicin
  - Acute: nausea and vomiting, diarrhea, red urine (not hematuria), anaphylaxis
  - Delayed: bone marrow depression, cardiotoxicity (may be delayed for years)

- Doxorubicin (Adriamycin)
  - Acute: nausea and vomiting, red urine, transient EKG changes, ventricular arrhythmia
  - Delayed: cardiotoxicity (most would get a MUGA scan prior to infusion), bone marrow depression
- Etoposide (VP-16) (topoisomerase inhibitor)
  - Acute: nausea and vomiting, diarrhea, fever, hypotension
  - Delayed: bone marrow depression
- Fluorouracil (FU)
  - Acute: nausea and vomiting, diarrhea
  - Delayed: oral and GI ulcers, bone marrow depression
- Flutamide
  - Acute: nausea and vomiting, diarrhea, hot flashes
  - Delayed: gynecomastia, hepatotoxicity
- Ifosfamide
  - Acute: nausea and vomiting, nephrotoxicity, Fanconi's syndrome
  - Delayed: bone marrow depression, hemorrhagic cystitis (prevented by concurrent mesna)
- Interferon α-2a, 2b, n3
  - Acute: fever, chills, myalgias, nausea, diarrhea, headache, arthralgias, hypotension
- Irinotecan (Camptosar)
  - Acute: nausea and vomiting, early diarrhea (< 24 hours)
  - Delayed: late diarrhea (> 24 hours), anorexia, stomatitis
- Isotretinoin (Accutane)
  - Acute: fatigue, headache, nausea and vomiting
  - Delayed: teratogenicity, cheilitis, hypertriglyceridemia, pseudotumor cerebri
- Leuprolide (luteinizing hormone–releasing hormone [LH-RH] analogue —leupron)
  - Acute: transient increase in bone pain or tumor mass
  - Delayed: impotence, testicular atrophy, peripheral edema
- L-Asparaginase (depletes tumors of asparagine)
  - Enzyme-consuming asparagine in tumor cells; has no marrow toxicity
- Levamisole
  - Acute: nausea and vomiting, diarrhea, flu-like symptoms, metallic taste
  - Delayed: agranulocytosis

10

- Melphalan (alkylator)
  - Acute: mild nausea, hypersensitivity reaction
  - Delayed: bone marrow depression
- Methotrexate (blocks folate metabolism)
  - Acute: nausea and vomiting, diarrhea, fever, hepatic necrosis, hypersensitivity reaction
  - Delayed: oral and GI ulceration, bone marrow depression, hepatic toxicity, renal toxicity, pulmonary infiltrates, and fibrosis
- Paclitaxel (Taxol)
  - Acute: hypersensitivity reactions, myocardial ischemia
  - Delayed: bone marrow depression, peripheral neuropathy
- Tamoxifen
  - Acute: hot flashes, nausea and vomiting, hypercalcemia, transient increase in bone or tumor pain
  - Delayed: vaginal bleeding and discharge, rash, thrombocytopenia, depression
- Vinblastine (Vinca alkaloids prevent microtubule disassembly)
  - Delayed: bone marrow depression, alopecia, peripheral neuropathy (blastine blasts the marrow)
- Vincristine
  - Delayed: peripheral neuropathy (cristine crushes the nerves)
- Leucovorin (folinic acid)
  - Used to rescue normal cells from methotrexate
  - Used to enhance 5-FU binding in tumor cells

SPECIFIC CANCERS

Leukemia, lymphoma, GI cancers, myeloma, brain tumors, lung cancer, and renal cancer are discussed in other chapters.

Breast Cancer

See Table 10–3 for risk factors.

Notes on Risk Factors

- The most important risk factor is family history (especially if in first-degree relatives). Twenty to 25% of women diagnosed with breast cancer have a positive family history.
- Overexposure to estrogen.

Table 10–3. Risk Factors for Breast Cancer

Family history

Early menarche

Late menopause

Nulliparity

Atypical lobular or ductal hyperplasia

Early exposure to ionizing radiation

Long-term postmenopausal estrogen replacement

Alcohol consumption

Carcinoma in situ (lobular or ductal)

Benign breast disease (marginal risk)

- Ductal carcinoma in situ is a precursor lesion for invasive cancer in the same breast. (Treat with wide excision plus radiotherapy but not node dissection.)
- Lobular carcinoma in situ has a 1% annual incidence of cancer in either breast (so treatment is expectant or bilateral mastectomy, not wide excision).
- Oral contraceptive use does not increase risk.

Biology/Genetics

All breast cancers have somatic genetic abnormalities. The most recently discovered genes are *BRCA1* and *BRCA2*. These women often have early onset of disease, disease in multiple generations, increased incidence of breast and lung cancer, and ovarian cancer. Areas of mutation have been discovered: deletion at codon 185 in *BRCA1* and deletion at codon 6179 in *BRCA2*. These deletions are present in 1% of Ashkenazi Jewish women.

Sporadic breast cancers also have abnormalities in certain genes: *p53, bcl-2, c-myc,* and *c-myb.* In some breast cancers, normal genes or gene products are overexpressed: HER-2/*neu* and cyclin D1.

Screening

- The American Cancer Society and National Cancer Institute recommend annual screening mammography for women over 40 years with a standard risk of breast cancer.

- Women who are high risk, or those with *BRCA1/2* mutations, should start screening at age 25, or 5 years before the earliest age that breast cancer was diagnosed in a family member.
- A woman with a normal mammogram but a palpable breast mass should undergo fine-needle aspiration (FNA) or core needle biopsy (the standard methods). A negative FNA or core biopsy of a palpable mass requires open biopsy.
- For women with suspicious, nonpalpable masses on mammogram, ultrasound-guided core needle biopsy, stereotactic biopsy, and MRI-guided biopsy may be useful.

Therapy

Primary Breast Cancer. These women usually have their disease detected early, usually by screening mammography. Early-stage disease is usually stages I and II (think tumor size, nodes, metastases [TNM]). Lumpectomy (wide excision of the tumor) with radiation therapy is equal to modified radical mastectomy (MRM). Radiotherapy is an essential part of therapy for breast conservation and is appropriate for patients with aggressive histology even after MRM. The only follow-up that is needed is examination and mammography for early-stage disease. The difficulty lies in assessing which women have micrometastasis and will eventually develop metastatic disease. The decision whether to give adjuvant therapy is based on

1. Axillary lymph node status
2. Tumor size and histology
3. Estrogen and progesterone receptor status
4. Age
5. Menopausal status

Axillary lymph node dissection gives some prognostic information but does not provide therapeutic benefit. However, for lack of better methods, *axillary lymph node dissection is the standard of care for all women with invasive breast cancer or large noninvasive tumors (> 2.5 cm).*

Systemic hormone or chemotherapy is indicated in the following situations:

- Invasive ductal or lobular cancer ≥ 1 cm in largest diameter
- Invasive carcinoma ≥ 3 cm in largest diameter with favorable histology (pure tubular, mucinous, papillary)

- Invasive breast cancer with positive axillary lymph nodes (any tumor regardless of size or histology)

Adjuvant chemotherapy reduces the annual risk of death by 20 to 30%. The most common regimen is cyclophosphamide, methotrexate, and FU (CMF). Doxorubicin can be an adjunct. Treatment is started within 1 to 3 months of surgery and consists of 4 to 6 monthly cycles. When given preoperatively, it is termed neoadjuvant therapy. Radiation and chemotherapy are employed consecutively, not concurrently.

Hormonal therapy for estrogen receptor-positive tumors consists of tamoxifen or ovarian ablation (premenopausal women). Current recommendations are to administer tamoxifen for 5 years. There is no added benefit in treating for longer periods. The beneficial effects of tamoxifen (decreased cancer, decreased osteoporosis) outweigh its side effects (ie, increase in thromboembolic effects and endometrial cancer).

The combination of hormonal therapy and chemotherapy is more effective than either alone. Some simple guidelines for women with operable breast cancer on adjuvant treatment are outlined in Table 10–4.

Metastatic Breast Cancer

Metastatic breast cancer has a variable clinical course. The main goals of treatment are palliation and prolongation of life. Most recurrences or metastases are diagnosed by symptoms and physical examination. Imag-

10

Table 10–4. Guidelines for Adjuvant Therapy in Breast Cancer

Age (yr)	Estrogen Receptor	Risk Level	Indicated Treatment
< 50	Negative	Any	Chemotherapy
	Positive	Low	Chemotherapy, hormonal, or both
		Moderate/high	Chemotherapy + hormonal, or investigational treatment
	Unknown	Any	Chemotherapy + hormonal
> 50	Negative	Any	Chemotherapy
	Positive	Low	Tamoxifen ± chemotherapy
		Moderate/high	Chemotherapy + hormonal, or investigational treatment
	Unknown	Any	Chemotherapy + hormonal

ing and extensive testing often do not improve survival. For women with limited or non–life-threatening disease, hormonal therapy is the treatment of choice. Those with hormone-unresponsive or life-threatening disease require first-line chemotherapy (CMF). Second- and third-line regimens include taxanes and vinorelbine. Taxane-containing salvage regimens improve overall survival.

Bone is the most common site of metastases. Bisphosphonates reduce pain and complications. *In fact, some studies show that they actually reduce the rate of skeletal and perhaps visceral metastases.*

Prostate Cancer

Prostate cancer is the most common cancer detected in American men. In 1995, 72,000 new cases were diagnosed. At autopsy, 40% of men over age 50 have prostate cancer. The average 50-year-old man has a 9.5% risk for developing clinically apparent cancer. He has a 2.9% risk of death (which raises questions about utility of screening; the vast majority of those with prostate cancer will die of something else; further, will interventions cause more trouble than asymptomatic cancers?).

Risk Factors

There aren't many.
- African-American race
- Family history of prostate cancer

Signs and Symptoms

- Usually asymptomatic
- Abnormal digital rectal examination (DRE)
- Rarely, the patient may experience urinary retention, other neurologic symptoms, or urinary obstruction (more common with BPH)
- Back pain or fracture (secondary to skeletal disease)

Screening

The goal is to detect and treat those patients in whom prostate cancer will cause morbidity and mortality. The DRE has approximately a 1.5 to 7% detection rate (usually lesions > T3). The next screening tool is the PSA. There are age-specific normal references for the PSA (Table 10–5).

Table 10–5. Age (Years) versus Prostate-Specific Antigen (ng/mL)

Age (yrs)	Prostate-Specific Antigen (ng/mL)
40–49	< 2.5
50–59	< 3.5
60–69	< 4.5
70–79	< 6.5

Laboratory Tests

- PSA is a glycoprotein produced in the cytoplasm of benign and malignant prostate cells. It correlates with the volume of tissue. PSA is used in detection, staging, and monitoring response to treatment. It is also used to detect recurrence. PSA is the first-line screening test. Approximately two-thirds of men with a PSA >10 ng/mL have cancer. Those with advanced disease have a PSA > 40 ng/mL (approximately 90% of those with metastatic disease will have a PSA this elevated). An increase in PSA velocity of more than 0.3 ng/mL per year is suspicious.
- Serum acid phosphatase is more predictive of metastatic disease. However, prostate acid phosphatase is normal in 25% of patients with metastatic disease.
- Imaging of choice is transrectal ultrasonography.
- Biopsy is transrectal ultrasonography guided. You may biopsy the apex, midportion, or base.
- MRI is valuable for evaluation of lymph nodes.
- Bone scan is done to rule out bone metastases.

Pathology and Staging

The majority of prostate cancer is adenocarcinoma. Most occur in the peripheral zone. A small percentage (5–10%) are in the central zone. Approximately 20% are in the central zone.

Gleason Grading System. A primary grade is given for the architectural pattern. A secondary grade is assigned to the pattern in the second largest area. Grading is based on the following:

- A small, well-differentiated cancer (grades 1 and 2) is usually localized to the prostate.

- Large volume (> 4 mL) or poorly differentiated (grades 4 and 5) are commonly locally metastatic. If the seminal vesicles are involved, there is an increased incidence of metastases.
- Gleason score = primary + secondary score.

Staging Points

- Just remember that a T3a (unilateral extracapsular extension) versus a T3c (seminal vesicle involvement) is an important distinction.
- Lymphatic metastases are usually through the obturator nodes.
- The most common site of bone metastases is the axial skeleton. They are both blastic and lytic.
- In terms of distant metastases, the order is the following: lung > liver > adrenals.

Treatment

1. Local disease treatment options are controversial. If the patient's anticipated survival is greater than 10 years, treatment is radiation and surgery (radical prostatectomy).
- Radical prostatectomy involves removal of the prostate, seminal vesicles, and ampullae of vas deferens. With nerve-sparing surgery (trying to avoid pudendals), there is improved urinary continence and erectile function. Local recurrence is uncommon. The ideal treatment option is for T1, T2, and select T3. If the margins are positive, adjuvant therapy is needed (radiation). If there are lymph node metastases, androgen deprivation is indicated.
- Radiation therapy options include external beam radiation and transperineal implantation. Survival is 65% over 10 years.
- Observation may be appropriate in those of advanced age or with well-differentiated cancer.
2. Locally and regionally advanced disease requires combination therapy: androgen deprivation ± surgery or radiation.
3. Seventy to 80% of metastatic disease responds to androgen deprivation. Testosterone is produced by Leydig's cells (95%). A smaller amount is produced by peripheral conversion of other steroids. Androgen ablation options are as follows:
   - LH-RH agonist (leuprolide, goserelin [Zoladex], buserelin) works at the level of the hypothalamus. Side effects include impotence, hot flashes, gynecomastia, and, rarely, anemia.

- Orchiectomy works at the level of the testes. Side effects are the same as above.
- Antiandrogens (flutamide) work at the prostate cell by competitively binding the receptor for dihydrotestosterone. The most common side effects are diarrhea and nausea.

Patients with limited disease and good performance status do well with combined androgen blockage (leuprolide and flutamide). Pamidronate and radiation are used to treat bone disease.

Bladder Cancer

Quick Points
- Risk factors
  - Male sex
  - Cigarette smoking
  - Exposure to industrial agents (especially aniline dyes)
  - Spinal cord compression with chronic urinary retention
  - Schistosomiasis (causes squamous cell carcinoma of bladder, unlike usual transitional cell carcinoma)
- Symptoms. Hematuria (gross or microscopic) is the presenting symptom in 85 to 90% of patients with bladder cancer. They may also present with dysuria, increased frequency, or nocturia. Occasionally, patients may present with features of urinary outflow obstruction, constipation, perineal pain, or flank pain.
- Transitional cell carcinoma represents 90% of cases (the remainder are mostly squamous).

Initial Management
- Work-up includes careful H&P, urine cytology, cystoscopy, and appropriate radiologic studies (eg, ultrasonography, IVP).
- If cystoscopy confirms the presence of bladder cancer, then the patient undergoes transurethral resection under general or regional anesthesia. A careful bimanual examination is performed at the start and end of the procedure.
- Superficial cancers are associated with a good prognosis, and 5-year survival rates are greater than 80%. These are usually treated by endoscopic surgical resection. Another option is intravesical therapy with

10

cytotoxic agents. Intracystic fulguration with bacille Calmette-Guérin (BCG) has been shown to be superior to chemotherapeutic agents.
- Invasive bladder cancer has a far worse prognosis, with 5-year survival rates of 50% (patients treated with radical radiotherapy or radical cystectomy with lymph node resection). The standard of care is radical cystectomy with placement of a continence device. If there is residual disease, chemotherapy (methotrexate, vinblastine, doxorubicin, cisplatin [MVAC]) is used.
- Remember, transurethral resection is the initial form of treatment for all bladder cancers. It is diagnostic, allows for staging, and controls superficial tumors.
- Approximately 15% of patients newly diagnosed with bladder cancer have metastatic disease. The current chemotherapy regimen of choice is MVAC.

Malignant Melanoma

See Table 10–6 for risk factors.
Signs of early melanoma:
- A — asymmetric lesion
- B — border irregularity
- C — color variation within the lesion
- D — diameter enlarging

Types of melanoma:
- Superficial spreading melanoma
- Lentigo maligna melanoma

Table 10–6. Risk Factors for Melanoma

Lightly pigmented skin

> 200 melanocytic nevi

History of excessive sun exposure

Family history of melanoma or atypical nevi

Country of childhood

Age > 15 yr

Dysplastic nevi (precursor lesions)

- Acral—letiginous melanoma most often affects the palms, soles, nail beds, and mucous membranes
- Nodular melanoma—no radial/horizontal growth phase, with rapid growth (weeks to months)

Excision and Staging

If a lesion is suspicious, a full-thickness biopsy that excises the entire lesion should be performed (1- to 2-mm margin). Never shave, curettage, or needle biopsy.

The staging system (think TNM, American Joint Committee on Cancer) is roughly as follows:

- Stage I—tumor thickness ≤ 1.5 mm
- Stage II—tumor thickness 1.51 to 4.0 mm
- Stage III—tumor thickness > 4.0 mm or with spread to in-transit sites or regional lymph nodes
- Stage IV—metastatic disease

Management and Prognosis

1. Thin primary tumors need 1-cm margins on excision, whereas thicker tumors require approximately 3-cm margins.
2. If lymph nodes are obviously involved, node dissection is indicated.
3. Sentinel lymph node biopsy using preoperative lymphoscintigraphy and intraoperative node mapping may be effective for staging.
4. Node dissection is beneficial for the intermediate-risk group (0.75–3.5 mm).
5. IFN-α and vaccine therapy may reduce recurrence in the high-risk group. IFN is indicated for 1 year in those patients with lymph metastasis.
6. Metastatic melanoma is generally incurable, and the goal of treatment should be palliation. Dacarbazine is commonly used.
7. After surgery, these patients require regular follow-up since they are at increased risk for recurrence or a second primary.

Prognostic indicators include tumor thickness, anatomic site of melanoma, age, histologic features, ulceration, and presence of metastases. *Tumors < 0.76 mm thick have an excellent prognosis. Sixty percent of patients with tumors > 3.65 mm thick have metastases.* The current 5-year survival rate is approximately 81%.

Testicular Cancer

Quick Points
- Testicular tumors are the most common neoplasms in men aged 18 to 30 years. Ninety to 95% of all primary testicular tumors are germ cell.
- Germ cell tumors have two major histologic types: seminomatous and nonseminomatous (malignant teratoma, embryonal carcinoma, endodermal sinus tumor, or choriocarcinoma).
- Risk factors include cryptorchidism, infertility, and genitourinary (GU) anomalies.
- The usual presentation is a scrotal mass, often painless.

Initial Management
- Do *not* do a biopsy. Perform ultrasonography, CT of abdomen and pelvis, and metastatic work-up as indicated.
- Measurement of tumor markers is essential, as seminomas do not produce them, and these markers (AFP), produced by endodermal sinus tumor (and by hepatocellular carcinoma) and human chorionic gonadotropin (hCG) (produced by choriocarcinoma), can be useful in finding residual disease.
- The staging system is as follows:
  - Stage I—restricted to the testis and surrounding adnexa
  - Stage II—involves draining lymphatics up to the diaphragm
  - Stage III—involves mediastinal or supraclavicular nodes
  - Stage IV—extranodal sites (lung, liver, bone, brain)

Management Points
1. Seminoma. Stage I is treated with inguinal orchiectomy with adjuvant radiotherapy. Stage II can be cured by orchiectomy and radiotherapy as well. Stages III and IV are treated with chemotherapy, with cure rates > 80%. Metastases to the lung (which can present in young men with new dyspnea on exertion) are called "cannonball" infiltrates.
2. Nonseminomatous germ cell tumors. Stage I tumors are treated with orchiectomy in combination with prophylactic retroperitoneal lymph node dissection or active surveillance. Cisplatin-based chemotherapy is essential for the treatment of Stages II to IV. Cure rates are greater

than 80%. This high cure rate can be achieved in metastatic germ cell tumors with bleomycin, etoposide, and cisplatin (BEC).

Head and Neck Cancer

Quick Points

- The male-to-female ratio is 3:1. Over 95% of squamous cell cancer of the head and neck is associated with tobacco and alcohol. As many as 15% of patients may have a viral etiology (think EBV and nasopharyngeal cancer).
- Cancers of the head and neck include the following areas: upper aerodigestive tract, paranasal sinuses, major and minor salivary glands, parapharyngeal space, thyroid, parathyroid, and the skin, soft-tissue, bone, and neurovascular structures in the head and neck.
- Squamous cell carcinoma compromises 90% of all head and neck cancers. The remaining are adenocarcinoma (salivary glands), melanomas, and soft-tissue tumors.
- Precancerous lesions may present as leukoplakia or erythroplakia.
- Clinical signs and symptoms may be pain, ulcers, or ill-fitting dentures for oral cancers. Cancer of the oropharynx, hypopharynx, and supraglottic larynx can present as a sore throat, ear pain, hoarseness, or dysphagia. Nasopharyngeal cancers present as unilateral otitis media or cranial nerve deficits (III, VI).

Initial Management

- Mirror or endoscopic examination of the nasal cavity, nasopharynx, hypopharynx, and larynx is necessary (call Otolaryngology). Panendoscopy and work-up should be done before biopsy of new, unknown head/neck mass (always look for a primary).
- A diagnostic biopsy must be performed.
- A CT scan is useful in assessing cervical lymph nodes and bony infiltration. An MRI better defines infiltration of soft tissues.
- Usually, a CXR and LFTs are adequate for staging.
- Early-stage disease (no nodes) can be treated with surgery or radiation (equivalent outcome).
- Radiation is the preferred modality for nasopharyngeal and most vocal cord tumors.

10

- In stage III/IV laryngeal cancer, chemotherapy + radiation has an equivalent survival rate to surgery + radiation but preserves the voice.
- For advanced, potentially resectable disease, patients usually need combined surgery and radiotherapy (the cure rate is approximately 40%).
- Neoadjuvant chemotherapy has not been shown to improve survival.
- Initial follow-up examination should be performed every 2 months for the first 2 years and every 3 to 4 months for the following 2 years.

Miscellaneous

- Li-Fraumeni syndrome is a *p53* mutation causing sarcoma, breast, bone, lung, larynx, leukemia, and adrenal cancers.
- Ovarian germ cell cancer is essentially the same as testicular cancer, so do cisplatin/etoposide.

BIBLIOGRAPHY

Reviews

Armstrong K, et al. Assessing the risk of breast cancer. N Engl J Med 2000; 342:564–71.

Bataille R, Harousseau JL. Multiple myeloma. N Engl J Med 1997;336:1657–64.

Bhatia S, et al. Breast cancer and other second neoplasms after childhood Hodgkin's disease. N Engl J Med 1996;334:745–51.

Bishop JF. The treatment of adult myeloid leukemia. Semin Oncol 1997; 24:57–69.

Bosl GJ, Motzer RJ. Testicular germ-cell cancer. N Engl J Med 1997;337:242–53.

Cannistra SA. Cancer of the ovary. N Engl J Med 1993;329:1550–9.

Cannistra SA, Niloff JM. Cancer of the uterine cervix. N Engl J Med 1996; 334:1030–8.

DeGroen PC, et al. Biliary tract cancers. N Engl J Med 1999;341:1368–78.

Falk RH, et al. The systemic amyloidoses. N Engl J Med 1997;337:898–909.

Fuchs CS, Mayer RJ. Gastric carcinoma. N Engl J Med 1995;333:32–41.

Grunberg SM, Hesketh PJ. Control of chemotherapy-induced emesis. N Engl J Med 1993;329:1790–6.

Hainsworth JD, et al. Treatment of patients with cancer of unknown primary site. N Engl J Med 1993;329:257–62.

Harris JR, et al. Breast cancer. N Engl J Med 1992;327:319–28, 390–8, 473–80.

Hortobagyi G. Treatment of breast cancer. N Engl J Med 1998;339:974–85.

Ihde DC. Chemotherapy of lung cancer. N Engl J Med 1992;327:1434–41.

Kulke MH, Mayer RJ. Carcinoid tumors. N Engl J Med 1999;341:858–68.

Levy MH. Pharmacologic treatment of cancer pain. N Engl J Med 1996; 335:1124–32.

Motzer RJ, et al. Renal cell carcinoma. N Engl J Med 1996;335:865–75.

Raghavan D, et al. Biology and management of bladder cancer. N Engl J Med 1990;322:1129–38.

Rose PG. Endometrial carcinoma. N Engl J Med 1996;335:640–9.

Rozman C, Montserrat E. Chronic lymphocytic leukemia. N Engl J Med 1995; 333:1052–7.

Rustgi AK. Hereditary gastrointestinal polyposis and nonpolyposis syndromes. N Engl J Med 1994;331:1694–702.

Schlumberger MJ. Papillary and follicular thyroid carcinoma. N Engl J Med 1998; 338:297–306.

Spechler SJ. Barrett's esophagus. Semin Oncol 1994;21:431–7.

Spiers AS. Clinical manifestations of CML. Semin Oncol 1995;22:380–95.

Tsukama H, et al. Risk factors for hepatocellular carcinoma among patients with chronic liver disease. N Engl J Med 1993;328:1797–801.

Vokes EE, et al. Head and neck cancer. N Engl J Med 1993;328:184–94.

Guidelines

American College of Obstetrics/Gynecology. Tamoxifen and the prevention of breast cancer. Int J Gynecol Obstet 2000;68:73–5.

American College of Physicians. Screening for prostate cancer. Ann Intern Med 1997;126:480–4.

American Society of Clinical Oncology. Clinical practice guidleines for the use of tumor markers in breast and colorectal cancer. J Clin Oncol 1996; 14:2843–77.

American Society of Clinical Oncology. Recommended breast cancer surveillance guidelines. J Clin Oncol 1997;15:2149–56.

American Society of Clinical Oncology. Update of recommendations for the use of hematopoietic colony-stimulating factors: evidence-based clinical practice guidelines. J Clin Oncol 1996;14:1957–60.

Burke W, et al. Recommendations for care of individuals with inherited predispositions to cancer. Part I—hereditary nonpolyposis colon cancer. JAMA 1997;278:915–9.

Burke W, et al. Recommendations for care of individuals with inherited predispositions to cancer. Part II—*BRCA1* and *2*. JAMA 1997;997–1003.

Carter HB, et al. Recommended PSA testing intervals. JAMA 1997;277:1456–60.

Cheson BD, et al. Guidelines for chronic lymphocytic leukemia. Blood 1996; 87:4990–7.

Chlebowski RT. Reducing the risk of breast cancer. N Engl J Med 2000; 343:191–8.

Markowitz AJ, Winawer SJ. Screening and surveillance for colorectal carcinoma. Hematol Oncol Clin North Am 1997;11:579–608.

National Institutes of Health. Consensus statement: treatment of early-stage breast cancer. Monogr Nat Cancer Inst 1992;11:1–15.

Studies and Trials

Breast Cancer

Delozier T, et al. Delayed adjuvant tamoxifen. Ann Oncol 2000;11:515–9. (*Delayed adjuvant tamoxifen improves survival in early breast cancer patients with receptor-positive tumors, even if started 2 or more years after treatment.*)

Diel IJ, et al. Reduction of new metastases in breast cancer with adjuvant clodronate. N Engl J Med 1998;339:357–63. (*Clodronate for 2 years decreased bony and visceral metastases by half.*)

Fisher B, et al. Tamoxifen for prevention of breast cancer. J Natl Cancer Inst 1998; 90:1371–88. (*Tamoxifen for 5 years in women at increased risk for breast cancer reduced risk of development by 50%.*)

Gastrointestinal Cancer

Giovannucci E, et al. Aspirin and the risk of colorectal cancer in women. N Engl J Med 1995;333:609–14. (*A case-control study of women in the Nurses' Health Study, showing that regular aspirin intake significantly reduces colorectal cancer rate after 10 years of aspirin consumption.*)

Greenberg ER, et al. A clinical trial of antioxidant vitamins to prevent colorectal adenoma. N Engl J Med 1994;331:14–7. (*An RCT showing that neither antioxidants nor beta-carotene reduced adenoma formation.*)

Lagermen J, et al. Symptomatic gastroesophageal reflux as a risk factor for esophageal cancer. N Engl J Med 1999;340:825–31. (*Gastroesophageal reflux disease increased the risk of esophageal adenocarcinoma by seven times.*)

Lieberman DA. Use of colonoscopy to screen asymptomatic adults. N Engl J Med 2000;343:162–8. (*Colonoscopy detected colonic cancer when sigmoidoscopy would not and should be offered to first-degree relatives of colon cancer patients.*)

Schatzkin A, et al. Lack of effect of a low-fat, high-fiber diet on recurrence of colorectal adenomas. N Engl J Med 2000;342:1149–55. (*Adopting a diet low in fat and high in fiber after diagnosis of colorectal adenomas did not affect the rate of recurrence of colorectal adenomas.*)

UK Coordinating Committee on Cancer Research. Epidermal anal cancer. Lancet 1996;348:1049–54. (*An RCT showing combined chemoradiotherapy to be better than radiotherapy to spare the sphincter.*)

Willett WC. Relations of meat, fat, and fiber intake to the risk of colon cancer in a prospective study among women. N Engl J Med 1990;323:1664–72. (*From *the Nurses' Health Study, this case-control study showed that colon cancer risk is related to high intake of animal, but not vegetable, fat.*)

Winawer SJ, et al. Prevention of colorectal cancer by colonoscopic polypectomy. N Engl J Med 1993;329:1977–81. (*Polypectomy significantly reduced later development of colorectal cancer.*)

Genitourinary Cancer

Malmstrom PU, et al. Five year follow-up of a prospective trial of radical cystectomy and neoadjuvant chemotherapy. J Urol 1996;155:1903–6. (*Neoadjuvant doxorubicin plus cisplatin improved survival when used together with cystectomy.*)

Messing EM, et al. Immediate hormonal therapy compared with observation after radical prostatectomy and pelvic lymphadenectomy in men with node-positive prostate cancer. N Engl J Med 1999;341:1781–8. (*Immediate antiandrogen therapy [either bilateral orchiectomy or goserelin] improved survival and reduced recurrence in patients with node-positive prostate cancer.*)

Walsh PC. Immediate vs. deferred treatment for advanced prostatic cancer. J Urol 1997;158:1623–4. (*Early intervention with hormonal therapy for asymptomatic advanced prostate cancer improves survival.*)

Leukemia and Lymphoma

Dighiero G, et al. Chlorambucil in indolent CLL. N Engl J Med 1998; 338:1521–6. (*Chlorambucil does not prolong survival if given in stage A CLL. Thus, one can defer therapy until the disease progresses to stage B or C.*)

Guilhot F, et al. Interferon alfa-2b combined with cytarabine versus interferon alone in CML. N Engl J Med 1997;337:223–9. (*An RCT showing that interferon is effective and more so when combined with low doses of cytarabine for improving survival in CML.*)

Mayer RJ, et al. Intensive postremission chemotherapy in adults with acute myeloid leukemia. N Engl J Med 1994;331:896–903. (*An RCT showing that postremission intensification prolongs remission and increases the chance for cure in patients younger than 60.*)

Philip T, et al. Autologous BMT as compared with salvage chemotherapy in relapses of chemotherapy-sensitive non-Hodgkin's lymphoma. N Engl J Med 1995;333:1540–5. (*Relapsing patients with NHL had a higher survival rate with autologous BMT.*)

Somers R, et al. A randomized study in stages IIIB and IV Hodgkin's disease comparing eight courses of MOPP versus an alternation of MOPP and ABVD. J Clin Oncol 1994;12:279–87. (*MOPP/ABVD improved response but not survival in advanced Hodgkin's.*)

Tallman MS, et al. All-*trans* retinoic acid in acute promyelocytic leukemia. N Engl J Med 1997;337:1021–8. (A seminal report confirming that use of all-*trans* retinoic acid improves outcome in patients with acute promyelocytic leukemia.

Zittoun RA, et al. Autologous or allogeneic bone marrow transplantation compared with intensive chemotherapy in acute myeloid leukemia. N Engl J Med 1995;332:217–23. (*An RCT showing that allogeneic BMT improves outcome slightly.*)

Lung Cancer

Pritchard RS, Anthony SP. Chemotherapy plus radiotherapy compared with radiotherapy alone in the treatment of locally advanced, unresectable, non-small-cell lung cancer. Ann Intern Med 1996;125:723–9. (*A meta-analysis showing that combined-modality treatment improves survival in stage IIIB [advanced, unresectable, nonmetastatic] NSCLC patients.*)

Roth JA, et al. A randomized trial comparing perioperative chemotherapy and surgery with surgery alone in resectable stage IIIA non-small cell lung cancer. J Natl Cancer Inst 1994;86:673–80. (*An RCT showing that chemotherapy plus surgery improved survival over surgery alone in stage IIIA patients.*)

Melanoma

Harris MN, et al. Malignant melanoma: primary surgical management based on pathology and staging. Cancer 1995;75:715–25. (*An overview of trials suggesting lymph node dissection for intermediate-thickness melanoma with intraoperative lymphatic mapping and selective lymphadenectomy.*)

Kirkwood JM, et al. Interferon alfa-2b adjuvant therapy of high-risk resected cutaneous melanoma. J Clin Oncol 1996;14:7–17. (*An RCT showing that IFN-α improved survival for high-risk melanoma patients after resection.*)

Tucker MA, et al. Clinically recognized dysplastic nevi. JAMA 1997; 277:1439–44. (*One dysplastic nevus doubles melanoma risk; 10 such nevi increase risk by 12 times.*)

Multiple Myeloma

Attal M, et al. A prospective, randomized trial of autologous BMT and chemotherapy in multiple myeloma. N Engl J Med 1996;335:91–7. (*An RCT showing that BMT benefited survival of myeloma patients, especially those under 60.*)

Berenson JR, et al. Efficacy of pamidronate in reducing skeletal events in patients with advanced multiple myeloma. N Engl J Med 1996;334:488–93. (*An RCT showing pamidronate to decrease fractures and bone pain in these patients.*)

Chapel HM, et al. Randomized trial of IVIg as prophylaxis against infection in plateau-phase multiple myeloma. Lancet 1994;343:1059–63. (*An RCT showing IV gamma globulin to decrease risk for life-threatening or recurrent infections.*)

Kyle RA. Benign monoclonal gammopathy. Mayo Clin Proc 1993;68:26–36. (*Most MGUS patients remain asymptomatic throughout life.*)

Skinner M, et al. Treatment of 100 patients with amyloidosis. Am J Med 1996; 199:290–8. (*An RCT showing that melphalan plus prednisone plus colchicine was superior to colchicine alone.*)

Other

Kyle RA, et al. A trial of 3 regimens for primary amyloidosis. N Engl J Med 1997;336:1202–7. (*Melphalan plus prednisone was better than colchicine-based regimens.*)

Sorenson HT, et al. The risk of cancer after DVT or PE. N Engl J Med 1998; 338:1169–73. (*DVT/PE conferred a cancer risk of 1.3. Forty percent of such patients had distant metastases. Thus, aggressive work-ups after DVT/PE are not warranted.*)

11

HIV Medicine

How far you go in life depends on your being tender with the young, compassionate with the aged, sympathetic with the striving, and tolerant of the weak and the strong. Because someday in life you will have been all of these. — George Washington Carver

Practice balances on a perilously imperfect point, between detachment and compassion. — Deborah Blum, *The New York Times*

CHARACTERIZE HISTORY

1. Date and route of infection, CD4 count, and date of draw
2. Opportunistic infections (ask each one specifically): PCP, toxoplasmosis, CMV, MAC, TB, HSV, thrush, *Cryptococcus* and *Cryptosporidium*, meningitis, endocarditis, pneumonia
3. Review of symptoms: fever, chills, night sweats, nausea/vomiting/diarrhea, cough, SOB, pain, weight loss, lethargy, headache, visual changes, lymph nodes, rash
4. Past medical and surgical history/allergies/medications; also alcohol, tobacco, drug use; sexual history; travel history

KEY POINTS TO THINK ABOUT ON PHYSICAL

1. General description, temperature, weight, hydration status
2. Visual acuity, pupils, fundus examination (dilate everybody's eyes) — rule out CMV retinitis (can see retinal hemorrhages, exudates, atrophy)
3. Mucosal discharges, ulcers, exudates, thrush
4. Neck stiffness, nodes, JVD
5. Chest: PCP, TB, bacterial pneumonia
6. Heart: cardiomyopathy — displaced point of maximal impact, abnormal sounds, endocarditis, murmurs
7. Abdomen: liver and spleen size, obstructions, tenderness

8. GU: ulcers, discharge, inguinal nodes. Rectalize everyone.
9. Skin and extremities: rashes, Kaposi's sarcoma
10. Neurology: cognitive status, neuropathy

LABS

- CBC, platelet, differential, CXR, urinalysis SMA-20, PT/PTT on *everyone* within 24 hours (ER is a sieve, as are direct admits)
- Look for neutropenia, anemia, MCV, thrombocytopenia, any infectious process, albumin, alkaline phosphatase, coagulation abnormalities
- LP indications: persistent fevers, mental status changes, headaches, meningeal signs
- Cultures: don't just get blood but also wounds, urine, and cultures for fungus and acid-fast bacilli (TB, MAC), especially in patients with low CD4 and persistent fevers
- Viral cultures of open lesions (rule out herpes)

MEDICATIONS

Antivirals

See Tables 11–1 and 11–2 for an overview and toxicities.

Notes on Antivirals

These block viral packaging.

Table 11–1. Antiviral Names and Dosages

Nucleoside analogue reverse transcriptase inhibitors	Zidovudine (AZT, Retrovir)	100–200 mg PO tid (maximum 1 g/d)
	Didanosine (Videx)	200 bid
	Zalcitabine (Hivid)	0.75 tid
	Stavudine (Zerit)	40 bid
	Lamivudine (Epivir)	150 bid
	Abacavir (Ziagen)	300 bid
Non-nucleoside reverse transcriptase inhibitors	Nevirapine (Virammune)	400 qd
	Delavirdine (Rescriptor)	400 tid
	Efavirenz (Sustiva)	600 qd
Protease inhibitors	Saquinavir (Invirase)	600 tid
	Ritonavir (Norvir)	600 bid
	Indinavir (Crixivan)	800 tid
	Nelfinavir (Viracept)	750 tid

Table 11–2. Selected Toxicities of Antiretroviral Agents

Drug	Toxicity
Zidovudine	Nausea/vomiting, bone marrow suppression, myopathy
Didanosine	Pancreatitis, peripheral neuropathy
Zalcitabine	Peripheral neuropathy, pancreatitis
Abacavir	Rash
Nevirapine	Rash
Efavirenz	Rash, fever, dizziness, lethargy for 2–14 days
Ritonavir	Blocks cytochrome P-450 (multiple drug interactions), diarrhea, abdominal pain
Nelfinavir	Diarrhea
Indinavir	Kidney stones if patient is not well hydrated

1. Reverse transcriptase inhibitors block viral integration into the genome, whereas protease inhibitors (PIs) block viral packaging.
2. Saquinavir is best tolerated but is least potent due to poor absorption.
3. Ritonavir is least tolerated but is effective; increases saquinavir level.
4. Indinavir is the most effective and is fairly well tolerated.
5. Nelfinavir can be given to children but don't confuse it with nevirapine (Virammune).
6. Adefovir is an experimental reverse transcriptase (RT) inhibitor (guanosine analogue) and has a qd dosing.
7. Amprenavir is an experimental protease inhibitor and causes lipodystrophy and insulin.

Therapeutics

- Patients should never be on one drug alone; if the patient is on a PI, he or she should also be on two RT inhibitors.
- Zidovudine and stavudine have better CNS penetration and work on activated lymphocytes, whereas didanosine, zalcitabine, and lamivudine work on resting cells; it is best to use one of each rather than two from the same set, as they would antagonize each other (Combivir = zidovudine + lamivudine; dose is 1 tablet (300 mg zidovudine plus 150 mg lamivudine bid).

- PIs actually allow CD4 counts to increase; older drugs just slowed CD4 decline.
- Two PIs can be used together at lower doses to avoid toxicity.
- All PIs have some effect on P-450, so avoid use with terfenadine (Seldane), astemizole (Hismanal), cisapride (Prepulsid), and rifampin.
- Non-nucleoside inhibitors and PIs require strict patient compliance, so don't give them to unreliable patients or active drug users; non-nucleoside inhibitors (nevirapine and delavirdine) may decrease PI levels.
- Resistance to nelfinavir does *not* confer resistance to previous PIs but resistance to previous PIs *does* give resistance to nelfinavir, so nelfinavir is better as first-line treatment.
- Antivirals are used if viral loads (number of viral copies in blood) shoot up (measured by PCR on blood specimen), if the patient deteriorates clinically, or has HIV cerebritis, or, depending on who you talk to, on diagnosis or at different CD4 cutoffs (see below).
- If the patient is on zidovudine, use ganciclovir (which also causes neutropenia), with caution.
- PIs are expensive; check with social work to ensure the patient has Medicaid or insurance before starting them (lest you start something that won't be continued after discharge).
- When the patient has failed the initial agents, switch to two RT inhibitors (at least one being a nucleoside analogue) plus a PI, all of which should be new to the patient. See Table 11–3 for approaches.

Table 11–3. Approaches to Starting Antiviral Therapy

	Conservative	*Aggressive*
Indication to start therapy	CD4 < 400/µL	At diagnosis
Initial agents	Zidovudine + another reverse transcriptase inhibitor	Protease inhibitor + zidovudine + lamivudine
Indications to change therapy	CD4 drops below 200/µL	Increase in viral load or 10% drop in CD4 count

COMMON OPPORTUNISTIC INFECTIONS

Remember that, in general, patients require lifelong suppression after therapy for most HIV-related opportunistic infections. See Table 11–4 for an overview of the clinical course.

Table 11–4. Clinical Course of HIV Infection

CD4	Illnesses
1,000	Acute retroviral syndrome (30–70% of patients)— pharyngitis, nodes, rash, fever
> 500	Lymphadenopathy Recurrent vaginal candidiasis Kaposi's sarcoma
200–500	Pneumococcal pneumonia Tuberculosis Herpes zoster Thrush Anemia Non-Hodgkin's lymphoma Cervical intraepithelial neoplasia
100–200	*Pneumocystis carinii* pneumonia Wasting AIDS dementia complex
50–100	Cytomegalovirus retinitis Cryptococcosis Cryptosporidiosis Histoplasmosis Toxoplasmosis
< 50	*Mycobacterium avium-intracellulare* complex Progressive multifocal leukoencephalopathy Primary central nervous system lymphoma Cryptosporidiosis

Pneumocystis carinii Pneumonia

Quick Points
- Patients with CD4 < 200 or a history of AIDS-defining illness are at risk.
- *Pneumocystis carinii* most commonly causes pneumonia, manifestations of which include cough, wheezing, and SOB.

- X-ray classically shows reticulonodular infiltrate; ABG classically shows exercise-induced oxygen desaturation.
- Definitive diagnosis is on bronchoalveolar lavage and/or bronchial biopsy.
- PCP can affect the retina, bone marrow, intestines, and other organs.

Initial Management

1. TMP-SMX (Bactrim) PO (if mild) or IV (if severe) (based on trimethoprim 15–20 mg/kg/d in three or four divided doses); each ampule of TMP-SMX has 80 mg and each double strength (DS) tablet has 160 mg
2. IV pentamidine (can cause pancreatitis; watch glucose carefully)
3. Trimetrexate + leucovorin
4. IV clindamycin + primaquine (primaquine also requires G6PD level)
5. Dapsone + TMP
6. Atovaquone 750 mg bid
7. Prednisone taper (beginning at 40 mg PO bid) useful if $pO_2 < 70$

Prophylaxis (by order of efficacy) (for patient with CD4 < 200 or a history of AIDS-defining illness):

1. Bactrim double strength (TMP-SMX) 1 tablet qd/three times a week
2. Dapsone 100 mg PO qd (± pyrimethamine or pentamidine)
3. Aerosolized pentamidine every month via Respirgard II
4. Atovaquone (Mepron) (often with dapsone or pentamidine)

- Agents other than TMP-SMX are used if the patient is allergic to TMP-SMX (which causes rashes, Stevens-Johnson syndrome, interstitial nephritis [seen by urine eosinophilia], hepatitis), or otherwise can't tolerate it.
- Before starting dapsone, always check the G6PD level (dapsone can cause hemolysis if the patient is deficient).

Cytomegalovirus

Quick Points

- The most commonly affected organ is the eye (specifically retinitis), manifestations of which are floaters, decreased vision, retinal hemorrhages, and exudates.

- CMV is diagnosed by retinal lesions or intranuclear lesions (owl eye inclusions) on tissue biopsy, not by CMV titers or antigenemia, as it is a ubiquitous infection.
- CMV also commonly causes pneumonia, colitis, adrenalitis, and esophageal ulcers in HIV patients.

Initial Management

See Table 11–5 for CMV treatment.

- When using ganciclovir, watch for neutropenia; you may need G-CSF; avoid simultaneous zidovudine.
- Use foscarnet if the patient failed ganciclover or really needs zidovudine; give good hydration; watch for renal failure.
- Patients requiring long-term IV maintenance will need a Hickmann or Broviac catheter.
- The new maintenance drug is cidofovir (Vistide—biweekly infusions in the clinic; very nephrotoxic and expensive; you may need G-CSF).

Table 11–5. Cytomegalovirus Treatment Regimens

	Induction	Maintenance
Ganciclovir based	5 mg/kg IV bid × 2–3 wk	5 mg/kg IV qd or 1 g PO tid + intraocular implant
Foscarnet based	90 mg/kg IV q12h × 2–3 wk	90 mg/kg IV qd

Herpes

Quick Points

- Causes skin vesicles on erythematous, ulcerated base; encephalitis is also common.
- Diagnosis is by Tzanck preparation of skin lesion or viral culture (special isolator from the Microbiology lab).

Initial Management

- Acyclovir PO or IV (dose based on severity, weight, renal status); prevent with 200 mg 5×/d.
- Patient does not need acyclovir if on ganciclovir or foscarnet.
- Can give topical trifluridine (Viroptic) solution for herpes as well.

Mycobacterium avium-intracellulare Complex

Quick Points
* Commonly causes persistent fevers, hepatomegaly, rising isolated alkaline phosphatase, and bone marrow suppression.
* Diagnosis is based clinically on bone marrow biopsy.

Initial Management
* Treat with two or three drugs from those listed in Table 11–6.

Table 11–6. Drugs for *Mycobacterium avium-intracellulare* Complex

Agent	Dose	Toxicity
Clarithromycin (Biaxin)	500 mg PO bid	Gastrointestinal upset
Rifabutin (Mycobutin)	300 mg PO qd	Uveitis
Ciprofloxacin	500 mg PO bid	Well tolerated
Ethambutol	800–1,000 mg PO qd	Retrobulbar optic neuritis
Azithromycin (Zithromax)	1.2 g PO qwk	Well tolerated

Candidiasis (Thrush, Esophagitis, Fungemia)

1. Mycelex troche 10 mg PO 5×/d
2. Fluconazole (Diflucan) 100 mg PO qd up to 400 mg PO qd (well tolerated)
3. IV fluconazole (same dose but very expensive)
4. Amphotericin IV (see discussion below)
5. Amphotericin PO (Fungizone) 1 cc qid

Cryptococcus (Meningitis, Encephalitis, Fungemia, Pneumonia)

* Amphotericin ± 5-flucytosine (for severe), then fluconazole (up to 800 qd) or amphotericin maintenance

Cryptosporidium

* Diarrhea, cholangitis, diagnosed on stool, colonoscopy, endoscopic retrograde cholangiopancreatography (ERCP)
* Paromomycin (Humatin) 1 g bid or azithromycin (Zithromax) 600 bid

Toxoplasmosis

Quick Points
- Toxoplasmosis typically causes ring-enhancing lesions in the brain with corresponding focal neurologic deficits.
- Patients negative for toxoplasmosis should avoid cat litter and raw, uncooked meats.

Initial Management
- If the patient has an intracranial mass, treat toxoplasmosis empirically with pyrimethamine (Daraprim) 25 to 100 mg PO qd plus (sulfadiazine 1–2 g PO qid or clindamcyin 300–900 mg PO tid) or atovaquone 750 mg qid.
- Watch for neutropenia (toxicity of pyrimethamine); give folate (leucovorin) to minimize bone marrow toxicity.
- If there is no response clinically or on CT/MRI, consider a brain biopsy to rule out lymphoma.
- Steroids are useful for mass effect or significant local edema.

Table 11–7 lists the primary propylaxis for opportunistic infections.

Table 11–7. Primary Prophylaxis for Opportunistic Infections in HIV Patients

Opportunistic Infection	Recommended First-Line Prophylaxis
Pneumocystis carinii pneumonia	TMP-SMX 1 DS tab PO bid for CD4 < 200
Mycobacterium avium-intracellulare	Azithromycin 1.2 g PO qw for CD4 < 100
Tuberculosis	Isoniazid 300 mg PO bid × 1 yr for PPD > 5 mm
Bacteria (*H. influenzae, S. Pneumococcus*)	Appropriate vaccines
Fungi (*Candida, Cryptococcus*)	Fluconazole 100 mg PO qd for CD4 <100
Cytomegalovirus	Ganciclovir 1 g PO tid for CD4 < 50 in patients with cytomegalovirus viremia
Toxoplasmosis	TMP-SMX 1 DS PO bid for CD4 < 200

COMMON ISSUES AND ENTITIES

Never forget that the same pathogens that affect normal people, as well as others, can affect AIDS patients. Manage accordingly.

Amphoterrible

- Amphotericin dosing: 0.3 to 1 mg/kg qd over 4 hours based on severity and renal function.
- Give 500 cc NS over 3 hours pre- and posthydration.
- Meperidine (Demerol) 25 mg IV prn for rigors, amphotericin fever.
- If meperidine fails, give hydrocortisone 50 mg to run with amphotericin in bag.
- Acetaminophen (Tylenol), diphenhydramine (Benadryl) as premedications.
- Follow BUN, creatine, magnesium, potassium.
- Liposomal amphotericin (very expensive) if the patient can't tolerate IV amphotericin but needs it.

Bone Marrow Suppression

- If the patient has absolute neutropenia (absolute neutrophil count [ANC] < 1,000), G-CSF improves survival if ANC < 500 or if the patient is septic.
- If neutropenic and febrile, cover with ticarcillin-clavulanate (Timentin) gentamicin/tobramycin.
- Always check the medication list.
- Thrombocytopenia in HIV is usually due to idiopathic thrombocytopenic purpura (ITP); treat with zidovudine, steroids, IV gamma globulin, and splenectomy. ITP is diagnosed after marrow biopsy to rule out MAC.
- Anemia is commonly due to HIV or to medication; check the reticulocyte count to assess bone marrow activity. Conduct iron studies if the MCV is low. High MCV actually indicates compliance with zidovudine. If the erythropoietin level is < 500, then epoetin alfa (Epogen) is of benefit.
- Check the testosterone level (if low, it can be replaced with oxandrolone or testosterone).

11

Diarrhea

- Differential diagnosis includes *Shigella, Yersinia, Entamoeba, Campylobacter, Salmonella*, and *Giardia* (all of which also occur in normal people). *Cryptosporidum, Isospora, Microsporidium*, CMV colitis, and MAC are also in the diagnosis. Consider ciprofloxacin to cover traditional bugs after the work-up is performed.
- Send stool for AFB, culture and sensitivity, ova and parasites, *Giardia, Cryptosporidium, Microspora, Isospora* (see the Parasitology section in Chapter 5 for more information); remember guaiac and blood culture. Send for *C. difficile* if on any antibiotic.
- Consider a Gastroenterology consult for colonoscopy.

Esophagitis (Dysphagia, Odynophagia)

- Differential diagnosis (in order of frequency): *Candida*, HSV, CMV, aphthous ulcers (first three treated with antimicrobials; last treated with steroids and/or thalidomide)
- Consider an upper gastrointestinal series or esophagogastroduodenoscopy

Line Sepsis/Endocarditis

- Differential diagnosis: *Staph.* (especially MRSA), *Strep., Pseudomonas, Candida*.
- Check Hickmann/Broviac catheter for inflammation.
- When giving drugs, you can alternate infusion through ports of the Hickmann catheter (you don't have to pull the line immediately unless it is *Candida*).

Meningitis/Encephalitis

- Differential diagnosis
  - Bacterial (treat with ampicillin + ceftriaxone)
  - *Cryptococcus* (get India ink, serum, and CSF crypt antigen)
  - HIV cerebritis (isolated elevated WBC and protein in CSF)
  - Herpes encephalitis (bloody CSF in all tubes; temporal lobe enhancement on contrast CT)
  - CMV encephalitis (periventricular enhancement on contrast CT)
- Intracranial enhancing masses (in order of frequency): toxoplasmosis, lymphoma, tuberculoma, cryptococcoma, progressive multifocal leukoencephalopathy (PML)

Nausea/Vomiting/Abdominal Pain

- Assess medex, ethanol use, swallowing, bowel movements, liver function, nutrition/hydration, and amylase level.
- Beware of dystonic reactions to prochlorperazine (Compazine)/metoclopramide (Reglan).
- Trimethobenzamide (Tigan) 250 mg PO tid PO/PR is a good antiemetic without many side effects.
- Chronic nausea may respond to dronabinol (Marinol).

Ocular Complications

- Occurs in 70 to 90% of AIDS patients
- Acute retinal necrosis (blurry vision, pain) usually due to VZV
- Have a low threshold for an Ophthalmology consult
- Differential diagnosis
  - Cotton-wool spots (most common; asymptomatic, benign, resolve spontaneously)
  - CMV (cottage cheese and ketchup appearance) (floaters, blurry vision are symptoms but not pain, redness, or photophobia)
  - Toxoplasmosis (> 50% of ocular toxoplasmosis patients have CNS disease, so a head CT is mandatory) (floaters, photophobia, blurry vision, redness, pain)
  - Herpes zoster ophthalmicus (V1 rash; treatment is acyclovir [IV or PO] or famciclovir (Famvir) 500 mg PO bid)
  - Syphilis
  - HSV (keratitis — severe pain, redness)
  - Lymphoma

Peripheral Neuropathy

- Exquisite pain in glove and stocking distribution seemingly without reason.
- Can be due to HIV, medications (didanosine, zalcitabine, etc), or deficiencies of carnitine, folate, or vitamin B_{12}.
- Treatment: tricyclic antidepressants (nortriptyline [Pamelor], amitriptyline [Elavil]), warm soaks, massages, pain medications.
- Check carnitine level; can replace with levocarnitine (Carnitor) 330 mg PO tid or over-the-counter L-carnitine.

Pneumonia

- Differential diagnosis: bacterial, PCP, TB, CMV, fungal, Kaposi's sarcoma.
- Check ABG, pulse oximetry, LDH, CXR.
- Consider a bronchoscopy if there is no response to initial empiric treatment.
- CMV pneumonia is diagnosed if the bronchoscopy finds no other pathogen (remember that intranuclear inclusions indicate CMV pathogenesis).

Rashes

- Differential diagnosis: drug rashes, prurigo nodularis ("itchy bumps"), eosinophilic pustular folliculitis, Kaposi's sarcoma, herpes, shingles, scabies, molluscum contagiosum.
- Have a low threshold for a Derm consult. Don't be afraid to call them.

HOUSEKEEPING

- Ophthalmologic examination: dilate with tropicamide (Mydriacyl) and phenylephrine (Mydfrin) and/or get an Ophthalmology consult on any and every patient with CD4 < 100.
- Nutrition:
  - Give Ensure 1 can PO tid (if fluid is restricted, give Ensure pudding)
  - Megestrol (Megace) (40 mg/cc) 20 cc PO qd or oxandrolone for weight loss without nausea.
  - Nutrition consult on everyone.
- If the patient can't eat, get a PEG or Hickmann catheter (Interventional Radiology/Surgery) for nutrition (enteral nutrition is preferable to TPN; TPN also requires a dedicated port of a Hickmann or triple-lumen catheter). Get these done as soon as possible for long-term nutrition, hydration, or IV medications. Use a PICC line for short-term IV drugs (a few weeks of amphotericin, vancomycin, etc). PICC lines can be put in by the IV team or Interventional Radiology, but they only last a few weeks to a few months and you can't get blood off them (unlike Hickmanns).
- Never forget social work and physical therapy.
- DNR orders are obtained as soon as possible for those who need them.
- *Don't get depressed; despite all of the death and destruction on this floor, you are helping these patients in the length, quality, or comfort of life. You may not be able to cure them, but you can make them feel better.*

REGULAR ANTIBIOTICS COMMONLY USED

1. Vancomycin 1 g IV q12h (for MRSA, refractory *Enterococcus*) — adjust for renal function; slow infusion over 1 hour prevents red man syndrome (not a true allergy).
2. Ticarcillin-clavulanate 3.1 g IV q4–q8 (adjust for severity, neutropenia, and cardiac/renal status, as ticarcillin-clavulanate is a heavy salt load) — given for broad-spectrum coverage (includes gram-positive and gram-negative organisms, especially *Pseudomonas*, but not *Enterococcus* or MRSA).
3. Gentamicin/tobramycin: 1 mg/kg q8h (see Chapter 5 for once-daily dosing); good for gram negative or *Enterococcus*. Use old q8h dosing in endocarditis/line sepsis to clean all ports.
4. Cefazolin (Ancef) 1 g IV q8h (cellulitis, gram positive); switch to cephalexin (Keflex) 500 mg PO bid.
5. Cefuroxime 750 mg to 1.5 g IV q8h (depending on severity) — pneumonia, UTI; switch to cefuroxime (Ceftin) 500 PO mg bid.
6. Ciprofloxacin 500 PO bid (MAC, UTI, gram negative, *Pseudomonas*): remember that PO = IV bioavailability.
7. Ceftriaxone 1 g IM/IV bid — good for gram negatives except *Pseudomonas*.
8. Ceftazidime 1–2 g IV q8h (for *Pseudomonas*).

BIBLIOGRAPHY

Reviews

Antman K, Chang Y. Kaposi's sarcoma. N Engl J Med 2000;342:1027–39.

Coodley GO, et al. The HIV wasting syndrome. J AIDS 1994;7:681–94.

Cunliffe NA, Denning DW. Uncommon invasive mycoses in AIDS. AIDS 1995;9:411–20.

Cunningham ET, Margolis TP. Ocular manifestations of HIV. N Engl J Med 1998;339:236–44.

Fernandez SM, et al. Rheumatological manifestations of HIV infection. Semin Arthritis Rheum 1991;21:30–9.

Flexner C. HIV protease inhibitors. N Engl J Med 1998;338:1281–92.

Kahn J, Walker BD. Acute HIV-1 infection. N Engl J Med 1998;339:33–40.

Kovacs JA, Masur H. Prophylaxis against opportunistic infections in HIV infection. N Engl J Med 2000;342:146–29.

Rao TK. Renal complications of HIV disease. Med Clin North Am 1996;80:1437–51.

Sepkowitz KA, et al. Tuberculosis in the AIDS era. Clin Microbiol Rev 1995;8:180–99.

Simpson DM, Tagliati M. Neurologic manifestations of HIV infection. Ann Intern Med 1994;121:769–85.

Guidelines

Ammasari A, et al. AIDS-associated cerebral toxoplasmosis: an update on diagnosis and treatment. Curr Top Microbiol Immunol 1996;219:209–22.

Carpenter CC, et al. Antiretroviral therapy for HIV infection in 1998. JAMA 1998;280:78–86.

Johanson JF, Sonnenberg A. Efficient management of diarrhea in AIDS. Ann Intern Med 1990;112:942–8.

Kaplan JE, et al. USPHS/IDSA guidelines for the prevention of opportunistic infections in persons infected with HIV. Clin Infect Dis 1995;21:S12–31.

Lederman MM, Valdez H. Immune restoration with antiretroviral therapy: implications for clinical management. JAMA 2000;284:223–8.

Saag MS, et al. HIV viral load markers in practice. Nat Med 1996;2:625–9.

Simonds RJ, et al. Preventing *Pneumocystis carinii* pneumonia in HIV patients. Clin Infect Dis 1995;21:S44–8.

Studies and Trials

Antiviral Therapy

Connor EM, et al. Reduction of maternal-infant transmission of HIV-1 with zidovudine treatment. N Engl J Med 1994;331:1173–80. (*Antepartum and intrapartum zidovudine use cut transmission of HIV to infants by 67%.*)

Landonio G, et al. Comparison of two dose regimens of zidovudine in a randomized multicenter study for severe, HIV-related thrombocytopenia. AIDS 1993;7:209–12. (*High-dose zidovudine [1,000 mg/d] more rapidly and more durably raised platelet counts in patients with HIV-related thrombocytopenia.*)

Staszewski S, et al. Efavirenz + AZT + 3TC, efavirenz + indinavir, and indinavir + 3TC + 3TC in the treatment of HIV infection. N Engl J Med 1999;341:1865–73. (*Efavirenz + zidovudine + lamivudine was the most effective and best tolerated of the three regimens in suppression of viral load and had the least adverse events in this RCT.*)

Cytomegalovirus Treatment

Martin DF, et al. Oral ganciclovir for patients with CMV retinitis treated with a ganciclovir implant. N Engl J Med 1999;340:1063–70. (*Oral ganciclovir was comparable in efficacy to IV in suppression of CMV retinitis when used in conjunction with an intraocular ganciclovir implant.*)

Whitcup SM, et al. Discontinuation of anti-CMV therapy in patients with HIV infection and CMV retinitis. JAMA 1999;282:1633–7. (*Maintenance anti-CMV medications were safely discontinued in 14 patients who had inactive, non–sight-threatening, CMV retinitis, HIV infection, and CD4 > 150 and were on highly active antiretroviral therapy. No recurrence occurred over a mean of 16 months.*)

Pneumonia

Bozzette SA, et al. A randomized trial of 3 antipneumocystis agents in patients with advanced HIV infection. N Engl J Med 1995;332:693–9. (*At 19%, patients on TMP-SMX had the lowest risk of developing PCP prophylaxis versus 22% for dapsone and 33% for pentamidine.*)

Hirschtick RE, et al. Bacterial pneumonia in persons infected with HIV. N Engl J Med 1995;333:845–51. (*Low CD4 counts and smoking were risk factors for bacterial pneumonia. Pneumonia quadrupled mortality rates. TMP-SMX prophylaxis reduced bacterial pneumonia by 67%.*)

Hoover DR, et al. Clinical manifestations of AIDS in the era of *Pneumocystis* prophylaxis. N Engl J Med 1993;329:1922–6. (*PCP prophylaxis delayed the first AIDS-defining illness by 6 to 12 months. MAC, wasting, CMV, and esophageal* Candida *occurred more frequently in prophylaxed patients. Twenty-eight percent of prophylaxed patients developed PCP anyway.*)

Saah AJ, et al. Predictors of failure of PCP prophylaxis. JAMA 1995;273:1197–202. (*Fever and CD4 [< 75] predicted failure of PCP prophylaxis.*)

Other

Case-control study of HIV seroconversion in health-care workers after percutaneous exposure to HIV-infected blood—France, UK, and US. MMWR Morb Mortal Wkly Rep 1995;44:929–33. (*Seroconversion risk factors were deep injury, visible blood contamination of needle, vascular placement of needle, and patient's terminal illness. Zidovudine reduced the risk by 80%.*)

Henry DH, et al. Recombinant human erythropoietin in the treatment of anemia with HIV infection and zidovudine therapy. Ann Intern Med 1992;117:739–48. (*An RCT showing that erythropoietin therapy decreased transfusion requirements and increased hematocrit in those HIV patients with erythropoietin levels < 500 IU/L.*)

Schambelan M, et al. Recombinant human growth hormone in patients with HIV-associated wasting. Ann Intern Med 1996;125:873–82. (*An RCT showing that human growth hormone improved weight and body mass but not quality of life, days of disability, or use of health care.*)

Shafran SD, et al. A comparison of 2 regimens for the treatment of *Mycobacterium avium*-complex bacteremia in AIDS. N Engl J Med 1996;335:377–83.

(*Clarithromycin-containing regimens were superior to those without it. Rifabutin had a significant rate of uveitis.*)

van der Horst CM, et al. Treatment of AIDS-associated acute cryptococcal meningitis. N Engl J Med 1997;337:15–22. (*Flucytosine used in the first 2 weeks of therapy along with amphotericin decreases the rate of relapse relative to amphotericin alone. Fluconazole [don't confuse it with flucytosine] use from weeks 2 to 10 increased the rates of achieving negative cultures.*)

Wilcox CM, et al. Fluconazole compared with endoscopy for HIV-infected patients with esophageal symptoms. Gastroenterology 1996;110:1803–9. (*Empiric fluconazole for 2 weeks was safe and effective in this population.*)

12

Chemical Dependency

Charity in the broad spiritual sense—the desire to relieve suffering...is the most precious possession of medicine. —Dr. Edward Churchill

Struggle now and enjoy later, or enjoy now and suffer later. —Prof. Ambati M. Rao

HOUSEKEEPING

1. Although most substance abuse wards are locked wards, they are not prisons. The patients that you see here are only here because they carry a medical diagnosis and abuse legal/illegal drugs; they were not sentenced to the floor by the justice system. Given this, their only desire is to get better so that they can leave the hospital. This desire is usually quite secondary to the need for more of their favorite drug, and you must not get frustrated when they (often) sign out against medical advice (AMA), despite your best efforts toward reaching and treating them. They are adults. They are free people. Treat them as such even when they appear to be shortsighted or irrational.

2. Don't take it personally. There will be many times when an ignorant, dirty, smelly, homeless, ugly, stupid, and drunken individual will be openly hostile to you, often calling you a bad doctor or less printable things. Freaking out and getting into yelling matches is not worth it; calmly realize just who is who in the dynamic. You are the physician with 8+ years of college and training, whereas the one insulting you shoots up in the park. Keep your perspective and maintain a professional demeanor in the face of overwhelming annoyance. Remember, you only lose if you sink to their level.

3. Be sympathetic. Don't forget that of all of the patients you are going to deal with, these people, in many ways, need your help the most. The folks on the cardiac floor usually have jobs, money, and families, great assets in their fight with illness. That is rarely the case here. No matter

how irritating or obnoxious a patient can be, remember that, at base, these people are pathetic and desperate. Try, when you can, to be kind.

4. Drugs are #1 to many of these patients. No matter how bad the disease, no matter what the weather, no matter how compassionate the doctor, the drug wins most of the time. Regardless of their health problems, these patients will always have, in the back of their minds, the constant nagging of their need. This will cause them to sign out and leave at inopportune times (from your standpoint), but you must remember that when it comes to the list of priorities, the drug comes first. This does not mean you shouldn't offer detoxification and rehabilitation, but just bear it in mind.

5. The weather is neither a sensitive nor a specific indicator of the number of admissions you will get; however, check day (social security/ disability) is.

6. A word on racism and classism. You may find some ugly thoughts bubbling up in your head during the rotation. Depending on the ethnic make-up in your area and the general socioeconomic level, you may find that your clients seem to fit specific racial or ethnic molds. *Do not confuse the floor with reality.* Never forget that there are just as many, if not more, drug addicts who are Caucasian, employed, or whatever, and that 99% of African Americans and Hispanics are not drug users. Social status is not a protection from abuse; it is only protection from admission to a locked floor. It's wrong, but it's the way it is in our society. Just try to keep your perspective; the last thing we need is another socially cynical doctor.

7. Beware of burnout. You will find yourself initially trying to be very kind and accommodating to your patients on the floor. After repeated failures to build a doctor-patient bond, you become frustrated and back off. You then may find yourself laughing it all away, ridiculing patients behind their backs in defense of just how awful their situation is. Finally, even this becomes impossible, and you become depressed and sick of the whole thing. If this describes you, remember (a) it's only 1 month, and (b) there but for the grace of God go I. If this does not happen to you, you may well be one of the rare and patient few who could actually go into substance abuse as a career—and people are needed here.

8. What to read. When reading while working on this floor, in addition to the topics presented below, we suggest you bone up on AIDS and general infectious diseases. You will see these a lot.

9. *Scary stuff.* As will often happen, there are times when a patient becomes either physically or sexually threatening. This is actually a rarity, but it can occur. In the case of a physical threat, remain calm and try to calm the patient down as quickly as possible. Usually, this involves promising them medications, drugs, or whatever. *Placate, then evacuate.* Once out of the room or situation, tell Nursing and have security escort the individual out of the hospital. Physical threat is an automatic ticket back to the park; if the violence is actual, then the patient must be arrested and brought up on charges. Sexual innuendo or worse (groping, harassment) should be handled the same way. If possible, change to a male intern or resident in minor cases (verbal only), but anything else is prosecutable and grounds for discharge. There is no need to confront or fight with a threatening patient; if they are acting that way (and are not insane), they are not overly interested in their health.

WITHDRAWAL AND OVERDOSES

See also Appendix A.

Heroin Withdrawal and Overdose

Quick Points

1. Signs and symptoms of withdrawal: diaphoresis, mydriasis, diarrhea, pruritus, irritability, anxiety, lacrimation, salivation, pleas for more medication, tachycardia, and piloerection.

2. Signs and symptoms of overdose: unresponsiveness, respiratory depression, pinpoint pupils, and sleep/coma.

3. The heroin high is described as like being in a warm, sort of quiet, womb-like place, insulated from hurt and want. I've also heard it described as like being in a hot tub. This drug is used by those who primarily desire escape and who are chronically unable to cope with the stimulation of their lives.

4. The usual route of administration these days is intranasal (which is good) due to an increase in the potency and purity of street heroin.

Other ways are injection and skin popping. Some people take a "speedball," which is a mix of cocaine and heroin together.

5. In history, quantify use: 1 bag of heroin is $10 to 20. The number of days of detoxification is, as a rule of thumb, the number of bags used/day + 2.

Initial Management

1. Treatment for withdrawing from opiates. The only adequate way to treat opiate withdrawal is to give the patient opiates. Normally, when patients are not on a methadone program (see below), they are placed on a "methadone detox," in which they are gradually weaned off the drug in lowering increments. We normally start at 40 mg PO bid and taper by about 10 mg per day for heavy users and 20 mg bid for light ones. You will, however, find that everyone is a heavy user and that no one will really tolerate the 20 mg bid schedule.

2. Clonidine 0.1 mg PO is effective to take the edge off heroin withdrawal.

3. Treatment for overdose. Overdose is life threatening as respiratory arrest, severe aspiration, and coma can result. As such, those in overdose from opiates must have an MICU evaluation first to see if they are stable enough to "sleep it off" on the floor. In the meantime, the emergency room will have tried naloxone 1 mg IV × 1 or naltrexone on the patient to see if they can get a response.

   a. A word or two about naloxone. This medicine is a competitive inhibitor of opioids (including natural endorphins and enkephalins) at the receptor site. When given, patients not only lose their present heroin high but also their methadone protection and are plunged very rapidly into complete withdrawal.

   b. Patients do not like this; it makes them ornery. Be careful when you do this as there may be a lot of screaming and flailing. No one is put on a naloxone drip; the drug is only used to see if it can reverse a coma that is suspected to be opiate induced. If it reverses the state, then the patient is either intubated if in respiratory collapse or allowed a nice long nap if not.

Further Discussion

1. Opiate receptors in their brain (read lymbic system) and in the periphery (GI tract, autonomic NS) are all well downregulated in these people, so the loss of a constant wash of opiates makes cotton feel like sandpaper, pencil tapping seem like jackhammers, and a 40-watt bulb look like the sun. The philosophical debate is this: nursing on substance abuse floors has been so jerked around by patients seeking drugs that they have become very hostile and stingy toward those seeking opiates. You will likely find yourself pressured to not give these drugs when asked for the patient's "own good." This usually results in the person leaving AMA as his or her main concern is not his or her medical condition but the avoidance of withdrawal symptoms.

   a. Methadone is highly controlled, and it is not possible to simply order it outside of the regimens of an approved methadone program or a scheduled detoxification system. However, you may keep the patient at a stable dose in the short term or even write for additional methadone if the detoxification is too fast; just be sure to verify withdrawal symptoms as objectively as possible or you will face severe flack from the powers that be.

   b. If you don't want to give more methadone or if you are bullied into not doing so, lorazepam (Ativan) or other benzodiazepines will help with some of the withdrawal symptoms, as will diphenhydramine (Benadryl). Patients are usually not too thrilled about using alternative medications but will take what they can get for relief in the end.

   c. But how do you tell if they are really withdrawing? This is tough because these people are very good at personal manipulation, fakery, and other shenanigans. The rule of thumb is basically to ignore their actual complaints (they long ago learned the symptoms first hand, and this test is no longer a sensitive one) and focus on the physical. It is hard, although not impossible, to fake sweating and mydriasis. Constipation can be faked, and, if they are really upset, tachycardia is also not reliable, but the physical exam should give you at least a gestalt as to whether this person is really withdrawing.

   d. Above all, you must remember that these are your patients and you are their doctor and therefore in charge. They have enough needless suffering in their lives, and, honestly, giving them more methadone

12

will not in any way alter their addiction state. On the other hand, no one likes to be manipulated or bullied, so a polite and objective stance is the best to take.

2. Long-term treatment is best done in a supervised living system for 6 months. Also, groups like Narcotics Anonymous may offer some benefit. Another extremely effective treatment is methadone therapy in a methadone clinic. Despite the stigma of being on methadone, it is a wonderful drug. It has a relatively low euphoric and sedative effect while it satisfies craving and prevents withdrawal. Better yet, it saturates opioid receptors so that use of heroin while on methadone is futile; the addict gets no real kick from the drug anymore. Add to this the fact that it is supervised and needleless and it makes for an excellent, albeit misunderstood, intervention.

Cocaine Withdrawal and Overdose

Quick Points
1. Cocaine withdrawal. Symptoms include hypersomnia, hyperphagia, depression, lethargy, anxiety, and craving. In general, the high lasts about 2 days, and once off it, the addict really only wants to sleep first, then eat, and, in general, to be left alone.
2. Cocaine high/overdose. Symptoms include all of the symptoms of amphetamine overdose, tachycardia, increased BP, paranoia, hypervigilance, insomnia, mania, and loss of appetite/weight loss (long term).
3. Note that routes of use are not only nasal but also smoking (crack) and "skin popping."

Initial Management
Treatment for withdrawal is basically to watch patients for agitation and give a benzodiazepine if needed to control this. Otherwise, all one can do is let them sleep and provide food and rest. Counseling and rehabilitation may or may not prove helpful; success is probably greater in a supervised living setting over a long period (ie, 6 months).

Further Discussion
1. Cocaine is a different story in many ways; some have suggested that the underlying addiction is far more psychological than truly physical.

Regardless, cocaine is probably the most addictive drug there is, especially when used as crack or freebasing. The upshot is that it stimulates all of the pleasure centers simultaneously so that normal urges for food, sex, sleep, and water are all well suppressed. Typical users are stuck in a constant and escalating chase for the needed high and generally are under-aroused, often (but by no means always) with character pathology.

Ethanol Withdrawal and Overdose

This is quite similar to withdrawal from benzodiazepines, barbiturates, and CNS depressants.

Quick Points

See Table 12–1 for questions to ask on history.

1. Signs and symptoms of withdrawal: nervousness; tremor; increased pulse, BP, and temperature; insomnia; tachycardia; ethanol craving; seizures ("rum fits"); hallucinations; occasionally delirium tremens (see below).

 a. Look out for the reverse of ethanol CNS depressant effects.

 b. Symptoms start 5 to 10 hours after the last drink (important to assess this in H&P).

 c. Symptoms will peak on days 2 to 3.

 d. The patient will get better by days 4 to 5.

 e. Severe withdrawal occurs in 5% (ie, hallucinations, psychosis, and seizures).

 f. Delirium tremens is a more severe symptom of the above, including confusion, agitation, generalized seizure, and fever/tachycardia.

 g. Wernicke's triad = ataxia, amnesia, ophthalmoplegia/nystagmus.

Table 12–1. CAGE Questions for Alcohol Abuse (and Examinations)*

Have you ever wanted to *C*ut down on your drinking?

Have you gotten *A*ngry when others asked about your drinking?

Have you felt *G*uilty about your drinking?

Do you ever need an *E*ye opener in the morning?

---

*With a cutoff of two or more positive answers, sensitivity = 80% and specificity = 85%.

2. Signs and symptoms of overdose: coma, unresponsiveness, vomiting, agitation.
3. Signs of chronic alcoholism:
   - Cognitive impairment (memory loss)
   - Mood disturbance (anxiety, depression)
   - Worsening grooming, appetite, sleep, gait
   - Refractory seizures, refractory hyperglycemia, refractory HTN
   - Recurrent gastritis
4. Complications include
   a. Ethanol hepatitis
   b. Pancreatitis
   c. Upper GI bleeding
   d. Holiday heart (atrial or ventricular arrhythmias in the absence of other cardiac pathology, especially paroxysmal SVT)
   e. Ethanol cardiomyopathy
   f. Mouth/stomach/liver/laryngeal cancer
   g. Macrocytic anemia (not necessarily B_{12}/folate deficiency)
   h. Wernicke's encephalopathy (anterograde amnesia often associated with VI nerve palsy due to thiamine deficiency)
   i. Multiple psychologic disorders

Initial Management
1. Treatment for ethanol withdrawal:
   a. At Beth Israel, we used a phenobarbital detoxification system consisting of as-needed doses of 130 mg of phenobarbital IM q4h over the first 24 hours followed by a standard detoxification of 60 mg PO qid for the first day, then tid, then bid, and then qd each day thereafter.
   b. It should be noted that benzodiazepines are also equally effective. In essence, the most important thing is to watch the patient, making sure that signs of withdrawal are promptly treated with either benzodiazepines or barbiturates.
   c. Most patients require 25 to 50 mg of chlordiazepoxide or 10 mg of diazepam every 4 to 6 hours the first day.
   d. Severe withdrawal requires much higher doses; up to 300 mg of chlordiazepoxide can be used per day, and this may still not be adequate to fully control agitation.

2. Treatment for ethanol overdose:
   a. In most cases, all the alcoholic needs is to "sleep it off" to regain full consciousness and coherence. This is why many lie in the ER for hours until you finally get called to admit them.
   b. In acute ethanol poisoning, the patient can be lavaged and the airway must be protected, but, in general, such measures are rarely necessary.
   c. Never forget to administer some thiamine 100 mg qd and folate 1 mg qd (either PO or IV) to that patient on admission; if you give them IV glucose without it, it will destroy their brains.

Further Discussion

- Oddly, no one seems to be resistant to giving these people more phenobarbital, the way some are with methadone; usually, the ethanol abusers are less manipulative than their compatriots, and ethanol withdrawal is a bit easier to establish with objective findings (elevated vitals, tremor, etc).
- Alcoholics tend to be malnourished, so don't be surprised at macrocytic anemia, low albumin, and wasting on examination.
- These guys tend to be a bit more gregarious and friendly than the other types of abusers. They also tend to be a bit older than the usual addict; as such, they often have more typical medical problems concomitant to their drinking, like HTN or COPD.
- Note that while inpatient detoxification is all well and good, no program has been shown to work as well as Alcoholics Anonymous for long-term abstinence. In any case, all patients should be offered long-term treatment and detoxification (ethanol withdrawal symptoms can last for up to 6 months and craving a lifetime).
- Naltrexone reduces long-term cravings for ethanol when used in conjunction with a long-term psychosocial program.

COMMON MEDICAL PROBLEMS

See Chapters 5 and 11 as well.

12

Cellulitis

Quick Points
1. A skin infection usually due to group A *Strep.* and *S. aureus* is quite common in injection drug users and the homeless as poor hygiene and drug delivery methods such as skin popping and injections without sterile technique predispose to infection.
2. This infection is characterized by redness, minimal swelling, heat, and prickly pain on palpation. Fever is usually present, but not in every case.
3. Erysipelas is similar to the above but tends to be better demarcated, is caused by group A *Strep.*, and often has an orange peel texture to it.

Initial Management
1. Treatment is usually with a cefazolin 1 g IV q8h for at least 10 days, and response is prompt. Patients in this particular setting tend to want to leave as soon as their symptoms abate, and you may find yourself treating them with oral medications; use cephalexin 500 mg PO bid or other oral first-generation cephalosporins.
2. Major complications include spread into fascial layers (necrotizing fasciitis) and osteomyelitis, both of which can be appreciated on x-ray film or CT and which are suspected when the patient does not respond to therapy, has a particularly severe case, or has symptoms suggestive of either (see below).

Osteomyelitis

Quick Points
1. This infection of the bone is usually caused by seeding from a distant infected source (ie, endocarditis), surgical or traumatic introduction (gunshot or stab wound), or spread from another infected site (cellulitis).
2. Pathogens are identical to those in endocarditis and cellulitis, with a preponderance of *S. aureus*, but *Strep.*, fungi, and gonorrhea all occur.
3. The most common sites to see this disease in IV drug users are (1) vertebral sites (seeding); (2) trauma sites, especially gunshot and stab wound areas; and (3) sites infected with repeated cellulitis.

4. Vertebral involvement usually involves two adjacent vertebral bodies, resulting in disk death and joint space narrowing. This can also lead to spinal abscess from contiguous spread.

5. Symptoms include (for vertebral) back pain, low-grade fever, and spine tenderness. Beware of any signs of epidural abscess: paresis, bowel and bladder dysfunction, and sensory loss. This is a surgical emergency, and prompt action will be needed to preserve function. Note that local cellulitis is very common in trauma-related osteomyelitis, as are poor wound healing and drainage.

6. Diagnosis is radiographic: vertebral involvement looks like disk space narrowing initially, followed by destruction of the cortex at adjacent end plates. In other sites, you will see periosteal thickening, lytic lesions (in hematogenous seeding), and sclerosis of the bone in chronic cases.

7. MRI and bone scan are also helpful, but bone scans, although sensitive, are not specific.

Initial Management

1. Blood cultures are usually not helpful in adult osteomyelitis, and culture is usually obtained surgically.

2. Treatment is, of course, dependent on the susceptibility of the offending organism. Bugs are basically the same spectrum as in endocarditis and cellulitis in the IV drug user population, and treatment, just as with subacute bacterial endocarditis (SBE), is long (4–6 weeks). However, oral agents can be used if the bug is sensitive and the patient's GI tract (and compliance) can be ensured.

3. In chronic osteomyelitis, there are multiple avascular foci in the bone that are impenetrable to antibiotics. In these cases, surgery must be consulted for resection of these areas.

12

Endocarditis

See also Chapter 5.

1. Endocarditis is defined as an infectious, usually bacterial, vegetation on a (usually) damaged valve. Age and male gender increase the risk, as do transient bacteremic states such as various medical procedures and IV drug abuse. Basically, any change or defect in the surface or integrity of a

valve causes a turbulent flow state downstream, predisposing to thrombosis. This can also occur when a person has systemic disease like lupus or wasting disease, causing Libman-Sacks disease or marantic vegetations, respectively, in the absence of infection. Overall, the left heart is more susceptible to infection than the right, probably due to higher pressures (and thence flow) and poorer PML performance in these high-flow areas.

2. *Symptoms* include fever (usually above 101°F), weight loss, malaise, CVA, septic emboli signs, new murmur, and CHF (in severe cases).

3. *Risk factors* (common):
   a. MVP (with murmur)
   b. Degenerative heart disease
   c. Rheumatic heart disease
   d. Congenital heart disease (previous surgical correction will not reduce the risk to 0)
   e. Prosthetic valves (metallic valves have the same risk as porcine)
   f. Previous SBE
   g. IV drug abuse (right heart)

4. *Risk factors* (uncommon): syphilitic aortitis, isolated secundum atrial septal defect, CABG, MVP without murmur, pacer, old rheumatic heart disease without valve damage

5. *Causes of transient bacteremia*:
   a. Dental/periodontal procedure
   b. Tonsil/adenectomy
   c. Rigid bronchoscopy
   d. Respiratory/intestinal mucosal surgery
   e. Cholecystectomy
   f. Esophageal dilation/sclerotherapy
   g. Prostate surgery/TURP/cystoscopy
   h. Vaginal hysterectomy/gynecologic procedures
   i. Catheterizing a bladder with UTI
   j. Incision and drainage of infected tissue

6. *Criteria for diagnosis*:
   a. Remember, one blood culture = 90%, two blood cultures = 94%, and three blood cultures = 97% for yield.
   b. Definitive diagnosis: biopsy, two major criteria, one major and three minor, or five minor (see below). All of the below criteria apply if it is suspected.

   c. Major criteria: two separate, positive blood cultures for the same organism; positive echocardiogram for vegetation.

   d. Minor criteria: preexisting heart condition or IV drug use, fever > 38°C, signs of systemic emboli, glomerulonephritis, Roth's spots, Osler's nodes, Janeway's lesions, increased Rh factor on serology, "soft" echo results, "soft" culture results

7. *The bugs*:

   a. IV drug use: 57% *S. aureus*, 13% *Strep. spp*, 7% *Enterococcus*, 8% gram-negative rods, 5% fungi, 5% polymicrobial, 5% culture negative

   b. Native valve: 50% *Strep.*, 10% *Enterococcus*, 20% *S. aureus*, 5% HACEK, 10% other, 5% culture negative

   c. Prosthetic valve (early): 33% coagulase negative *Staph.*, 15% *S. aureus*, 17% gram-negative rods, 13% fungi, 9% *Strep.*, 9% diptherioids, 4% other

   d. Prosthetic valve (late): 29% coagulase negative *Staph.*, 36% *Strep.*, 11% *S. aureus*, 11% gram-negative rods, 5% fungi, 3% diptherioids, 5% other

   e. HACEK, by the way, refers to a weird group of fastidious, slow-growing bugs and stands for Haemophilus, Acinetobacter, Cardiobacter, Eikenella, and Kingella. Remember to save the cultures for a few weeks (4–6) in case one of these grows out.

8. *Cardiac manifestations*:

   a. Murmurs (new or increased)

   b. Valve ring abscess can involve endocardium and cause heart block

   c. Pericarditis/hemopericardium due to burrowing abscess

   d. MI (coronary artery embolus)

   e. Myocardial abscess

   f. Diffuse myocarditis leading to CHF

   g. CHF (usually due to subacute *Strep.* endocarditis but also seen in *Staph.*)

9. *Embolus*: usually to the spleen, kidneys, and brain and to the lung in right-sided SBE (shows up as a circular infiltrate on x-ray, usually cavitary/empyemic) or body abscess

10. *Immunologic reactions*:

   a. Glomerulonephritis, sterile meningitis, polyarthritis, mucocutaneous petechiae, splinters, Roth's spots, and Osler's nodes

11. One to 5% of *Staph.*-infected patients with SBE develop frank cerebral abscess.

12. Mycotic aneurysm shows up much later in the course, found at major bifurcation sites in the aortic system (eg, splenic, superior mesenteric). Beware of signs of rupture and bleeding.

13. IDU:
    a. Younger patients
    b. Usually acute and not chronic SBE
    c. Infected but previously normal tricuspid valve
    d. Not usually CHF signs but rather embolic phenomenon
    c. Osteomyelitis is common
    f. Seventy-five percent develop septic pulmonary complications; watch out for misdiagnosing these people with pneumonia.
    g. Remember that 10% of febrile IDUs have endocarditis.

BIBLIOGRAPHY

The references for this chapter are included in Chapter 16.

13

Gastroenterology

Eliminate the impossible, and what is left, no matter how improbable, is the truth. — Sherlock Holmes

Common sense in matters medical is rare, and is usually in inverse ratio to the degree of education. — Sir William Osler

GASTROINTESTINAL BLEEDING

Quick Points
- Sometimes, it is difficult to determine if a patient is suffering from an upper versus a lower GI bleeding. The anatomic cutoff is at the ligament of Treitz.
- Classically, upper gastroinestinal bleeding (UGIB) presents as hematemesis, coffee-ground emesis, or melena.
- If there is rapid transit down the GI tract, UGIB may present as maroon stool or hematochezia.
- Your initial evaluation should include the insertion of a nasogastric (NG) tube. If clear or bilious return is obtained, an UGIB is less likely. Current recommendations do not support the uses of NG tube lavage.

Initial Management
- The critical first step is to determine the patient's hemodynamic status.
- Evaluate patient's volume status immediately (orthostatics).
- At least two large-bore needles should be inserted (16 to 18 gauge if possible). (Central lines are not optimal for GI bleeding since they are relatively long catheters.) Patients should be given crystalloid immediately (NS wide open).
- If patients show hemodynamic compromise, then an ICU evaluation should be obtained. Initial tests include a CBC, PT/PTT, and

BUN/Cr ratio (> 30 may indicate UGIB). The initial CBC may be normal because patients are so volume contracted.
• Call Gastroenterology for endoscopy.

Upper Gastrointestinal Bleeding

Quick Points
See Table 13–1 for common etiologies.
• Less common causes:
  • Scleroderma
  • Blue rubber bleb nevus syndrome
  • Osler-Weber-Rendu disease (AVMs)
  • Dieulafoy's lesion
• Diagnosis is usually obtained by endoscopy.
• Urgent endoscopy is indicated in patients with persistent or recurrent bleeding or high-risk patients.
• Risk factors for rebleeding: age > 60, coagulopathy, bleeding during hospitalization, major blood loss, and comorbidities (ie, cardiac).
• Certain endoscopic findings predict the risk of rebleeding. A clean ulcer base has the lowest risk of rebleeding, whereas a nonbleeding visible vessel or actively bleeding vessel is at highest risk. The presence of an adherent clot usually has a 20% chance of rebleed.

Initial Management
• The beauty of EGD is that it also allows for therapeutic maneuvers. Patients who are found to have an actively bleeding vessel or a visible vessel that is not actively bleeding should receive endoscopic therapy. Options include heater probe, cautery, laser, or sclerotherapy.

Table 13–1. Common Etiologies of Upper Gastrointestinal Bleeding

Peptic ulcer disease (PUD)

NSAID use

Cirrhosis with varices

Mallory-Weiss tear (usually after vomiting)

- Those with low-risk endoscopic stigmata and low clinical risk factors should be fed and discharged early.
- A 48- to 72-hour observation period is recommended in patients who are at high risk clinically but are low risk in terms of findings at EGD.
- Those at high risk for rebleeding should be admitted to the ICU.
- Remember that gastric ulcers need to be biopsied (if they are not actively bleeding) at least 10 times to rule out gastric cancer. An antral biopsy should be taken to rule out *Helicobacter pylori*.
- Pharmacologic therapy has not been shown to improve outcomes but is recommended for PUD. Acid reduction therapy is recommended (H_2 blockers, proton-pump inhibitors).
- *H. pylori*-positive patients should be treated; options are listed in Table 13–2.
- Management of Varices:
  - Sclerotherapy or band ligation
  - Nadolol 40 mg PO qd is useful to reduce portal HTN and may reduce mortality. Somatostatin or octreotide (25–50 µg/hr) IV should also be given.
  - Octreotide is equal to sclerotherapy and superior to vasopressin and tamponade in the management of varices.
  - If all else fails, balloon tamponade is an option in preparation for transjugular intrahepatic portosystemic shunting (TIPS).

Table 13–2. *Helicobacter pylori* **Treatment Regimens**

Acid Reduction	Antibiotics	Duration
Pepto-Bismol 2 tabs PO qid	Tetracycline 500 mg PO qid + metronidazole 250 mg PO tid	2 wk
Omeprazole 20 mg PO bid	Clarithromycin 500 mg PO bid + metronidazole 500 mg PO bid	1 wk

Lansoprazole (Prevacid) 15 mg PO qd can be substituted for omeprazole and amoxicillin 1 g PO bid for metronidazole.

Lower Gastrointestinal Bleeding

Quick Point
See Table 13–3 for common etiologies.)

Initial Management
- The first thing to do is rule out an upper GI source (insert an NG tube).
- Colonoscopy should initially be attempted. This is sometimes limited in patients who are bleeding.
- An angiogram is another option and also offers a therapeutic advantage (embolization option).
- A nuclear study (using labeled RBCs) requires rapid bleeding and is often nondiagnostic.
- Evaluation of the small bowel is extremely difficult. This should be considered in the bleeding patient who has had multiple negative EGDs and colonoscopy. Options include enteroclisis or intraoperative endoscopy.
- Treatment is of the cause and often requires surgery and supportive care (IV fluids, blood, bowel rest).

Table 13–3. Common Etiologies of Lower Gastrointestinal Bleeding

Diverticular disease

Arteriovenous malformations

Colitis

Bowel ischemia

Neoplasms

Upper gastrointestinal bleeding with rapid transit (don't forget this)

ESOPHAGUS

Quick Points
- Symptoms of esophageal disease may masquerade as cardiac disease (chest pain in patients with gastroesophageal reflux disease [GERD]) or pulmonary disease.
- The word "dysphagia" should ring alarm bells. These patients will likely need endoscopy to rule out carcinoma.

- Dysphagia may be divided according to its etiology: obstructive, nonobstructive, and functional (diagnosed when a structural or motor abnormality cannot be found).
- Dysphagia above the cricopharyngeus is often perceived as the food "sticking" in the throat. These patients may also regurgitate undigested foods.
- Nonobstructive dysphagia may be due to neuromuscular disorders such as Parkinson's, myasthenia gravis, or myopathies.
- Anatomic obstructions include strictures, webs, rings (Schatzki's), or carcinoma (adenocarcinoma or squamous cell).
- Patients with dysphagia must have endoscopy. Other methods of evaluation include cine-esophagram (to evaluate motility) and manometry. Treat the cause.
- Esophageal cancer. Adenocarcinoma and squamous cell carcinoma are the two most common esophageal carcinomas. Classic risk factors for squamous cell cancer are history of ethanol and tobacco use (see the Head and Neck section in Chapter 11 for more information).

Gastroesophageal Reflux Disease

Quick Points
- The etiology of GERD is unclear. It seems that an important component is an inappropriate transient relaxation of the lower esophageal sphincter (LES). This allows the reflux of acid, bile, and pepsin. The presence of a hiatal hernia may also play a role.
- Symptoms can be quite variable. Classic presentation is "heartburn" after eating or when lying down. Some patients may present with a chronic cough, noncardiac chest pain, asthma exacerbations (from microaspirations), or a hoarse voice.
- Besides causing symptoms, GERD may actually cause structural esophageal anomalies. The most harmful side effect is Barrett's esophagus. The esophageal mucosa resembles gastric mucosa, and on biopsy there is a specialized columnar epithelium with intestinal metaplasia. This is a premalignant condition. Barrett's esophagus is seen in 10% of patients with GERD.

13

Initial Management

The diagnosis of GERD is usually made on EGD, where typical esophageal erosions are seen. If upper endoscopy is nondiagnostic, a 24-hour pH monitoring can be performed.

- The key component of GERD therapy is lifestyle modification (the most difficult thing to do):
  - Patients should not eat meals before bedtime (try to eat at least 3–4 hours before lying down).
  - Patients should avoid fatty foods, alcohol, chocolate, and caffeine.
  - Weight loss is also recommended.
- First-line therapy is an H_2-blocker with or without prokinetics (cisapride [Propulsid]). Proton-pump inhibitors should only be used in refractory patients. Proton-pump inhibitors should not be used for an extended period of time because some patients may develop hypergastrinemia or atrophic gastritis (if they have concurrent *H. pylori*).
- Surgical management should only be considered in patients with severe disease who are refractory to medical therapy. The procedure of choice is Nissen fundoplication. However, there are no good long-term results.
- Patients with Barrett's esophagus should undergo surveillance endoscopy with biopsy every 2 to 3 years as it is associated with later adenocarcinoma of the esophagus.

Esophageal Dysmotility

Achalasia:

- Achalasia classically presents as dysphagia. Patients may also experience chest pain and regurgitation.
- On CXR, there is no gastric bubble.
- A characteristic finding on manometry is incomplete relaxation of the LES and decreased peristalsis in the esophageal body.
- Classic therapy is pneumatic dilation, but this may cause perforation.
- Current therapy is injection of botulinum toxin. Repeated injections are required, and some patients do experience relief.
- Surgical therapy is myotomy.

Diffuse esophageal spasm:

- These patients often complain of chest pain.

- The diagnosis is made by manometry, which demonstrates peristalsis interrupted by esophageal contractions.
- Therapy: bougie dilation, nitrates, and calcium channel blockers.

Esophagitis

Quick Points

- The characteristic complaint of esophagitis is odynophagia (painful swallowing).
- Immunocompromised patients are at increased risk for infectious esophagitis, especially *Candida albicans*, CMV, and HSV.
- Pills that induce esophagitis include NSAIDs, KCl, tetracycline, quinidine, zalcitabine, zidovudine (AZT), alendronate, iron, and vitamin C. Injury usually occurs when pills are swallowed without water or in the supine position.
- Caustic esophageal injury occurs from ingestion of alkali (eg, drain cleaners).

Initial Management

- Remove the offending agent (discontinue pills or start antibiotics).
- Patients usually require endoscopy. At the time of EGD, biopsy, brushings, and viral cultures are performed. Keep in mind that patients with oral thrush may have coexisting *Candida* esophagitis. They may need empiric therapy with fluconazole (Diflucan).
- In cases of caustic injury, treatment, at first, is supportive with IV fluids and pain medications. EGD is usually performed in the first 24 hours to assess the degree of injury. Patients with mucosal injury must be observed carefully for 24 hours. Surgery is needed with shock, sepsis, perforation, or deterioration.

STOMACH

Gastroparesis

Quick Points

- Gastroparesis is impaired gastric emptying without obstruction.
- The etiology of gastroparesis can be mutifactorial: CNS difficulty, enteric nervous system abnormality, or systemic diseases. Common

13

causes include diabetes and postoperative changes (vagotomy or after gastric resection).
- Patients usually present with nausea and vomiting, early satiety, bloating, and, sometimes, weight loss.
- Often, diabetics with gastroparesis will have peripheral neuropathy or nephropathy.

Initial Management
- First make sure there is no evidence of obstruction on EGD (may show retained food) or upper GI series.
- Diagnosis can be made by gastric scintigraphy (radiolabeled solid and liquid meals).
- Gastroparesis may be reversible in diabetics if sugars are better controlled.
- Prokinetic agents are widely used (cisapride 10–20 mg qid).

Peptic Ulcer Disease

Quick Points
- The two most common causes of duodenal and gastric ulcers are *H. pylori* and NSAIDs. Approximately 15% of patients with *H. pylori* develop PUD in their lifetime. Risk factors for bleeding on NSAIDs are given in Table 13–4.
- Both NSAIDs and *H. pylori* cause ulcers by different mechanisms. NSAIDs cause ulcers by causing a disruption in the milieu. There is an imbalance between mucosal protective factors and acid and pepsin. The defensive factors depend on prostaglandins, which are inhibited by NSAIDs. The mechanism by which *H. pylori* causes ulcers has yet to be uncovered. However, most patients with *H. pylori* have abnormal gastrin and acid production.
- NSAIDs account for 5 to 10% of duodenal ulcers and 20 to 40% of gastric ulcers.

Initial Management
- The most important therapy is prevention: try to avoid NSAIDs in those at risk or give prophylaxis to such patients along with NSAIDs. Newer

NSAIDs specific for the cyclooxygenase type 2 (Cox-2) enzyme (Celebrex, Vioxx) are available; these shouldn't affect gastric mucosa.

- The gold standard for diagnosis is EGD with biopsy. A surrogate marker for *H. pylori* is the presence of chronic active gastritis on antral biopsy.
- The current consensus is that all patients with documented duodenal or gastric ulcers, who are infected with *H. pylori*, should receive antibiotics to cure the infection. *H. pylori* has also been implicated in gastric cancer and lymphoma. There is a clear association between *H. pylori* and mucosa-associated lymphoid tissue (MALT) lymphoma. Treatment regimens for *H. pylori* are listed in Table 13–2.
- The gold standard for post-test evaluation is the urea breath test.
- Differential for stomach ulcers postulcer surgery: incomplete vagotomy, incomplete antrectomy, Zollinger-Ellison syndrome (islet cell tumor of pancreas producing great amounts of gastrin), ulcerogenic drugs, or *H. pylori*.

Table 13–4. Risk Factors for Bleeding on NSAID

Age > 76

History of peptic ulcer disease or gastrointestinal bleeding

Steroid use

Multiple comorbidities

Gastric Cancer

Quick Points

- At the time of presentation, the disease is locally advanced or metastatic. Anorexia and weight loss are common. Classic physical examination findings are Virchow's node (supraclavicular), Sister Mary Joseph's node (periumbilical), enlarged ovary (Krukenberg's tumor), or Blumer's shelf (mass in the cul de sac).
- There is a strong correlation between the prevalence of *H. pylori* and gastric cancer.
- Chronic atrophic gastritis and intestinal metaplasia are linked to gastric cancer.

- Atrophic gastritis is an autoimmune disease, which affects the body and fundus of the stomach (it spares the antrum). In this disorder, there is increased gastrin in response to decreased acid.
- Ménétrier's disease (hypergastric state, with hyperrugation of the gastric mucosa) is considered premalignant by some.
- Ninety-eight percent of gastric cancers are adenocarcinomas, and the remainder are non-Hodgkin's lymphoma or leiomyosarcomas.

Initial Management

- The first diagnostic test is usually an upper GI series. Less than 3% of all gastric ulcers evaluated by endoscopy and biopsy are malignant.
- CT scan of the abdomen will delineate tumor extent and metastasis.
- Screening is recommended in Japan for persons over age 50.
- Complete surgical resection is the only chance for cure.

SMALL BOWEL

Malabsorption

There are three phases of normal digestion and absorption:

- Intraluminal phase
- Mucosal phase
- Absorptive phase

The classic presentation of patients with intestinal malabsorption is diarrhea and weight loss. Patients may also show signs of nutritional deficiency. The stools are usually bulky (steatorrhea) and foul smelling. Patients may present with anemia (iron deficiency, megaloblastic). A Schilling test may need to be performed in the evaluation of vitamin B_{12} deficiency. The Schilling test has three parts:

1. Radioactive B_{12} ingestion
2. Radioactive B_{12} and intrinsic factor ingestion (if there is B_{12} uptake now, that indicates intrinsic factor deficiency)
3. Radioactive B_{12} + intrinsic factor + antibiotics (if uptake occurs with this, that indicates bacterial overgrowth)

Patients may even present with a bleeding tendency (poorly absorbed vitamin K). A stool weight should be performed (maximum 200 g/d), and a fat content should also be performed (maximum 7 g/d on a 100-g fat diet). A positive Sudan stain gives strong evidence of steatorrhea, and a quantitative assay may not be necessary (save the poor nurses).

The key is to determine which phase of digestion and absorption has been interrupted. A mucosal abnormality can be determined by measuring D-xylose absorption or the ratio of mannitol to lactulose absorption. A small bowel biopsy may be necessary to identify the cause of mucosal injury.

Celiac Sprue (Gluten-Sensitive Enteropathy)

Quick Points
- Genetic predisposition to develop T-cell–mediated enterocyte injury in response to gluten in the diet.
- This disorder is more commonly seen in diabetics.
- Symptoms include diarrhea, flatulence, weight loss, and weakness.
  - Stools are usually large, floating, greasy, and foul smelling.
  - Patients often suffer from vitamin deficiencies.
  - The characteristic skin rash is dermatitis herpetiformis (10%), the treatment for which is dapsone.
- Both this skin lesion and celiac sprue are associated with HLA-DR3 and HLA-Dw2.

Initial Management
- A small bowel biopsy is needed to confirm the diagnosis. The characteristic finding is loss of intestinal villi, hypertrophy of the intestinal crypts, and infiltration of the lamina propria with lymphocytes and plasma cells.
- A number of serologic tests are available for celiac disease to screen patients and monitor adherence with treatment (IgG and IgA antigliadin antibodies). A combination of both tests offers a sensitivity and specificity of over 95%.
- The removal of gluten from the diet is essential. Gluten is found in wheat, rye, barley, and oat products.
- Some patients may also require steroid therapy. If there is no response with the removal of gluten, then give a gluten challenge and re-biopsy to rule out lymphoma.

13

Whipple's Disease

Quick Points
- This is a rare multisystemic illness caused by infection with the bacillus *Tropheryma whippelii.*
- This disorder usually affects Caucasian men 30 to 60 years of age.
- Symptoms: malabsorption, fever, lymphadenopathy, and arthralgias.

Initial Management
- Diagnose by duodenal biopsy revealing periodic acid–Schiff (PAS)-positive macrophages with the characteristic bacillus.
- Treat with TMP-SMX (Bactrim) for 1 year; a response is usually evident in 1 to 3 months.
- If untreated, the disease is fatal.

Bacterial Overgrowth

Bacterial overgrowth in the small intestine may result in malabsorption. Causes of bacterial overgrowth include
- Gastric achlorhydria
- Anatomic abnormalities of the small intestine
- Small intestine motility disorders
- Gastrocolic or coloenteric fistula
- AIDS and pancreatitis

The breath test (an increase in hydrogen in the breath after xylose injection) is usually positive. Treatment should include correction of the anatomic defect (if possible). Empiric therapy with broad-spectrum antibiotics usually results in improvement.

Lactase Deficiency

Quick Points
- Lactase is a brush-border enzyme that hydrolyzes lactose into glucose and galactose. Deficiency affects 50 million people in the U.S.
- Symptoms: bloating, abdominal cramps, and flatulence. If higher concentrations of lactose are ingested, an osmotic diarrhea may occur.

Initial Management
- Diagnosis is made by the hydrogen breath test.

- Clinically, many physicians will empirically try a lactose-free diet for 2 weeks. Treatment is minimizing lactose intake (eg, avoid milk, ice cream, cottage cheese).
- There are lactase caplets available over the counter, as well as milk products that have been pretreated with lactase.

PANCREAS

Acute Pancreatitis

Quick Points
- Acute pancreatitis remains a serious illness, with a mortality of 5 to 10%.
- Gallstones and alcohol consumption are the most common causes.
- Hypertriglyceridemia-induced and postoperative pancreatitis tend to be very severe. Rarer causes are coxsackievirus B, HIV, drugs (didanosine, zalcitabine), pancreas divisum, pancreatic cancer, or a stenosed sphincter of Oddi.
- Patients classically present with abdominal pain (usually epigastric), radiating to the back. There is often associated nausea and vomiting.
- The first step in diagnosis is obtaining a serum amylase ± a serum lipase. Values of serum amylase or lipase three times above normal are characteristic of acute pancreatitis.
- It is important to keep in mind that other conditions can cause a hyperamylasemia. Sometimes a lipase and a spot urine amylase may be necessary. Keep in mind that hypertriglyceridemia artifically lowers amylase and lipase
- If the patient is severely ill and there is any doubt in the diagnosis, a CT (C+) scan should be obtained. Severe pancreatitis on CT scan will be evidenced by an enlarged, edematous gland, intraglandular necrosis (doesn't enhance with contrast), and surrounding edema, with or without fluid collections. A CT scan may not be necessary for mild cases. Ultrasonography is another option.

Initial Management
- Any alcohol consumption should be stopped immediately.
- If a common bile duct stone is suspected, then immediate endoscopic retrograde cholangiopancreatography (ERCP) is the procedure of choice.

13

- The cornerstones of therapy are aggressive fluid resuscitation, making the patient NPO, analgesia, and careful monitoring.
- Patients with severe pancreatitis should receive nutritional support (TPN).
- A CT scan should be obtained if a patient is severely ill or deteriorates within 72 hours. It is important to distinguish between interstitial disease and necrosis.
- All patients with pancreatic necrosis should receive antibiotic therapy (imipenem, ciprofloxacin, cefuroxime). If there is an abscess on the CT or evidence of infected necrosis, then an FNA should be performed. These patients may require débridement.

Further Discussion

The best definition is an acute inflammatory process of the pancreas that may involve peripancreatic tissues and other remote organ systems. The criterion of severity is based on the presence of multiorgan system failure and local complications.

The pathophysiology is complex. There has been a return to the theory that acute pancreatitis is caused by trypsinogen activation to trypsin. Trypsin then activates a cascade of mediators (kallikreins, phospholipases, elastases), resulting in localized inflammation, possible necrosis, and multiorgan system failure.

It is important to determine the cause of pancreatitis. The severity of the attack should be determined. Keep in mind that evidence of significant disease includes significant third space losses, hemoconcentration, oliguria, azotemia, and hemodynamic instability. Ranson's criteria can give you an early assessment of prognosis (Table 13–5).

Table 13–5. Ranson's Prognostic Criteria for Acute Pancreatitis

At Presentation	Over First 48 Hours
Age > 55	HCT ↓ by 30%
WBC > 16,000/µL	BUN ↑ by 5 mg/dL
Glucose < 200 mg/dL	Calcium < 8 mg/dL
LDH > 350 U/L	PaO_2 < 60 mm Hg
AST > 250 U/L	Base deficit > 4 meq/L
	Fluid sequestration > 6 L

The APACHE II and III scores (> 8 indicates severe disease) can also be used. It is very complex, and some critical care units have a computer program to generate the score.

Chronic complications include formation of phlegmons and pseudocysts, which present with nonresolving symptoms and are diagnosed on ultrasound or CT; they frequently require surgical intervention.

Chronic Pancreatitis

Quick Points
- Chronic alcoholism is present in 60 to 70%. Other causes are pancreatic duct obstruction, pancreas divisum, intraductal plugs, stones, cystic fibrosis, and hyperparathryroidism.
- Symptom: recurrent epigastric pain, especially after alcohol ingestion.
- Chronic changes: fibrosis, inflammation, and loss of exocrine tissue.

Initial Management
- Serum amylase or lipase may be normal.
- Pancreatic calcifications may be seen in up to 30% of plain abdominal x-rays.
- Ultrasonography may reveal pancreatic enlargement, ductal dilation, or pseudocysts.
- CT scan is approximately 70% and specificity is 90%.
- The gold standard for diagnosis is ERCP.
- Treat pain. Analgesia may even include nerve blocks. Clearly, patients must abstain from alcohol or other causative agents.
- Patients with persistent pain should undergo ERCP to define the caliber morphology of their pancreatic ducts, which may have a "chain of lakes" appearance.
- Some may need an internal surgical drainage procedure (eg, a longitudinal pancreatojejunostomy; Peustow procedure) or stent placement.
- Some advocate the use of pancreatic enzyme replacement (pancrealipase).
- Complications of chronic pancreatitis include malabsorption (when 90% of exocrine function is lost), pseudocysts, and an increased incidence of cancer.

13

Carcinoma of the Pancreas

A relationship to alcohol and tobacco is suspected in patients with pancreatic cancer. Most often there are no specific symptoms, and diagnosis is made in the late stages of disease. Diagnostic tests include CT scan, MRI, ultrasonography, or ERCP. An elevated CA 19-9 > 200 mg/dL is indicative of a poor prognosis. CA 19-9 should not be used for screening. The 5-year survival rate is extremely poor.

APUDomas

These are rare neuroendocrine tumors that secrete various gastric hormones. APUD stands for amine precursor uptake and decarboxylation. These tumors often present with diarrhea and include glucagonoma (DM with migrating necrolytic erythema), VIPoma (secretory diarrhea, hypokalemia, and flushing), gastrinoma (Zollinger-Ellison syndrome), and somatostatinoma (causes atreatorrhea, not secretory diarrhea). These tumors often have somatostatin receptors, so they can be imaged with octreotide radioisotopes. Eighty percent of these tumors are malignant and located in multiple sites. Treatment options vary according to the type of tumor. Gastrinomas should be treated with high-dose proton-pump inhibitors. The other tumors usually require surgical debulking.

COLON

Diarrhea

Quick Points
- Acute infectious diarrhea can be categorized as inflammatory versus noninflammatory.
- The key differences are that inflammatory diarrhea is usually small volume, bloody, and positive for fecal leukocytes.
- Noninflammatory diarrhea usually is small bowel in etiology and consists of nonbloody, large-volume stools.
- Acute diarrhea usually resolves in 5 to 7 days without therapy.
- *Special Situations:*
  - Traveler's diarrhea is frequently caused by enterotoxogenic *E. coli*. Remember to avoid contaminated water. Antibiotics are only needed in moderate to severe diarrhea. Therapy is usually ciprofloxacin or TMP-SMX.

- The classic causes of food poisoning are *S. aureus* and *C. perfringens.* Patients usually develop nausea and vomiting within 1 to 6 hours of food ingestion. This is usually self-limited.
- *E. coli* 0157:H7 can cause severe dysentery, HUS, and TTP (5–10% of patients—remember Jack in the Box?).
- *C. difficile* usually occurs in patients who have had recent antibiotic therapy. The organism can give off toxin A or B, producing pseudomembranous colitis. Stool studies for toxin B should be sent if the diagnosis is available. Treatment is either oral vancomycin or flagyl for 7 to 10 days.

Initial Management
- Initial studies should include stool for WBC (should be positive in infectious diarrhea) and stool for Gram's stain and culture.
- Immunocompromised patients should also have stool for ova and parasites (three sets) sent.
- Keep in mind that secretory diarrhea (ie, VIPoma, cholera) will have a stool osmolality equivalent to the serum osmolality.
- Steatorrhea, nausea, anorexia, and chronic diarrhea should prompt a search for *Giardia*.
- Chronic diarrhea with negative stool studies should undergo endoscopic evaluation and biopsy (initial flexible sigmoidoscopy with colonoscopy, if necessary).

Constipation

Quick Points
- Define the complaint: is it hard stools, straining with bowel movements, or less than three bowel movements per week?
- Common causes of constipation include irritable bowel syndrome, poor bowel habits, and a poor diet (no fiber).
- Irritable bowel syndrome can manifest as constipation (treat with psyllium), alternating constipation with diarrhea, or morning diarrhea. Weakness, stress, immobility, and dementia are factors.
- Serious causes include
  - Colonic obstruction (from cancer, strictures, foreign body, or diverticulosis)

13

- Neuropathies (multiple sclerosis, diabetes, Hirschsprung's mega-colon [congenital absence of the myenteric plexus], Chagas' disease)
- Hypothyroidism
- Scleroderma
- Inflammatory bowel disease
- Medications (opiates and anticholinergics most commonly)

Initial Management
- Once serious causes are ruled out (if there is a recent and abrupt change in bowel habits, consider a flexible sigmoidoscopy and/or barium enema), the options are
  1. Fiber supplements and plenty of fluids
  2. Bulk laxatives (psyllium)
  3. Emollients (docusate [Colace]) to soften the stool
  4. Hyperosmolar agents (sorbitol, lactulose) (commonly used in bowel cleansing)
  5. Stimulants (senna [Senokot; can cause melanosis coli] and phenolphthalein [Ex-Lax; may increase the risk for colon cancer])
  6. Cisapride (Propulsid)

INFLAMMATORY BOWEL DISEASE

Ulcerative Colitis

Quick Points
- Ulcerative colitis (UC) is idiopathic inflammation of the colon, characterized by bloody stool.
- Patients who present with bloody diarrhea should first be examined for infectious etiologies (amebae, *Campylobacter, Salmonella, Shigella*).
- UC is classified as follows:
  1. Mild: less than four bowel movements qd
  2. Moderate: > four bowel movements qd with mild toxicity
  3. Severe: six or more bloody bowel movements qd ± toxicity (fever, tachycardia, elevated ESR, anemia)

Management

- Mild to moderate distal colitis can be treated with topical mesalamine or steroids.
- Oral 5-aminosalicylate is the treatment with mild, more extensive disease.
- More severe disease is treated with a steroid taper.
- Patients with severe disease or who appear toxic require IV steroids.
- Cyclosporine has been used for steroid failures.
- The big acute risk of UC is toxic megacolon. These patients need to be hospitalized, with close monitoring. The classic x-ray is "thumbprinting." They must be kept NPO, NG tube to suction, and treated with IV steroids and broad-spectrum antibiotics.
- Maintenance therapy (5-aminosalicylate) is indicated for all patients with diffuse colitis. Azathioprine and 6-mercaptopurine may be needed to maintain remission in some patients.
- The risk for colon cancer increases after 10 years. These patients need colonoscopy at regular intervals, with segmental biopsies. If dysplasia is found, it needs to be confirmed by a second pathologist. Severe dysplasia is an indication for colectomy.

Crohn's Disease

Quick Points

- Crohn's disease can affect the entire GI tract (from the mouth to the anus) and is characterized by skip lesions and the formation of fistulas.
- Symptoms: These patients do not have bloody diarrhea. Patients present with chronic diarrhea and weight loss. Gallstones, hypocalcemia, and oxalate stones are more common in Crohn's than UC since it affects the ileum more often. Some patients may also have a palpable abdominal mass in the right lower quadrant.
- Extraintestinal problems include arthralgias, uveitis, erythema nodosum, anal fissure, and fever.
- Crohn's is characterized by a bimodal age distribution. It is also more commonly seen in Ashkenazi Jews.

13

Management
- Once again, these patients need to be evaluated for causes of infectious diarrhea.
- Those with mild disease can be treated with oral 5-aminosalicylate. Some patients may be unresponsive and require oral flagyl.
- Patients with moderate to severe disease need oral steroids. Steroids work better in Crohn's enteritis than colitis.
- Many of these patients require surgery for obstruction (caused by strictures), severe unremitting disease, fistula repair, and abscess drainage.

POLYPS

Polyps are an important clinical entity because of the risk of cancer they carry. Familial adenomatous polyposis (FAP) and Gardner's syndrome both carry a high risk of cancer. Both are autosomal-dominant disorders, with alteration in the *APC* gene on chromosome 5. These patients have multiple polyps throughout the GI tract. All patients with this disorder and their family members need annual flexible sigmoidoscopy from age 12 to 40. If no polyps are found by age 40, then the next screening should begin at age 50 (routine screening). If an adenoma is found, total colectomy must be performed.

Gardner's syndrome is polyps associated with osteomas. Turcot's syndrome is characterized by colonic polyposis and brain tumors, with an unknown risk of cancer. Lynch syndrome is a familial constellation of colon cancer without polyps, endometrial cancer, and ovarian cancer. Peutz-Jeghers syndrome is characterized by hamartomas of the intestine and mucus pigmentation with minimal risk of colon cancer.

COLON CANCER

Colorectal cancer is the second leading cause of death due to malignancy in the U.S. These cancers are almost all adenocarcinomas. The current belief is that they arise from malignant transformation of an adenomatous polyp. Risk factors are listed in Table 13–6.

Table 13–6. Risk Factors for Colon Cancer

Age > 50

Personal history of adenomatous polyps

Familial polyposis or nonpolyposis syndrome

Smoking

Family history of colon cancer

Streptococcus bovis bacteremia

Inflammatory bowel disease

Quick Points
- These tumors grow slowly and may be present for years before symptoms occur.
- Asymptomatic tumors may be detected by fecal occult blood.
- Usually, chronic blood loss occurs from right-sided tumors, whereas obstruction usually occurs on the left side.
- An important aspect of colon cancer is screening. According to the U.S. Preventive Services Task Force, all average-risk patients over the age of 50 should be offered screening with annual fecal occult blood testing and flexible sigmoidoscopy every 5 years.
- These guidelines do not apply to high-risk patients.
- False-negative guaiacs can be due to vitamin C. False positives are due to red meat, NSAIDs, and dietary peroxidase (turnips, horseradish).

Management
- Diagnostic tests include barium enema or colonoscopy.
- Carcinoembryonic antigen (CEA) levels should be drawn at the time of diagnosis. They are used to follow clinical response, not make a diagnosis.
- Surgical resection is the treatment of choice. Regional lymph node dissection should be done for staging. Most will get a preoperative CXR and abdominal CT to rule out metastasis.
- Adjuvant chemotherapy with 5-FU and either levamisole or leucovorin is recommended in stage II (node-positive) disease. Approximately 20% of patients will have stage IV disease at the time of diagnosis. The overall survival rate for colon cancer is 35%.

13

LIVER AND BILIARY TRACT

Evaluation of Liver Function Tests

A common problem faced is the evaluation of an abnormal SMA-20. It is important to understand what each tests reflects and take a systematic diagnostic approach. A simple classification is as follows:

- Hepatic synthetic function: albumin, cholesterol, and PT
- Impaired hepatic uptake and secretion of bile: bilirubin
- Cholestasis: alkaline phosphatase (keep in mind that this can also come from bone, intestine, kidney, or placenta. Sometimes a gamma-glutamyl transferase is necessary as well to confirm liver origin).
- Hepatocellular disruption: aspartame aminotransferase (AST) and alanine aminotransferase (ALT) (more specific). Keep in mind that high levels indicate viral, drug-induced, toxic, or ischemic liver injury. AST or ALT elevations that are less than 300, with an AST/ALT ratio > 2, are usually compatible with ethanol use.

Once again, a careful H&P is necessary. Pay special attention to risk factors for hepatitis B and C. Usually, the evaluation of abnormal LFTs requires that the following diseases be considered:

- *Hepatitis B*
  - Patients will usually give a history of parenteral drug use or unprotected sex.
  - Diagnosis is made by hepatitis B surface antigen (HBsAg) and IgM anti-hepatitis B core antigen.
- *Hepatitis C*
  - Risk factors: parenteral drug use, blood transfusions
  - Diagnosis is made by anti-hepatitis C virus (HCV)
- *Autoimmune Hepatitis*
  - Associated with autoimmune disorders. Occurs in women.
  - Diagnostic tests: ANA, anti–smooth-muscle antibodies
- *Fatty liver*
  - Alcohol classically causes fatty liver.
  - Nonalcoholic steatohepatitis (NASH) is seen with obesity, hyperlipidemia, and diabetes (these are not always seen with NASH).
    - NASH is distinct from fatty liver. These patients have chronic, mild elevations of the aminotransferases. The course is usually benign.

- These patients usually have ultrasonography consistent with fatty liver. Also, changes disappear with weight loss. Confirm with biopsy.
- *Wilson's disease*
  - Patients presents in the second or third decade with neuropsychiatric disorders.
  - Labs: ceruloplasmin, 24-hour urine copper, hepatic copper level
- *Hemochromatosis: "bronze diabetes"*
  - This is the most common autosomal-recessive metabolic disease seen in the U.S.
  - Laboratory tests include ferritin, iron studies, hepatic iron.

Viral Hepatitis

Currently, there are five types of hepatitis causing acute and chronic hepatitis:

- Hepatitis A. Hepatitis A virus (HAV) is an RNA virus transmitted via the fecal-oral route. Patients usually present with jaundice, nausea, and vomiting. Infection is self-limited (no chronic phase). Acute infection is diagnosed by anti-HAV IgM. Persons with hepatitis B (chronic), who are superinfected with hepatitis A, have increased mortality. The HAV vaccine is recommended in travelers to endemic areas.
- Hepatitis B. Hepatitis B is an enveloped DNA hepadnavirus. There is a protein coat (HBsAg) surrounding the core protein (HBcAg). HBsAg is the earliest marker of acute infection, and its presence indicates ongoing infection. Recovery is usually indicated by loss of HBsAg and the presence of hepatitis B surface antibody (HBsAb). HBeAg correlates with infectivity. Those who are vaccinated have HBsAb.
  - The actual virus does not cause hepatocellular damage. Instead, it is the cytotoxic lymphocyte-mediated reaction against hepatitis B core (HepBcAb).
  - Heterosexual activity accounts for 40% of transmission of hepatitis B (HBV). HBV accounts for almost 50% of the cases of acute viral hepatitis.
  - The risk for chronic infection depends on the age of acquisition of the virus. Approximately 90% of infants with hepatitis B go on to chronicity, whereas less than 5% of adults develop chronic disease. The risk of hepatocellular carcinoma is 1 to 3% yearly in patients with HBV-related cirrhosis.

13

- Hepatitis C. Hepatitis C is a small RNA virus. The highest rates of hepatitis C are among injection drug users and hemophiliacs (before better blood screening). Sexual transmission is rare (there is a theoretic risk). Persistent infection develops in 85 to 100% of infected patients. Chronic hepatitis occurs in 60 to 70%. Approximately 25 to 30% of infected patients progress to cirrhosis over 20 years.
  - Extrahepatic manifestations include mixed cryoglobinemia, lichen planus, porphyria cutanea tarda, lymphocytic silaoadenitis, immune thrombocytopenia, and membranoproliferative glomerulonephritis.
- Hepatitis D. Hepatitis B is required for co-infection. These patients are at risk for fulminant hepatitis.
- Hepatitis E. This is more common in developing countries. The method of transmission is fecal-oral. Pregnant females may develop fulminant hepatitis (10%).

Management of Acute Hepatitis

Indications for hospitalization are inability to tolerate PO intake or signs of liver failure (encephalopathy, elevated PT). Travelers to endemic (for hepatitis A) areas should be vaccinated 4 weeks before departure. Contacts of patients with hepatitis B should be vaccinated. Hepatitis C patients should be aware that they can infect others via body fluids.

Management of Chronic Hepatitis

Current available therapy for hepatitis B and C is IFN-α. IFN-α terminates viral replication. In chronic HBV, using IFN-α transiently increases AST and ALT (this is a marker of response). In chronic HCV, the reverse occurs. The use of IFN-α in HCV has a 40% response rate at 6 months. Sustained response rates are higher if it is continued for 12 to 18 months.

Drug-Induced Liver Injury

Drug-induced injury is idiosyncratic. Most hepatotoxic effects involve cell necrosis. Some of the drugs may injure the biliary system or sinusoidal or endothelial cells. Acetaminophen is a direct hepatotoxin (causes centrilobular liver necrosis). Early treatment with *N*-acetylcysteine is effective. Isoniazid, viruses, methyldopa, and halothane cause mononuclear liver infiltration. Valproate, tetracycline, asparaginase, and alcohol cause fatty liver. Steroids, oral contraceptives, and chlorpromazine cause portal inflammation. Carbon tetrachloride causes necrosis and fatty liver.

Cholestasis

Cholestasis must be classified into intrahepatic or extrahepatic obstruction. Intrahepatic cholestasis usually results from hepatocellular injury. Extrahepatic cholestasis usually results from biliary obstruction due to stones, strictures, inflammation, or tumors. The initial test should be ultrasonography of the liver or biliary tree. If the biliary system is dilated, the next test is ERCP.

Primary Biliary Cirrhosis

Primary biliary cirrhosis is due to autoimmune destruction of the interlobular and septal bile ducts in the liver. Patients are usually female, aged 35 to 60. Hashimoto's thyroiditis and scleroderma may be associated. These patients usually have the picture of hyperlipidemia, elevated ESR, jaundice, and pruritus. This is a progressive disease. Patients often suffer from osteopenia. Treatment is with ursodeoxycholic acid, methotrexate, or both.

Primary Sclerosing Cholangitis

The etiology of this disease is unknown, but it is commonly seen in the setting of inflammatory bowel disease (typically UC). It is more common in males. There is inflammation and fibrosis of the extrahepatic biliary tree. Diagnosis is made by ERCP, where multiple strictures are seen ("beads on a string"). There is no medical therapy. These patients will need a liver transplant.

Cirrhosis and Portal Hypertension

Quick Points
- Presenting findings: ascites, spontaneous bacterial peritonitis (SBP), gastric or esophageal varices, hepatic encephalopathy
- Hepatorenal syndrome: serum creatinine > 1.5 mg/dL, urine output < 500 cc qd, urine sodium >10 meq/L, and creatinine clearance < 40 mL/min.

Management
- Ascites:
  - Diagnostic paracentesis (serum/ascites albumin gradient > 1 indicates portal HTN)

- Treatment includes sodium restriction and diuretics (spironolactone [Aldactone] + furosemide [Lasix]). Patients should lose approximately 0.5 kg per day.
- Spontaneous bacterial peritonitis. Common pathogens are enteric gram-negative rods and *S. pneumoniae*. Use quinolones for prophylaxis. Treat with cefotaxime.
- Varices. See the section on UGIB for a discussion of endoscopy, sclerotherapy, nadolol, and shunts.
- Hepatic encephalopathy. Treat with lactulose 30 cc PO qid. Flumazenil can briefly reverse lethargy in these patients.

Hepatocellular Carcinoma

Hepatocellular carcinoma is much more frequent in Asia and Africa. It is associated with HBV and HCV. Other risk factors are aflatoxins, drugs, and cirrhosis of any etiology. Patients with suspected hepatocellular carcinoma should have ultrasonography or dynamic CT and an alpha-fetoprotein drawn. These patients have a poor prognosis.

Evaluation of a Liver Mass

These are often discovered in asymptomatic patients. The initial tests include an SMA-20; hepatitis B surface antigen, HCV, and alpha-fetoprotein. If these tests are abnormal, a biopsy is needed. If LFTs are only mildly abnormal, then imaging with ultrasonography, dynamic CT, or MRI is needed. If the mass appears to be a hemangioma, observation is suggested. If not, an FNA should be done. If there is evidence of hepatic defect, there is increased suspicion of hepatocellular carcinoma.

BIBLIOGRAPHY

Reviews

Bennett WF, Bova JG. Review of hepatic imaging and approach to liver masses. Hepatology 1990;12:761–5.

Camilleri M. Appraisal of medium and long-term treatment of gastroparesis. Am J Gastroenterol 1994;89:1769–74.

Cook DJ, et al. Stress ulcer prophylaxis in critically ill patients. JAMA 1996; 275:308–14.

D'Amico G, et al. The treatment of portal hypertension. Hepatology 1995; 22:332–54.

Dusheiko GM. Treatment and prevention of chronic viral hepatitis. Pharmacol Ther 1995;65:47–73.

Ferzoco LB, et al. Acute diverticulitis. N Engl J Med 1998;338:1521–6.

Fisher RS, Parkman HP. Management of nonulcer dyspepsia. N Engl J Med 1998;339:1376–81.

Fregia A, Jensen DM. Evaluation of abnormal liver tests. Compr Ther 1994; 20:50–4.

Herrera JL. Serologic diagnosis of viral hepatitis. South Med J 1994; 86:677–84.

Kaplan MM. Medical approaches to primary sclerosing cholangitis. Semin Liver Dis 1991;11:56–63.

Laine L, Peterson WL. Bleeding peptic ulcer. N Engl J Med 1994;331:717–27.

Lee WM. Drug-induced hepatotoxicity. N Engl J Med 1995;333:1118–28.

Lieberman D. GI bleeding. Gastroenterol Clin North Am 1993;22:723–36.

Lindor KD, et al. Ursodiol in primary sclerosing cholangitis. N Engl J Med 1997; 336:691–5.

Lowenfels AB, et al. Prognosis of chronic pancreatitis. Am J Gastroenterol 1994; 89:1467–71.

Park SI, Giannella, RA. Approach to the adult patient with acute diarrhea. Gastroenterol Clin North Am 1993;2:483–97.

Ransohoof DF, Gracie WA. Treatment of gallstones. Ann Intern Med 1993; 119:606–19.

Ranson JH, et al. Prognostic signs and the role of operative management in acute pancreatitis. Surg Gynecol Obstet 1974;13:69–81.

Riordan SM, Williams R. Treatment of hepatic encephalopathy. N Engl J Med 1997;337:473–9.

Runyon BA. Care of patients with ascites. N Engl J Med 1994;330:337–42.

Runyon BA, et al. The serum-ascites albumin gradient is superior to the exudate-transudate concept in the differential diagnosis of ascites. Ann Intern Med 1992;117:215–20.

Saini S. Imaging of the hepatobiliary tract. N Engl J Med 1997;336:1889–94.

Steer ML, et al. Chronic pancreatitis. N Engl J Med 1995;332:1482–90.

Steinberg W, Tenner S. Acute pancreatitis. N Engl J Med 1995;330:1198–210.

Trier JS. Celiac sprue. N Engl J Med 1991;325:1709–19.

Zein NN, Rakela J. Interferon therapy in hepatitis C. Semin Gastrointest Dis 1995; 6:46–53.

Guidelines

American Gastroenterological Association. Guidelines on the use of esophageal pH recording. Gastroenterology 1996;110:1981–2.

American Gastroenterological Association. Technical review on the clinical use of esophageal manometry. Gastroenterology 1994;107:1865–84.

Bond JH. Polyps guidelines. Ann Intern Med 1993;119:836–43.

Camilleri M, et al. Clinical management of intractable constipation. Ann Intern Med 1994;121:520–8.

Hanauer SB, Meyers S. Management of Crohn's disease in adults. Am J Gastroenterol 1997;92:559–66.

Kornbluth A, Sachar DB. Ulcerative colitis practice guidelines in adults. Am J Gastroenterol 1997;92:204–11.

Winawer SJ, et al. Screening for colorectal cancer with fecal occult blood testing and sigmoidoscopy. J Natl Cancer Inst 1993;85:131–8.

Studies and Trials

Gastrointestinal Cancer

Fuchs CS, et al. Dietary fiber and the risk of colorectal cancer in women. N Engl J Med 1999;340:169–76. (*Fiber intake was not associated with a decreased risk of colon cancer in women.*)

Gastrointestinal Bleeding

Besson I, et al. Sclerotherapy with or without octreotide for acute variceal bleeding. N Engl J Med 1995;333:555–60. (*An RCT showing that octreotide reduced rebleeding in variceal bleeding.*)

Imperiale TF, et al. A meta-analysis of somatostatin versus vasopressin in the management of acute esophageal variceal hemorrhage. Gastroenterology 1995; 109:1289–94. (*A meta-analysis showing that somatostatin was superior to vasopressin in safety and efficacy in this situation.*)

Laine L, et al. Prospective evaluation of immediate vs. delayed refeeding and prognostic value of endoscopy in patients with upper GI hemorrrhage. Gastroenterology 1992;102:314–6. (*An RCT showing that immediate refeeding was okay in those with endoscopic criteria for low rebleeding risk [eg, no visible vessel present].*)

Richards RJ, et al. Can the BUN/creatinine ratio distinguish upper from lower GI bleeding? J Clin Gastroenterol 1990;12:500–4. (*The mean BUN/Cr ratio for UGIB was 35 and for lower bleeding was 18.*)

Silverstein FE, et al. GI toxicity: celecoxib vs. NSAIDS. JAMA 2000; 284:1247–55. (*Celecoxib decreases ulcers and GI complications by 50% relative to NSAIDs.*)

Silverstein FE, et al. Misoprostol reduces serious GI complications in patients with rheumatoid arthritis receiving NSAIDs. Ann Intern Med 1995;123:241–9. (*Misoprostol reduced serious complications by 40% in this RCT.*)

Peptic Ulcer Disease

Roggero E, et al. Eradication of *H. pylori* infection in primary low-grade gastric lymphoma of mucosa-associated lymphoid tissue. Ann Intern Med 1995; 122:767–9. (*This RCT showed that eradicating* H. pylori *was associated with regression of MALT lymphoma in 60% of patients.*)

Talley NJ, et al. Absence of benefit of eradicating *H. pylori* in patients with nonulcer dyspepsia. N Engl J Med 1999;341:1106–11. (*Eradicating* H. pylori *did not improve chronic gastritis or quality of life over 1 year.*)

Reflux Disease

Pasricho PJ, et al. Intrasphincteric botulinum toxin for the treatment of achalasia. N Engl J Med 1995;332:774–8. (*In this RCT, botulin produced remission of achalasia.*)

Vigneri S, et al. A comparison of five maintenance therapies for reflux esophagitis. N Engl J Med 1995;333:1106–10. (*Omeprazole + cisapride was the best regimen in this RCT.*)

Inflammatory Bowel Disease

Belluzzi A, et al. Effect of an enteric-coated fish oil preparation on relapse in Crohn's disease. N Engl J Med 1996;334:1557–60. (*Fish oil reduced relapse rates in Crohn's patients.*)

Feagan BG, et al. Methotrexate for the treatment of Crohn's disease. N Engl J Med 1995;331:836–41. (*Methotrexate alleviates Crohn's disease and spares steroids.*)

Greenberg GE, et al. Oral budesonide as maintenance treatment for Crohn's disease. Gastroenterology 1996;110:45–51. (*Oral budesonide prolongs remission but remission was not sustained after 1 year in this RCT.*)

McLeod RS, et al. Prophylactic mesalamine treatment decreases postoperative recurrence of Crohn's disease. Gastroenterology 1995;109:404–13. (*Mesalamine reduces recurrences after surgery.*)

Other

Rensch MJ, et al. Gluten-sensitive enteropathy in patients with insulin-dependent diabetes mellitus. Ann Intern Med 1996;124:564–7. (*Of IDDM patients, 6.4% had gluten-sensitive enteropathy, much higher than the 0.06% rate in the general population.*)

Wong JB, et al. Cost-effectiveness of interferon alfa-2b for chronic hepatitis B. Ann Intern Med 1995;122:664–75. (*A meta-analysis showing that IFN-α increases life expectancy by over 3 years and reduces lifetime treatment costs.*)

13

14

Endocrinology

Success is more a function of consistent common sense than it is of genius. —An Wang

Elegance is seeing and comprehending at once both the unseeable and the details. —Henri Poincare

PANCREAS: DIABETES MELLITUS AND HYPOGLYCEMIA

See also Chapters 15 and 16.

Classic symptoms are polydipsia, polyuria, and polyphagia. Reversible causes are listed in Table 14–1.

Type I: (formerly known as insulin dependent)
- Fifty percent monozygotic twin concordance
- Usually begins in teenage years; diagnosed soon after onset
- Possible viral trigger for autoimmune antibody response to beta cells and insulin
- Absolute insulin deficiency; allows development of diabetic ketoacidosis (DKA)

Type II: (formerly known as non-insulin dependent)
- One hundred percent twin concordance; 25% inheritance in primary relatives

Table 14–1. Reversible Causes of Diabetes Mellitus

Drugs	Niacin
	Thiazides
	Steroids
	Pentamidine
Endocrine	Cushing's disease
	Acromegaly

- Usually develops in middle-aged, overweight patients; diagnosed 5 to 10 years after onset.
- Relative insulin resistance (so patients are usually hyperinsulinemic, which increases heart disease, etc, as insulin is a growth factor for endothelium).
- Thus, patients rarely present with ketoacidosis but may present with nonketotic hyperosmolar coma (sugars in type II can go much higher than in type I because DKA doesn't occur and the patient doesn't present until sugars get really high).
- Many type II patients are maintained on insulin.
- Maturity-onset diabetes of youth is an autosomal-dominant (chromosome 7) variant of type II beginning in childhood.

Diagnosis

1. Normal fasting sugar is < 110 mg/dL and a normal 2-hour postprandial sugar is < 140 mg/dL.
2. Impaired glucose tolerance = normal sugar of 110 to 126 or 2-hour sugar of 140 to 200.
3. Diabetes = fasting sugar > 126 or 2-hour sugar > 200 (thus, if baseline fasting sugar is between 110 and 126, the patient should get a glucose tolerance test and check the 2-hour sugar).
4. In pregnancy, diabetes = fasting sugar > 105 or 2-hour sugar > 165.
5. Screen for type II (type I declares itself) using fasting sugar in patients at high risk:
   - Age > 45
   - Strong family history
   - Ethnicity: African American, Hispanic, Native American
   - Obesity
   - Prior gestational diabetes
   - History of HTN
6. Hemoglobin A_{1c} (HbA$_{1c}$) measures glycosylated hemoglobin (measures glucose control over the past 3 months; it is more useful for follow-up than diagnosis).

Management

1. The Diabetes Control and Complications Trial (DCCT) showed that
   - Risks for retinopathy, nephropathy, and neuropathy are cut by 35 to 75% with intensive treatment of type I patients (it is assumed that the same holds true for type II patients).

14

- The ADA recommends target goals of $HbA_{1c} < 7\%$ and fasting sugar of 80 to 120 for both types I and II.
2. Treat comorbidities (cholesterol, smoking, HTN, sedentary lifestyle).
3. Intensive monitoring requires qid fingersticks (mandatory for type I diabetics, who are more brittle). Type II patients need to be very motivated and cooperative for this to work. Watch out for hypoglycemia (occurs in obtunded, alcoholic, those who have had DM for a long time due to autonomic neuropathy, and those on beta-blockers).
4. Type I:
   - Insulin pump
   - Transplantation is usually done in conjunction with renal transplant; more recently, islet cell transplants have been shown to be successful in conjunction with nonsteroid-based immunosuppression, but this is still experimental.
   - Insulin management:
     - Long-acting forms include NPH, Lente, and Ultralente (NPH is a workhorse).
     - Short-acting forms are regular and Lispro (Lispro is very quick).
     - Initial regimens can kick off with morning and bedtime dosing of NPH and regular (regular insulin should be at least 40% of the total daily dose), with adjustments based on insulin (in postprandial hyperglycemia, go with regular or Lispro for coverage).
   - Suspect glucagonoma in patients with metastatic liver cancer and hyperglycemia (also presents with beefy red tongue and migratory necrolytic erythema).
5. Type II:
   - Reduce weight (a 15–20% calorie cut, with loss of 10 to 20 lbs, goes a long way).
   - Oral therapies:
     - Sulfonylureas include older agents (eg, chlorpropamide) that are basically not used anymore because of toxicity. Newer agents (glipizide [Glucotrol] and glyburide [Micronase]) are equivalent; they increase insulin production. Recall that type II diabetics have insulin resistance with hyperinsulinemia, so these are falling out of favor too. Toxicity is hypoglycemia.
     - Metformin (Glucophage) is becoming a mainstay. It decreases hepatic gluconeogenesis and increases insulin responsiveness.

Thus, not only does it decrease insulin requirement, but it also does not produce hypoglycemia (unlike sulfonylureas). The only problem is the toxicity of lactic acidosis; thus, it should not be used in liver/kidney disease, ischemic patients, anyone taking contrast dye, or anyone who is sick and at risk for sepsis/acidosis.

- Troglitazone (Rezulin) also increased insulin sensitivity and looked as if it might become the main drug; however, it has fallen dramatically off its pedestal due to hepatotoxicity.
- Repaglinide (Prandin) promotes insulin secretion after a meal, improving glycemic control, and works synergistically with metformin.
- Acarbose (Precose) is an adjunct, reducing α-glucosidase in the gut, thus delaying glucose absorption. It can bring down HbA_{1c} 0.5 to 1%; give it before meals.

- Insulin is indicated in patients who are refractory, are infected, or have urinary ketones.

Starting Insulin

1. Very often, you will have to start an insulin sliding scale (fingerstick qid) for new inpatients. Our personal standard when you don't have a patient's baseline medication history is as follows:

   0–80: orange juice, milk, and call a doctor
   80–200: nothing
   201–250: 2 U regular
   251–300: 4 U regular
   301–350: 6 U regular
   351–400: 8 U regular
   > 400: 10 U regular and call a doctor

2. If you know someone takes a lot of insulin to start off with, you may want to start the sliding scale at 4 or 6 U and add 2 or 4 U for every 50-point jump in sugar. But nurses often balk if you order > 10 U regular for a sugar under 400 (be diplomatic).

3. Don't leave someone on a sliding scale for their entire hospital stay. After ~2 days, calculate how much their daily insulin requirement is and order a standing dose: give two-thirds of their daily requirement in the morning and one-third in the evening. Of the morning dose, two-thirds is NPH and one-third is regular, whereas of the evening dose, both NPH and regular should be one half. For example, if some-

14

one is averaging 36 U of regular insulin a day on your sliding scale, his or her initial standing dose would be 16 U NPH and 8 U regular in the morning and 6 U NPH and 6 U regular in the evening. Continue to readjust as needed (with illnesses, new medications, etc).

For information on DKA and nonketotic hyperosmolar coma, see Chapter 16.

Diabetic Complications

- *Retinopathy* eventually occurs in all type I diabetics and most type II patients.
  - It may be present on diagnosis of type II (remember they've had it for 5–10 years before diagnosis). Thus, type II diabetics need an ophthalmologic examination on presentation, whereas type I diabetics can wait up to 5 years.
  - Nonproliferative retinopathy (hemorrhages, exudates, cotton-wool spots)
  - Proliferative retinopathy (neovascularization; worse) (panretinal photocoagulation can be of benefit)
  - Need an annual ophthalmologic examination and evaluation for laser
- *Neuropathy* occurs in most diabetics
  - Autonomic disease:
    - Gastroparesis, diarrhea/constipation, incontinence/urinary retention, impotence, orthostatic hypotension, etc.
    - Treat gastroparesis with cisapride (Propulsid), oral erythromycin, or metoclopramide (Reglan)
  - Loss of foot sensation leads to ulcers and chronic pain.
  - Screen with nylon monofilament.
  - Examine the feet on each visit and have the patient check them daily.
  - The patient should never walk barefoot.
  - Promptly refer foot ulcers to a podiatrist.
  - Tricyclic antidepressants may be of benefit (amitriptyline [Elavil] 20 mg qhs).
- *Nephropathy*. Thirty-five percent of type I diabetics develop nephropathy; 10% of type II patients do.
  - A Kimmelstiel-Wilson lesion is pathognomonic on biopsy.
  - Screen for urine microalbumin annually (predicts renal and heart disease).

- Kidney transplantation restores life expectancy (unlike dialysis); age is not a contraindication to kidney transplantation.
- ACE inhibitors should be given for diabetics with HTN or microalbuminuria. Losartan (Cozaar), diltiazem (Cardizem), and verapamil (Calan) are alternatives, as they also likely reduce albuminuria.
- Beta-blockers reduce hypoglycemia awareness and thiazides can increase glucose.

Gestational Diabetes

- Preexisting diabetes: the target for HbA_{1c} is < 6% to reduce maternal risk (preeclampsia, preterm labor, progression of diabetic retinopathy and nephropathology) and to reduce fetal risks (death, acute respiratory distress syndrome, hypoglycemia, macrosomia).
- If the patient has significant retinopathy, Ophthalmology should examine her often (at least every 2 months).
- Oral hypoglycemics are teratogenic; the patient should switch to insulin.
- New-onset gestational diabetes develops due to insulin resistance (thought to be due to human placental lactogen) that occurs in the seventh month in 2 to 4% of women. Half of them will get diabetes within 5 to 10 years (especially if they are obese or have family history).
  - Screen at 24 to 28 weeks, especially if patient is > 25, is not Caucasian, has a family history, or is obese.

Hypoglycemia

Work-up if the patient has sugar < 50 or is symptomatic with sugar < 80 (sweating, tachycardia, dizziness, syncope).

- C-peptide > 0.4 nM when sugar is < 50 implies insulinoma or ingestion of sulfonylureas (check urine sulfonylureas in patients who are health workers, relatives of diabetics, fakers, etc). Proinsulin is higher in insulinoma than sulfonylureas.
- Low C-peptide with high insulin indicates exogenous insulin use.
- Use MRI and selective angiography to localize insulinomas. The gold standard is laparotomy with intraoperative ultrasonography.
- Diazoxide or octreotide is used for unresectable lesions.
- Differential diagnosis includes cancers, wasting, adrenal failure, and severe malnutrition.

Thyroid Disease

Thyroid-releasing hormone from the hypothalamus causes pituitary thyroid-stimulating hormone (TSH) secretion and then thyroid release of thyroxine (T4), which is then converted to T3 in peripheral tissues. Feedback loops exist.

Tests

- Radioactive iodine uptake (RAIU) is increased in thyroid hyperfunction or iodine deficiency; it is decreased in iodine excess, hypothyroidism, thyroiditis, and factitious thyroid excess.
- TSH and free T4 are the main tests used. TSH is very sensitive (if abnormal, it indicates disease even if the free T4 is okay; thus, subclinical disease should generally be treated). Free T4 is needed only if pituitary disease is an issue.
- Forget about T3RU; it is useful only to grill medical students.
- Thyroxine-binding globulin is increased in pregnancy and estrogen use and is decreased by steroids and systemic illness.

Hypothyroidism

Quick Points
- Symptoms include edema, obesity, slowness, lethargy, cold intolerance, and carpal tunnel syndrome.
- It is usually due to Hashimoto's disease; other causes include drugs (lithium, amiodarone), postablation for Graves' disease, and thyroiditis.
- Hashimoto's patients have antimicrosomal or antithyroglobulin antibodies.
- Hashimoto's patients often have DM, Addison's disease, or pernicious anemia.

Initial Management
- Treat with thyroxine. The replacement dose is usually 1.7 µg/kg PO qd; check TSH 6 weeks later for response. In those who are old, have heart disease, or have a long history of hypothyroidism, start at 25 µg/kg, add 25 µg every 6 weeks, and check TSH every 6 weeks.
- The dose may need to be increased in pregnancy or in patients on sucralfate, cholestyramine, or aluminum hydroxide or after high-bran meals.

Hyperthyroidism

Quick Points
- Graves' disease = diffuse toxic goiter; Plummer's = toxic multi-nodular goiter.
- Other causes:
  - Choriocarcinoma and hydatidiform moles (TSH is similar to hCG)
  - Jodbasedow phenomenon (iodine intake in a deficient patient)
  - Amiodarone
- Symptoms include hyperactivity, ophthalmopathy (bug-eyes), dermopathy (pretibial myxedema, which usually occurs in hypothyroidism), heat intolerance, and weight loss.
- The elderly can have apathetic hyperthyroidism (weight loss, atrial fibrillation, and CHF).
- Graves' disease is the most common (usually in women 30–40), due to the long-acting thyroid stimulator antibody (which binds and stimulates TSH receptors). It can cause neonatal thyrotoxicosis. It does not cause thyroid cancer.
- RAIU is important to differentiate Graves' disease from subacute thyroiditis (de Quervain's disease; has a high erythrocyte sedimentation rate) and factitious disease (has a low thyroglobulin).

Initial Management
- Treatment: beta-blockers (to control pulse), antithyroid drugs (propylthiouracil [PTU] and methimazole [MMZ]; block T4 synthesis), radioactive ablation (for both Graves' and Plummer's), and surgery.
  - PTU is preferable to MMZ: both can cause agranulocytosis, and rash, but PTU blocks peripheral T4 conversion to T3 as well, whereas MMZ causes aplasia cutis in the fetus.
  - Radioactive iodine is the mainstay; 80% of patients eventually need thyroxine replacement.
  - Surgery is indicated for those with a coexisting cold nodule in Graves' disease (complications include hypoparathyroidism and injury to the recurrent laryngeal nerve).
- Pregnancy:
  - Avoid radiation and MMZ; avoid surgery in the first or third trimester.

14

- Use a minimum dose of PTU to control the mother's thyroid (you don't want to cause fetal hypothyroidism).
- Postpartum thyroiditis is self-limited and autoimmune; treat with beta-blockers.
- Thyroid storm:
  - Fever, tachycardia, and hypotension; occurs with surgery, anesthesia, and sepsis.
  - Treatment includes beta-blockers, digoxin, PTU, potassium iodide (Lugol's solution, which blocks thyroxine production and peripheral T4 deiodination to T3), and steroids (which block deiodination and provide adrenal support).
- *Do not convert atrial fibrillation due to hyperthyroidism prior to cardiac surgery.*

Goiter and Masses

Quick Points
- Can cause dysphagia, odynophagia, and tracheal compression (surgery is needed if severe).
- Risk factors for malignancy: neck radiation in childhood, cervical nodes, or recent or rapid growth of nodules.
- Papillary carcinoma has a good prognosis (if you had to have a cancer, this is it); it spreads by lymphatics, occurs in the young, and often occurs after radiation to the neck.
- Follicular carcinoma occurs in the elderly and spreads hematogenously.
- Medullary carcinoma (due to parafollicular C cells) causes hypercalcemia due to release of calcitonin; it occurs in multiple endocrine neoplasia (MEN) type 2 or 3 (see below).
- Anaplastic cancer is bad (0% survival at 1 year).

Management
- Ultrasonography or thyroid scans (classifies nodules as hot [uptake of radioiodine] vs. cold [no uptake]) are useful.
  - Use FNA for dominant nodules and all cold nodules.
  - Hot nodules are almost always benign; use radiation or surgery for hyperthyroid patients with hot nodules.

- Monitor euthyroid patients.
- Benign cold nodules may be reduced by thyroxine.
- Treat with surgery, lymph dissection, and radioiodine ablation; monitor thyroglobulin for recurrence.
- If TSH is detectable, using thyroxine to suppress TSH can prevent further enlargement.

Miscellaneous

- Subacute thyroiditis occurs often after viral URI; it is first hyperthyroid, then hypothyroid, and finally euthyroid. The ESR is high. Treatment is supportive: ASA or steroids to reduce inflammation.
- Sick euthyroid syndrome (normal TSH but low thyroxine) occurs in stress and sickness due to increased reverse T3 (inactive; produced when deiodinase is reduced). Care is supportive; there is no specific therapy.

Pituitary Disease

Tumors

Tumors are classified by micro- (< 1 cm) versus macroadenomas (> 1 cm), as well as functional versus nonfunctional. Nonfunctional tumors need therapy only if there are compressive symptoms (visual field loss, hydrocephalus).

Prolactinomas are the most common functional tumor.

- Prolactin is increased by drugs (metoclopramide, phenothiazines) as dopamine tonically inhibits its release and is increased by thyroid-releasing hormone (TRH) (which rises in hypothyroidism).
- Prolactin > 200 ng/mL implies prolactinoma.
- Signs and symptoms include infertility, oligomenorrhea, and galactorrhea; diagnose by prolactin level and CT/MRI.
- In women, these tumors are small and benign; treat with bromocriptine ± oral contraceptives.
- In men, they are aggressive. Treat with trans-sphenoidal resection.

Empty-sella syndrome is usually benign due to obesity in women where CSF displaces the pituitary.

Acromegaly is diagnosed with symptoms (large hands and feet, doughy skin, widely spaced teeth, big tongue, carpal tunnel syndrome), high somatomedin C (also known as insulin-like growth factor 1), and demonstrating that hyperglycemia does not suppress growth hormone. Treat with trans-sphenoidal surgery; use octreotide for palliation. Note that acromegalics often have precancerous colon polyps and need frequent colonoscopies.

TSH tumors and nonsecreting adenomas (which usually make gonadotropins but are asymptomatic) are rare and should be treated surgically with or without octreotide.

Hypopituitarism

Quick Points
- The anterior pituitary is the endocrine gland and the posterior pituitary is really an outgrowth of the brain.
- Signs of anterior hypopituitarism include growth failure, hypothyroidism, adrenal insufficiency, and hypogonadism.
- Causes of anterior hypopituitarism:
  - Pituitary tumors (compression of remaining gland)
  - Metastases (often from the breast or lung)
  - Other masses: craniopharyngioma, dysgerminoma, optic glioma
  - Radiation
  - Sheehan's syndrome (postpartum pituitary necrosis due to hypotension in labor; diabetes is a risk factor)
  - Infiltrative: autoimmune, sarcoidois, histiocytosis, and TB
  - Pituitary apoplexy (infarction of pituitary tumor leading to compression causing headache, visual disturbance, stiff neck, and fever)
  - Kallmann's syndrome (congenital midline defects, with cleft palate, anosmia, and pituitary-hypothalamus hypofunction) is another etiology.
- Posterior pituitary dysfunction causes diabetes insipidus (polydipsia + polyuria). It is usually due to infiltration (tumors, sarcoidosis, histiocytosis, etc).

Management
- Diagnose anterior hypopituitarism by TSH, free T4, and plasma cortisol response to adrenocorticotropic hormone (ACTH).
- Replace thyroid hormone and glucocorticoids.

- Pituitary apoplexy may require urgent decompression if visual signs are progressive; it may also need steroids and mannitol.
- Diagnose diabetes insipidus (DI) by high serum osmolality (> 290 mOsm/L) with dilute urine osmolarity (< 275 mOsm/L); if serum osmolality is < 280, then the patient has psychogenic polydipsia. Therapies are as follows:
  - Central DI will respond to fluid restriction plus intranasal desmopressin (an analogue of ADH, which, coincidentally, also treats von Willebrand's disease), whereas nephrogenic DI will not.
  - Nephrogenic DI: use a low-sodium diet plus thiazides (volume depletion lowers polyuria).

Adrenal Disease

Recall that

1. Corticotropin-releasing hormone (hypothalamus) stimulates ACTH, which stimulates cortisol.
2. Renin (kidney) stimulates angiotensin and, in turn, aldosterone.
3. ACTH contains melanin-stimulating hormone; thus, hyperpigmentation occurs with pituitary ACTH tumors (Cushing's disease) or adrenal insufficiency (Addison's disease), which causes a compensatory increase in ACTH.
4. There are three cortical zones (GFR): zonas glomerulosa (aldosterone), fasciculata (cortisol), and reticularis (androgens). Medulla produces catecholamines (epinephrine and norepinephrine).
5. 21-Hydroxylase deficiency causes congenital adrenal hyperplasia (low cortisol and aldosterone, high precursors that are androgenic and have some glucocorticoid effect). Signs and symptoms are virilization and salt wasting if severe. Diagnose by increased 17-OH progesterone.

ACTH is regulated by circadian rhythm, stress, and cortisol feedback. ACTH and cortisol are highest in the morning. Renin is regulated by intra-arterial volume, BP, and potassium.

Cushing's Syndrome (too much cortisol)

Quick Points
- Signs and symptoms: truncal weight gain, HTN, striae, ecchymoses, osteoporosis, hypokalemia, hypernatremia, buffalo hump, moon facies, and muscle weakness

14

- Differential: iatrogenic steroid use, pituitary tumor, ectopic ACTH production (eg, small cell of lung), and adrenal tumors

Management

- Diagnose with urinary free cortisol (not plasma level, which varies widely).
- Work-up by first checking ACTH (if high, this indicates pituitary or ectopic production).
  - Distinguish pituitary from ectopic ACTH by inferior petrosal sinus sampling.
  - With respect to the adrenal, carcinoma produces multiple hormones (cortisol, mineralocorticoids, and androgens), whereas adenomas produce only steroids.
- Treatment:
  - Trans-sphenoidal resection of pituitary tumors
  - Treatment of ectopic lesions
  - Unilateral adrenalectomy for adrenal tumors
  - Bilateral adrenalectomy (for bilateral micronodular dysplasia, incurable pituitary tumors, incurable ectopic masses)
- *You must replace cortisol for 3 to 12 months* to allow recovery of the pituitary-adrenal axis.
  - Florinef (fludrocortisone, mineralocorticoid) is essential after bilateral adrenalectomy.
  - Watch for Nelson's syndrome (after bilateral adrenalectomy, pituitary ACTH adenomas can go ballistic and be very aggressive).

Further Discussion

- The dexamethasone suppression test is not useful anymore, except to torture your medical students; the concept was that screening with low-dose dexamethasone would suppress physiologic hypercortisolemia but not pathologic conditions, would be confirmed with a repeat low-dose test, and that high-dose dexamethasone would suppress pituitary causes but not adrenal or ectopic sources.
- Metyrapone test (also esoteric). Metyrapone blocks adrenal 11 beta-hydroxylase (preventing cortisol formation); thus, if the pituitary is working (or hyperfunctional), it will crank out ACTH and increase

cortisol precursors, but that great rise in 11-DOC (11 dehydroxycortisol), will not occur in adrenal or ectopic tumors. It is also used to assess adrenal insufficiency to see if the pituitary is working.

Addison's Disease (too little cortisol)

Quick Points
- Signs: weakness, anorexia, nausea, hypotension, hyperkalemia, hyponatremia
- Differential: withdrawal of exogenous glucocorticoids, TB, autoimmune (associated with DM, vitiligo, pernicious anemia, Hashimoto's, etc), infiltration (CMV, histoplasmosis, amyloid, sarcoid), hemorrhage (meningococcemia, anticoagulation), drugs (ketoconazole, rifampin)
- In hypopituitarism, the aldosterone levels are okay, and hyperkalemia is absent.

Initial Management
- Diagnose on ACTH stimulation test (lack of cortisol rise indicates deficiency) and plasma ACTH level (which would be low if pituitary deficiency was the cause).
- Treat with cortisol (same as hydrocortisone) 20 to 25 mg/d and, if needed, fludrocortisone 50 to 100 μg/d.
- Stress-dose steroids (given when the adrenals are not working) = hydrocortisone 100 mg tid (this is basically the maximum amount the adrenals could produce if functional).

Conn's Syndrome

- Hyperaldosteronism causes hypokalemia, HTN, and, rarely, periodic paralysis.
- If renin is high, this can be due to juxtaglomerular hyperplasia (Bartter's syndrome) or volume depletion.
- Do imaging and surgery for adenomas or spironolactone for hyperplasia.

Pheochromocytoma

Quick Points
- Signs: episodic HTN, headache, palpitations, volume depletion (leading to hypotension that is postural or after surgery).

14

- Pheochromocytoma is the 10% tumor: 10% malignant, 10% bilateral, 10% extra-adrenal *(the most common extra-adrenal site is the organ of Zuckerkandl).*

Management
- Diagnosis: urinary vanillylmandelic acid and metanephrines (falsely elevated by cocaine, L-dopa, methyldopa, MAOIs, hypoglycemia, and exercise); localize by CT/MRI or MIBG scan.
- Treat with surgery under cover of medicines (phenoxybenzamine superior to phentolamine as the former's alpha-antagonism is noncompetitive) and preoperative volume repletion.
  - Use beta-blockers only after alpha-blockade is achieved.
- Metyrosine (blocks catecholamine synthesis) is palliative.

Incidentaloma   (ie, incidental adrenal masses)
- Nine percent of people at autopsy have nonfunctional adrenal adenomas (so commonly found on CT/MRI done for other reasons).
- Work-up includes urine free cortisol, upright renin, urine metanephrine, and plasma testosterone (depending on clinical signs and symptoms).
- Masses < 3 cm are unlikely to be adrenal tumors but have a ~15% chance of being metastases in patients not known to have cancer and a 75% chance in those with known cancer.
- Surgical removal should be done if the mass is > 6 cm.

Multiple Endocrine Neoplasia
Remember The Three Triangles (Figure 14–1).
- Autosomal dominant; type II due to *c-ret* proto-oncogene

Gonads
Recall that
1. Pulsatile gonadotropin-releasing hormone (Gn-RH) from the hypothalamus causes pituitary release of follicle-stimulating hormone (FSH) and LH (important because constant Gn-RH activity, as occurs with leuprolide administration for prostate cancer, causes inhibition of FSH/LH release).
2. In men, LH stimulates Leydig's cells to make testosterone (negative feedback on pituitary) and FSH stimulates Sertoli's cells to support spermatogenesis and make inhibin B (negative feedback on pituitary).

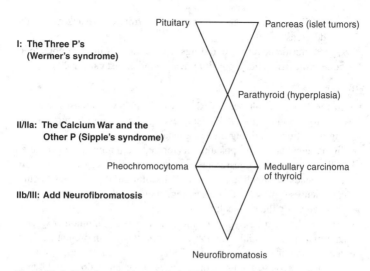

I: The Three P's (Wermer's syndrome)

Pituitary

Pancreas (islet tumors)

Parathyroid (hyperplasia)

II/IIa: The Calcium War and the Other P (Sipple's syndrome)

Pheochromocytoma

Medullary carcinoma of thyroid

IIb/III: Add Neurofibromatosis

Neurofibromatosis

Figure 14–1. Multiple endocrine neoplasia: The Three Triangles.

3. In women, LH stimulates release of androstenedione from thecal cells and FSH stimulates granulosa cells to convert that to estradiol, as well as produce inhibin.

Men

- Reproductive failure is manifest by low libido, impotence, small testes, and serum testosterone < 100 ng/dL.
- Causes: prolactinoma and craniopharyngioma as well as primary gonadal failure, Klinefelter's syndrome (XXY karyotype with high FSH), and idiopathic failure of pituitary to secrete gonadotropins at puberty.
- Treat with testosterone (300 mg IM q3wks; transdermal or trans-scrotal patches).
- Androgen insensitivity or testicular feminization syndrome (eg, Jamie Lee Curtis) patients have XY karyotype but look female due to the mutant androgen receptor. They present with amenorrhea. There is a higher risk of gonadal tumors, so the testes should be excised.

14

- Cystic fibrosis causes azoospermia and sterility due to absence of the vas deferens.
- Gynecomastia occurs due to drugs (isoniazid, heroin, spironolactone, cimetidine, tricyclics), physiologically, and breast cancer

Women

- In the follicular phase, Gn-RH pulse frequency increases, causing FSH to rise more than LH. Rising estradiol causes a LH surge, causing ovulation, heralding the luteal phase.
- In the luteal phase, corpus luteum (formed from remnants of ruptured follicle) secretes progesterone, estradiol, and inhibin A, which eventually leads to a decline in FSH/LH, dissolution of the corpus luteum, and menses (unless, of course, a pregnancy signal, in the form of hCG, is received by the corpus luteum).
- Amenorrhea can be hypothalamic (due to stress, strenuous exercise, anorexia, prior cranial radiation), hypopituitarisim, or premature ovarian failure (autoimmune disease). Treat with oral contraceptives (if the goal is to keep estrogen support, menses to prevent endometrial hyperplasia, and prevent pregnancy) or pulsatile Gn-RH, clomiphene, or gonadotropins to induce ovulation for fertility.
- Work-up:
  - Primary amenorrhea (never had menses)
    - If the FSH is high, think dysgenetic gonads (no secondary sex characteristics); if it is normal, look for an absent uterus (normal secondary sex characteristics); if it is low, there is probably a physiologic delay (no secondary sex characteristics).
  - Secondary (three missed menses)
    - *Always check hCG* (you must rule out pregnancy, even if the patient claims to be immaculate).
    - If progesterone causes withdrawal bleeding, then anovulation (likely polycystic ovary disease) is the cause of amenorrhea.
    - Then do cyclic oral contraceptives, if menses resumes, then there is estrogen deficiency; if there is no menses, then endometrial failure is present.
    - Consider the prolactin level.
  - Asherman's syndrome is a complication of dilation and curettage (D&C), abortions, etc.

- Polycystic ovary disease (Stein-Leventhal syndrome; can be autosomal dominant or X-linked): amenorrhea, infertility, hirsutism, and obesity due to adrenal androgen excess causing obesity and stimulating LH while inhibiting FSH, continuing a vicious cycle. Patients often have type II diabetes and acanthosis nigricans. Treat with oral contraceptives, weight reduction, and fertility treatments (clomiphene, FSH).

Parathyroids and Calcium

Recall that

1. PTH stimulates calcium absorption in the gut, resorption in the kidney, phosphaturia, and vitamin D production in the kidney. Calcitonin does the reverse. Calcium is intimately linked to PTH in the feedback loop.
2. Vitamin D (formed by conversion of 7 dehydrocholesterol to cholecalciferol in the skin by ultraviolet light, then to calcidiol in the liver, and then to calcitriol in the kidney) causes calcium absorption in the gut and kidney to hold on to both calcium and phosphate.

Hyperparathyroidism

See Chapter 3 for a discussion of hypercalcemia.

Quick Points
- Most cases are detected as asymptomatic hypercalcemia.
- Classic signs of hypercalcemia are "stones, bones, groans, and psychic overtones" (renal stones, bone loss and pain, abdominal pain [from pancreatitis or peptic ulcer disease], and lethargy).
- Differential:
  - Most commonly due to solitary parathyroid adenoma (~85%) and sometimes to diffuse hyperplasia (~15%)
  - Malignancy (metastases or paraneoplastic syndromes [squamous cell of lung/cervix and renal cell make PTH-related protein, whereas human T-cell leukemia/lymphoma virus (HTLV-1) lymphomas and B-cell lymphomas can make vitamin D])
  - Drugs (thiazides, lithium, vitamin D, antacids [milk-alkali syndrome])
  - Paget's disease (increased bone turnover leading to fractures, frontal bossing, deafness, and high-output CHF due to atrioventricular fistulas in new bone)

14

- Sarcoidosis
- Familial hypocalciuric hypercalcemia (benign; renal defect).
- Brown tumors of bone occur due to excess osteoclast activity stimulated by PTH (not malignant).

Management
Urinary calcium, pyridonoline (collagen crosslinks), cAMP, and phosphate are increased (although PTH stimulates calcium resorption, excessive serum calcium leads to kidney dumping anyway). So are alkaline phosphatase and, of course, PTH.

- Diagnose and treat on surgery (imaging is not helpful).
- Surgery is indicated for symptoms, subclinical osteoporosis, or kidney stones, and if calcium is more than 1 or 2 points above normal.
- The adenomatous gland is removed. In hyperplasia, 3.5 of 4 glands are removed.
- Risks include injury to recurrent laryngeal nerve and hypocalcemia (due to loss of glands and hungry bone syndrome, where bones try to make up for previous osteolysis).
- For Paget's disease (alkaline phosphatase and urinary hydroxyproline are elevated), use medications (steroids/alendronate/calcitonin) if the disease is progressive, painful, or widespread or if there are fractures or neurologic deficits.

Hypoparathyroidism
See Chapter 3 for a discussion of hypocalcemia.
- Can occur after thyroid surgery, radiation, autoimmune syndromes, infiltration (hemochromatosis).
- Differential diagnosis: pseudohypoparathyroidism (PTH resistance—Albright's syndrome), vitamin D deficiency (rickets in kids, osteomalacia in adults; bowing occurs only in rickets), acute pancreatitis.
- Treat with calcium and vitamin D. PTH will soon be commercially available.

Polyglandular Autoimmune Disease
Type 1: Mucocutaneous candidiasis, hypoparathyroidism, Addison's disease, alopecia, vitiligo

Type 2: Insulin-dependent diabetes mellitus, Addison's disease, Hashimoto's disease, hypogonadism, hypoparathyroidism

Finer Points of Metabolic Defects

Hemochromatosis is due to iron overload (excessive GI absorption), leading to liver failure, CHF, bronzing of the skin, diabetes, hypogonadism, and pseudogout (calcium pyrophosphate deposition—weakly positive birefringent crystals). Therapy helps all of those except pseudogout and hypogonadism.

Acute intermittent porphyria attacks are precipitated by alcohol, sulfonamides, anticonvulsants, and barbiturates. The defect is in hemoglobin synthesis. Signs and symptoms include abdominal pain and neuropathy. Diagnose by urine porphobilinogen and delta-aminolevulinic acid. Treat with blood transfusions.

Procollagen deficiencies cause osteogenesis imperfecta (type I; blue sclera); Ehlers-Danlos syndrome (type II; finger hyperextensibility), and chondrodysplasia (type III). Fibrillin deficiency causes Marfan syndrome.

Gout causes tophi, arthritis (negatively birefringent crystals), and uric acid stones. Treat with uricosurics (probenecid) if the urine urate is < 700 mg/d. Use allopurinol for high-production cases (urine urate > 700 mg/d). See Chapter 17 for more information.

Lesch-Nyhan syndrome (due to hypoxanthine-guanine phosphoribosyltransferase deficiency) causes gout, CNS problems, and self-mutilation.

Wilson's disease is due to deficient ceruloplasmin (copper transport), leading to deposits in the cornea (Kayser-Fleischer ring), liver, and basal ganglia. It can present with simultaneous fulminant hepatitis and Coombs'-negative hemolytic anemia. Treat with lifelong penicillamine (can cause pancytopenia) and sometimes liver transplant.

Gaucher's disease is an autosomal-recessive glucocerebrosidase deficiency. Signs and symptoms include liver and marrow failure. Diagnose on marrow biopsy (Gaucher's cells). Treat with aglucerase (synthetic enzyme).

Tay-Sachs disease is due to an autosomal-recessive deficiency (common in Ashkenazi Jews and French Canadians) of hexosaminidase A and causes accumulation of GM2 ganglioside, cherry-red spot, and death in infancy.

Fabry's disease is an X-linked deficiency of alpha-galactosidase. It causes heart and eye problems.

14

Glycogen storage disorders: Type 1 (von Gierke's) is G6PD deficiency and it affects the liver. Type 2 (Pompe's) affects the heart due to lysosomal alpha-glucosidase deficiency. Type 5 (McCardle's) affects muscles due to phosphorylase deficiency.

Niemann-Pick disease is due to sphingomyelinase deficiency. It causes a cherry-rod spot in the retina.

BIBLIOGRAPHY

Reviews

Adler RA, Rosen CJ. Glucocorticoids and osteoporosis. Endocrinol Metab Clin North Am 1994;23:641–54.

Andrews NC. Disorders of iron metabolism. N Engl J Med 1999;341:1986–95.

Baran DT. Osteoporosis. Obstet Gynecol Clin North Am 1994;21:321–35.

Clark CM, Lee DA. Prevention and treatment of complications of diabetes mellitus. N Engl J Med 1995;332:1210–7.

Conn PM, Crowley WF. Gonadotropin releasing hormone. N Engl J Med 1991; 324:93–103.

Cook DM, Loriaux DL. The incidental adrenal mass. Am J Med 1996;101:88–94.

Dayan CM, Daniels GH. Chronic autoimmune thyroiditis. N Engl J Med 1996; 335:99–107.

DeFronzo RA. The triumvirate: beta cell, muscle, liver. A collusion responsible for noninsulin-dependent diabetes mellitus. Diabetes 1988;37:667–87.

Delmas PD, Meunier PJ. The management of Paget's disease of bone. N Engl J Med 1997;336:558–61.

Hermus AR, Huysonans DA. Treatment of benign nodular thyroid disease. N Engl J Med 1998;338:1397–404.

Joshi N, et al. Infections in patients with diabetes mellitus. N Engl J Med 1999; 341:1906–12.

Kaye TB, Crabo L. The Cushing syndrome. Ann Intern Med 1990;112:434–44.

Kitabchi AE, Wall BM. Diabetic ketoacidosis. Med Clin North Am 1995; 79:9–37.

Kuhl C. New approaches for the treatment of pregnant diabetic women. Diabetes Rev 1995;3:621–31.

Lorber D. Non-ketotic hypertonicity in diabetes mellitus. Med Clin North Am 1995;79:39–52.

Marsh DJ. Medullary thyroid carcinoma. Thyroid 1995;5:407–24.

Melmed S, et al. Recent advances in acromegaly. J Clin Endocrinol Metab 1995; 80:3395–402.

Molitch ME. Pathologic hyperprolactinemia. Endocrinol Metab Clin North Am 1992;21:877–901.

Nathan DM. Long-term complications of diabetes mellitus. N Engl J Med 1993; 328:1676–85.

Oertel YC. Fine-needle aspiration and the diagnosis of thyroid cancer. Endocrinol Metab Clin North Am 1996;25:69–91.

Robertson GL. Diabetes insipidus. Endocrinol Metab Clin North Am 1995; 24:549–72.

Samuels MH, Ridgway EC. Gonadotropin-secreting pituitary adenomas. Baillieres Clin Endocrinol Metab 1995;9:337–58.

Santoro N, et al. Hypogonadotropic disorders in men and women. Endocrinol Rev 1986;7:11–23.

Sarne DH, Schneider AB. External radiation and thyroid neoplasia. Endocrinol Metab Clin North Am 1996;25:181–95.

Siris ES. Paget's disease of bone. J Clin Endocrinol Metab 1995;80:335–8.

Surks MI, Ocampo E. Subclinical thyroid disease. Am J Med 1996;100:217–23.

Surks MI, Sievert R. Drugs and thyroid function. N Engl J Med 1995; 333:1688–94.

Thai AC, Eisenbarth GS. Natural history of IDDM. Diabetes Rev 1993;1:1–14.

Weetman AP, McGregor AM. Autoimmune thyroid disease. Endocrinol Rev 1994; 15:788–830.

Wysolemerski JJ, Broadus AE. Hypercalcemia of malignancy. Annu Rev Med 1994;45:189–200.

Guidelines

American Diabetes Association. Standards of medical care for patients with diabetes mellitus. Diabetes Care 1994;17:616–23.

American Thyroid Association. Treatment guidelines for patients with hyperthyroidism and hypothyroidism. JAMA 1995;273:808–12.

Burch HB. Evaluation and management of the solid thyroid nodule. Endocrinol Clin North Am 1995;24:663–710.

Elliott WJ, et al. Drug treatment of hypertension in patients with diabetes. Diabetes Rev 1995;3:477–509.

Studies and Trials

Chandalia M, et al. Beneficial effect of high dietary fiber in Type 2 diabetes. N Engl J Med 2000;342:1392–8. (*High dietary soluble fiber improves glycemic control and reduces lipids and hyperinsulinemia in Type II diabetics.*)

Chiasson JL, et al. The efficacy of acarbose in the treatment of patients with non-insulin-dependent diabetes mellitus. Ann Intern Med 1994;121:928–35. (*An RCT showing that acarbose reduced HbA_{1c} by up to 0.9%.*)

DeFronzo RA, Goodman AM. Efficacy of metformin in patients with non-insulin dependent diabetes mellitus. N Engl J Med 1995;333:541–9. (*Metaformin reduced HbA$_{1c}$ by 1.5% and when combined with glyburide by 1.7%.*)

Diabetes Control and Complications Trial. Retinopathy and nephropathy in patients with Type 1 diabetes 4 years after a trial of intensive therapy. N Engl J Med 2000;342:381–9. (*The reduction in risk of nephropathy and retinopathy from intensive therapy persisted for at least 4 years, despite increasing hyperglycemia.*)

Diabetes Control and Complications Trial. The effect of intensive therapy of diabetes on complications in Type I diabetes. N Engl J Med 1993;329:977–86. (*Over 6.5 years, the risk of nephropathy and retinopathy was substantially lowered by intensive glucose control. Intensive treatment increased weight gain and tripled rates of hypoglycemia but did not increase mortality or impair quality of life.*)

Fonseca V, et al. Effect of metaformin and rosiglitazone combination therapy in Type 2 diabetics. JAMA 2000;283:1695–702. (*Once-daily combined metformin + rosiglitazone improved glycemic control and insulin sensitivity more than metformin alone. Side effects were not increased in the combination group.*)

Gress TW, et al. Hypertension and antihypertensive therapy as risk factors for Type 2 diabetes. N Engl J Med 2000;342:905–12. (*Beta-blockers increase the risk of subsequent diabetes by 28% [a risk that should be weighed against their beneficial cardiovascular effects], whereas thiazides and other antihypertensives had no effect.*)

Lewis EJ, et al. The effect of ACE inhibition on diabetic nephropathy. N Engl J Med 1993;329:1456–62. (*An RCT showing that captopril reduced decline in renal function by 48% [an effect independent of blood pressure control].*)

Liberman UA, et al. Effects of alendronate on bone mineral density and the incidence of fractures in postmenopausal osteoporosis. N Engl J Med 1995; 333:1437–43.

15

The Medical ICU

If you carry a lantern, you will not fear the darkness. — Anonymous

The ICU is a dangerous place if you don't need it. — Dr. Roslyn Schneider

This chapter will focus primarily on those elements of medicine specific to the ICU, although the rotation should also serve as an excellent opportunity to learn about just about any area of internal medicine in the acute setting.

LAWS OF THE INTENSIVE CARE UNIT

This is courtesy of Drs. Mark Rosen and Dana Lustbader.
1. The wedge is always 15.
2. If we know what's really going on 20% of the time, we're doing well.
3. You cannot kill someone in an ICU; you have total control over all parameters.

TIPS FOR A BETTER LIFE

1. When in doubt, do what the nurses tell you to.
2. Don't forget to eat, sleep, or answer calls of nature.
3. Keep track of vital signs, medications, etc., but if you obsess over each little thing and try to fix all of the numbers, you will do more harm than good (to the patient and yourself).
4. Don't be afraid of the machines. The only way you'll learn about them is to play with them (under the supervision of a good resident or fellow, of course). And if you don't learn about them, you've wasted a whole month.
5. It is the nurses' job to inform; it is your job to decide.
6. *Never lose your cool.* Patience, confidence, and flexibility are the keys to procedures, management, and diplomacy (which are what this month is all about). If you lose your nerve, your friends will lose faith in you and your enemies will pounce.

7. Don't be afraid to sit and talk with the family (about medical and non-medical stuff); it's nice, sometimes all you can do, and good for you and them.

VENTILATORS

The purpose of INTUBATION is EXTUBATION. Each day ask if the patient is ready to come off the ventilator. — Dr. Paul Mayo

Don't let anybody tell you not to touch the ventilator. You must become familiar with it; otherwise, both your education and the patient's care are done a disservice.

Ventilator Settings

Ventilator settings are mode, rate, oxygen concentration, tidal volume, and positive end-expiratory pressure (PEEP). The blue panel on the right has the settings; the green panel on the left shows what is actually happening.

Modes

1. Assist control = continuous mandatory ventilation. This means that the patient will get the set rate of breaths at the set tidal volume, plus with any additional breaths the patient triggers, the machine will give the full tidal volume. If the patient is passive, he or she doesn't have to do any work. This is what patients are started on at admission. Remember that with this mode, the patient must be fairly coordinated with the ventilator (ie, use as much sedation as necessary; if he overbreathes too much, there is a big risk of respiratory alkalosis).
2. Synchronized intermittent mandatory ventilation (SIMV). The patient gets the set rate at the set tidal volume. Any additional breaths that are triggered, the patient has to do all of the work; thus, the tidal volumes are variable on the extra breaths. This is a mode used by the surgeons during weaning (by slowly decreasing the set rate of breaths, eventually the patient will do almost all of the work of breathing). This is not used in the MICU, for several reasons. As an aside, the old intermittent mechanical ventilation was asynchronous, so sometimes the machine would blow air in when the patient was exhaling (very bad).
3. Continuous positive airway pressure (CPAP) is used by medicine to wean (see below).

Waveforms

These are the shapes under the modes on the blue panel.

1. Square: rapid inflow and outflow of air; used when high flow is needed (eg, asthmatics) and in recording peak pressures in order to measure respiratory mechanics.
2. Ramp: rapid and slow component to inflow; physiologic; used in most cases.
3. Sine: archaic; not used currently.

Rate

Generally start at 12 to 14 breaths/minute, but targeted to achieve the desired $PaCO_2$.

Tidal Volume

This should be 5 to 8 cc/kg (ideal body weight) (used to be 12, but that had worse outcomes). (Increase or decrease the rate and tidal volume depending on acid-base status and ventilation needs.)

Oxygen Concentration

Try to get under 60%; prolonged use of high oxygen is toxic (pulmonary fibrosis, etc). Always start the new patient on 100% until you are sure of adequate oxygenation; then reduce oxygen as soon as possible to the lowest safe level.

Positive End-Expiratory Pressure

By applying pressure to always keep intrathoracic pressure high, alveoli are recruited and kept open, improving gas exchange. PEEP of 5 cmH_2O is standard to improve physiologic function (overcomes resistance of tubing and counteracts work of breathing due to auto-PEEP [see below]). A PEEP up to 10 is usually no problem. Use PEEP to reduce oxygen needs and improve pulmonary function. *The dangers of PEEP include barotrauma (pneumothorax, etc) and decreased venous return (and thus less cardiac output).*

Basic Mechanics

"Mechanics, Frank? Assist control 14 over 12, tidal volume 500, peak 40, plateau..." (meanwhile, everyone's eyes are glazed over).

Most of what is said on morning rounds is just a recital. So, once you know the terms, you're set.

Peak Pressure

This is maximum pressure during inspiration, the index of risk of barotrauma and decreased cardiac output. When doing mechanics, record during the square waveform. Most alarms don't go off below 50.

Plateau Pressure

Record by setting a plateau of 1 sec. Observe on the viewscreen that flow is stopped just after inspiration for that time; thus, the lung is not moving and pressure equilibrates to the plateau pressure.

Compliance

This is the change in volume for a given change in pressure (ie, tidal volume divided by [plateau – PEEP]). Normal is 50 to 70 for a ventilated patient. Below 20 is very bad (stiff lung; probably ARDS). Compliance is one indicator of the health of the lung parenchyma. Remember that emphysema patients have high compliances to start with.

Resistance

This is the change in pressure for a given flow (ie, [peak – plateau]/flow rate). Measure with the flow rate of 60 L/min (ie, 1 L/sec). Normal is under 20. Resistance is an indicator of the function of the larger airways. Remember that high PEEP will artificially lower resistance, and severe ARDS sometimes pulls the airway walls outward, lowering resistance as well.

Auto-PEEP

In patients with obstructive airway disease (asthma, emphysema), expiration takes a long time, and inspiration may occur prior to expiration being over (ie, breath stacking). Just like PEEP, this has the risk of barotrauma and decreased venous return. Measure auto-PEEP through the auto-PEEP button, which involves a 1-sec pause prior to inspiration (a stop in flow preinspiration will cause a sudden rise in pressure if there is auto-PEEP). Like plateau pressure, auto-PEEP requires a passive patient to be measured.

Sedation/Paralysis

Sedation is critical to good ventilation (reduced work of breathing, improved coordination, patient comfort). Lorazepam (Ativan) (20 mg/100 cc D_5W) and midazolam (Versed) (100/100) are commonly used (the former is less expensive). Fentanyl (narcotic: 2.5 mg/50 cc D_5W) can be added. For intubation, use etomidate (0.2–0.6 mg/kg; usually 20–30 mg).

If sedation is not adequate for safe ventilator use, paralysis may be needed. *It is extremely critical for the patient to be sedated while paralyzed (remember, you're basically locking them in; assess sedation by heart rate and blood pressure).* Atracurium is the main paralytic used here. (The main side effect is histamine release, so try to avoid it in asthmatics; it also causes tachycardia. The main advantage is plasma metabolism, so you can give it in those with liver or renal failure.) Vecuronium can be used (liver metabolism; can be used in renal failure as it doesn't have atracurium's side effects). The ER likes succinylcholine (too short acting even for a drip; the side effect is hyperkalemia, so avoid it in renal failure, muscle crush, and burn patients). Succinylcholine also has prolonged effects in patients with low plasma cholinesterase (some patients are homozygous for this trait). Pancuronium is an older agent.

Remember that neuromuscular blockading agents can lead to prolonged myopathy, especially if used more than 24 hours, and also in patients who are concomitantly on steroids or aminoglycosides.

Troubleshooting

The most common ventilator alarm is high peak pressure. Ninety-nine percent of the time, this is due to a mucus plug in one of the airways, which requires suction. To buy time, turn the PEEP off. Bronchodilators may also help in the obstructive lung disease patients.

The next most common alarm is low volumes being given. This is often due to a cuff leak (the endotracheal tube is held in place by a balloon, which keeps air from leaving the lung). Deflate the cuff and reinflate with 5 to 7 cc (more may cause mucosal ischemia). Check the ET tube's position as well. Note that when peak pressure goes off, the low tidal volume alarm goes off as well due to the safety pop of the valve.

Also common is the patient overbreathing the ventilator. This is bad because of the risk of barotrauma, work of breathing, etc. Further, high rates can lead to breath stacking, leading to auto-PEEP. This may be due to inadequate sedation, increasing ventilation requirement, or, quite commonly, inadequate volumes being given (cuff leak, etc). So assess and act accordingly.

15

Anybody on a ventilator who gets a pneumothorax has a high risk of tension pneumothorax (due to positive-pressure ventilation) and thus needs a chest tube.

Auto-PEEP may be present in patients with high pressures or over-breathing. You need to increase the time of expiration, so decrease the rate, increase sedation, and increase the inspiratory flow rate. You may need to allow permissive hypercapnia (ie, allow CO_2 to rise to avoid other risks).

Weaning

Sometimes, if you want to learn to fly, you have to jump off a cliff. — Dr. Bala Ambati

CPAP is used to wean patients in the ICU and stepdown. Notice that CPAP and PEEP are the same analog dial on the ventilator. CPAP (of x amount of pressure) keeps the alveoli open. When on this mode, the patient has to breathe at his or her own rate and do his or her own work. The ventilator will assist with CPAP and also pressure support, which will provide x amount of pressure with each breath. If pressure support is 20 or 30, the patient is not really doing any work. So, the patient is a candidate for extubation if he or she tolerates CPAP with low pressure support.

Prior to weaning, assess the patient's work of breathing, work capability, CO_2 production, dead space fraction, and central driver. The patient is a candidate for a weaning trial based on clinical context. Ask the following:

- Is what got the patient on the ventilator getting better?
- Is the lung status (as assessed by gas exchange and mechanics) good?
- Is the patient neurologically alert enough (off sedation, good gag reflex, etc)?
- Is the patient's musculature strong enough?

Toleration of CPAP is assessed by the rate and tidal volume (tidal volume/rate > 100 is great), gas exchange, and the patient's perception. On occasion, after CPAP, the patient can be put on a T-piece (connection of tube to wall O_2): if the patient is okay on this, he is overcoming the extra work of breathing and is ready to come off.

Newly intubated patients can be rapidly weaned. Stepdown is for those who need to be weaned over the long term. Such patients should have a tracheotomy, which lets them eat and speak, and patients can come off sedation.

Ventilatory Strategies and Advanced Mechanics

Acute Respiratory Distress Syndrome

There are many areas of the lung perfused but not ventilated (ie, lots of shunt). Avoid high tidal volume and keep the patient passive (sedated and coordinated to reduce barotrauma and CO_2 production and improve gas exchange, thus reducing the ventilation requirement). Assess PEEP by inflection point analysis: change the viewscreen to the pressure volume curve with zero PEEP and observe at which pressure the compliance (the slope of the curve) increases, which is the inflection point and the "best PEEP" (achieve maximum compliance, which represents optimal alveolar recruitment and thus mechanics and gas exchange, while leaving room for as much tidal volume as possible). Also, in this setting, keep oxygen as low as possible (with PEEP and medical management).

Obstructive Lung Disease

Go up on peak flow as needed and reduce the rate to control auto-PEEP. Use heavy sedation. Avoid paralysis (such patients are often on steroids). Keep track of auto-PEEP: if > 10 to 15, decrease the rate or tidal volume, or increase the peak flow, or use a square waveform.

Unilateral Lung Disease

Because one lung is perfused but not ventilated, there is a high shunt, leading to refractory hypoxia. The temptation to use PEEP to improve oxygenation is counterproductive, as PEEP goes only to the good lung, decreasing perfusion there and worsening the situation. Management is as follows:

- Lateral decubitus (put the good lung down, thereby increasing perfusion there preferentially by gravity). There is a risk of decubitus and lateral thoracic nerve injury (winged scapula), and if the bad lung is purulent, it can cause drainage of pus into the good lung.
- Place the Swan catheter into the proximal pulmonary artery of the bad lung and cause partial occlusion by inflating the balloon (if you get wedge tracing, you're too far in for this, as you will cause pulmonary infarction).
- Double-lumen endotracheal tube: ventilate only the good lung and optimize its mechanics.

15

Assessment of Coordination

- Rate (a high rate is uncomfortable and causes auto-PEEP).
- Triggering (if the patient initiates a breath but is not able to generate the minimum pressure to trigger a machine breath, this indicates weakness).
- Tidal volume starvation (the patient wants more volume than given) leads to double triggering and faster rate, etc. If the tidal volume is too low, increase it; otherwise, sedate the patient.
- Flow volume starvation (the patient wants a faster flow than given), usually central neurologic disease, causes up-concave waveform (artificially reduces peak pressure). However, this increases the risk of barotrauma. It also increases the work of breathing, reduces cardiac output, and cuts the efficiency of gas exchange. Don't try to match it with a higher flow rate (doesn't work); you need to sedate or paralyze.

Pressure Waveforms

You need a visual aid; look at the ventilator viewscreens, books, etc.

1. The pressure-time curve should be down-concave; if it is up-concave, there is an increased risk of barotrauma (see above).
2. Emphysema has a two-component expiratory phase (fast and slow, representing the difficulty of parenchyma to exhale).
3. Auto-PEEP has a sudden increase in pressure preinspiration if the flow is stopped.
4. Triggering difficulty: you can see on the monitor that the patient is trying to trigger with very weak breaths

HEMODYNAMICS

Types of shock:

- Hypovolemic
- Cardiogenic
- Distributive (includes sepsis, anaphylaxis, neurogenic)
- Obstructive (PE, tamponade)

Key hemodynamic parameters focus on volume status, cardiac function, vascular tone, and oxygen delivery.

Parameters include (see Table 15–1 for normal values)

- Central venous pressure (CVP) — measured in the superior vena cava; gives right atrial filling pressure and is a good marker of volume status, assuming that the right ventricle is okay.

- Pulmonary capillary wedge pressure (PCWP, or wedge)—we will explain how to measure this below; it is used for volume status and gives left atrial filling pressure.
- Cardiac index—cardiac output/body surface area
- Systemic vascular resistance—(mean arterial pressure – CVP)/cardiac output (basically pressure gradient caused by flow of cardiac output).
- Oxygen delivery—DO_2 (oxygen delivery) = cardiac index $\times$ arterial O_2 content; VO_2 (oxgyen consumption) = cardiac index $\times$ (arterial – venous O_2 content); oxygen extraction ratio = DO_2/VO_2 (or [arterial – venous O_2 content]/arterial O_2 content).

A central line can be hooked up to a pressure transducer to yield CVP. For further measurements, you need a Swan-Ganz catheter.

A Swan is needed based on the clinical context; its use has decreased since literature over the past few years has cast doubt on its safety and efficacy. Basically, one would consider it if close monitoring of cardiac output, volume status, and/or oxygen delivery is required (eg, if the patient has both CHF and sepsis or is in cardiogenic shock). Always ask how the Swan is guiding management (in terms of volume, inotropes, pressors, etc).

Once the Swan introducer is placed, float the Swan. You know where its position is by looking at the pressure waveform (initially, CVP tracing, then right atrium tracing, then right ventricle tracing, which looks like ventricular tachycardia, then pulmonary artery tracing, which is the same as right ventricle except for dicrotic notch; once in the pulmonary artery, inflate the balloon and advance it until the pulmonary artery tracing converts to a wedge tracing, which is very similar to CVP tracing).

Table 15–1. Normal Hemodynamic Values

Central venous pressure	5 mm Hg
Pulmonary capillary wedge pressure	< 12 mm Hg
Cardiac index	2.6–4.2 L/min/m^2
Systemic vascular resistance	700–1,600 dynes $\times$ s/cm^5
Oxygen extraction ratio	25–30%

15

How Do You Get the Wedge?

This is the essence of looking good on rounds.

Look at a wedge tracing and line it up with the EKG tracing. There are a (atrial), c (early systolic isovolemic contraction after closure of atrioventricular valves), and v (ventricular) waves, each of which increases pressure. The a wave occurs just after the P wave, and the v a bit after the QRS (often during the T wave in the right atrium tracing but after T is in the wedge position). The a wave drops into the x descent, and the v wave drops into the y descent. The c wave is a blip on the x descent. The true wedge (end-diastolic pulmonary artery occlusion pressure) is the z point, which is the nadir of the valley between the a and c waves (if not obvious, pick the middle of the x descent).

If you look carefully at a wedge tracing, you will see that the baseline gently swings up and down, due to respiratory variation (Tracing 1, Appendix H). Wedge measurements should be done at end expiration, the relative valley in patients on ventilators and a relative hump on self-breathers. See Table 15–2 for special patterns.

If you're really paying attention, you'll see that the wedge is pretty close to the pulmonary artery diastolic. You can generally cheat and say that the PCWP is about 2 to 4 points below the pulmonary artery diastolic pressure (PADP). You can't use this rule of thumb in tachycardia (pulmonary artery diastolic is elevated due to lack of time to relax) or in pulmonary HTN. *If the wedge is higher than the PADP, that means the balloon is overinflated. Always deflate the balloon once you've taken the wedge tracing.*

Special Cardiac Catheter Patterns

- Equalization of end-diastolic pressures on all chambers occurs in constrictive pericarditis, effusion, and tamponade.
- A square root sign occurs in constrictive pericarditis and restrictive myopathy (this sign is also known as y greater than x pattern, seen in the Swan tracing).

How Do You Use the Numbers?

For cardiovascular assessment of interventions needed (ie, do you give volume, inotropes, or pressors?), look at PCWP, cardiac index (CI), and systemic vascular resistance, each of which can be low, normal, or high. Classic patterns of shock are listed in Table 15–3 (often you see mixed, which is when you need a Swan).

Table 15–2. Special Hemodynamic Patterns

Pattern	Causes
Cannon a waves	Atrioventricular dissociation (pacemaker, complete heart block)
	Mitral stenosis (see waves on Swan) (Tracing 2, Appendix H)
	Tricuspid stenosis (see on jugular pulse, central venous pressure tracing)
Cannon v waves	Mitral regurgitation (see on Swan) (Tracing 3, Appendix H)
	Ventricular septal defect
	Tricuspid regurgitation (see on jugular pulse, central venous pressure tracing)
Dampened x descent	Atrial fibrillation
Prominent x descent	Cardiac tamponade
Dampened y descent	Cardiac tamponade, mitral stenosis
Prominent y descent	Constrictive pericarditis, restrictive myopathy
Absent a wave	Atrial fibrillation, flutter, or standstill
Wedge not equal to left ventricle end-diastolic pressure	Mitral stenosis, left atrial myxoma, poor placement of Swan, decreased left ventricle compliance
Elevated mean pressure	Volume overload, ventricular failure, tamponade, atrial myxoma

Mixed venous O_2 gives an indication of oxygen delivery; it may be falsely high in septic states when peripheral tissues have impaired oxygen uptake.

Specific Interventions (ie, The Dreaded Drips)

- Pressors (the idea is to preserve cerebral and cardiac perfusion at the other's expense):
  - Dopamine (400 mg/250 cc D_5W): mild inotrope and pressor (has both alpha and beta receptor activity); definite chronotrope. Doses of 2 to 5 μg/kg/min are considered renal doses (due to dopaminergic receptors in the kidney). The main disadvantage is tachycardia.

Table 15–3. Classic Patterns of Shock

Pressure	Wedge Index	Cardiac Resistance	Systemic Vascular	Type
Hypovolemic	Low	Low	High	
Cardiogenic	High	Low	High	
Distributive	Low	High	Low	

- Norepinephrine (Levophed; 16 mg/250 cc D_5W): mostly pressor; much less tachycardia. This is the workhorse pressor.
- Phenylephrine (Neo-Synephrine): pure alpha agonist. Not used often (they say because it doesn't work, although we've never seen it used, so we couldn't say).
  - Inotropes (use in low cardiac output states; beware of ischemic risk):
  - Dobutamine: workhorse inotrope; also causes tachycardia and sometimes hypotension; used as a dobutamine "holiday" for chronic CHF patients.
  - Amrinone, milrinone (phosphodiesterase inhibitors, increase cAMP): not used much because of a concern over mortality; these are pure inotropes (no increase in heart rate, which is a theoretical plus).
- Vasodilators (for malignant HTN, etc):
  - Nitroprusside (tachyphylaxis after 2–3 days; also a risk of cyanide toxicity)
  - Labetalol
- Rate control (see Chapter 6).

ACID-BASE STATUS

Respiratory disturbances will be taken care of by the ventilator (adjust the rate and tidal volume as needed). Ventilator settings can also be used to compensate for metabolic disturbances. See Chapter 3 for a full discussion of metabolic acidosis and alkalosis.

Diabetic Ketoacidosis

Quick Points
1. Usually (but not always) in type I diabetics.
2. Can be precipitated by illnesses or not taking medications, or can be how the patient presents.

Initial Management
1. *Most important is hydration with NS of at least 1 to 2 liters in the first 2 hours* (if you're alone with a DKA patient and had to pick between saline and insulin, pick saline).
2. Insulin drip: give 10 U regular insulin IV bolus and then 0.1 U/kg regular insulin/hr.
3. Need fingerstick glucose q1h, frequent input and output, ABGs, and SMA-7 (monitor potassium, bicarbonate, anion gap, and phosphate closely) (need A-line and MICU for such frequent blood draws).
4. Start D_5 once glucose is < 250 mg/dL.
5. Patients will usually have high potassium on admission due to acidosis but are likely potassium depleted. Thus, begin fluid replacement with 10 to 20 mEq KCl/L of NS and continue as long as the patient is on IV insulin. Actively replete potassium when it goes below 5 mEq/L.
6. Give bicarbonate only if the pH is < 6.9, bicarbonate is < 5 mEq/L, or potassium is > 7 mEq/L, or if the patient has hyperkalemic EKG changes, hypotension refractory to fluids (acidosis can impair vasoconstriction), or extreme air hunger.
7. Once the bicarbonate is > 18 mEq/L or the anion gap is < 15, you can cut the insulin drip to 1 to 2 U/hr. When the patient can eat, give subcutaneous regular insulin 1 hour before discontinuation of drip (otherwise, the patient can lapse immediately back into DKA).

Nonketotic Hyperosmolar Coma

1. Sugars can be astronomical (sometimes over 900 mg/dL). Patients are often very dehydrated and elderly. Hyperviscosity can cause DIC.
2. You need aggressive hydration as above. But be careful with free water (a too rapid correction can cause cerebral edema as in the management of hypernatremia).

15

HOUSEKEEPING

1. Get on the nurses' good side (they run the place and can make life heaven or hell).
2. Renew drips each day
3. Get TPN orders down early; TPN requires a dedicated clean port (internal jugular vein/subclavian, not femoral).
4. Do a system-by-system assessment each day (don't forget weaning and feeding).
5. Organ transplant team: nice people but slavedrivers.
6. Overnight intern: make sure labs and x-rays are in for *all* patients.
7. *Learn how to use the IV pumps and to suction the patients* (the latter can be a lifesaver).
8. Remember that you're running the case, not the privates (but keep them informed).
9. Be aware of transfusion-related lung injury and post–re-expansion pulmonary edema.
10. Don't forget famotidine (Pepcid) and heparin (especially in A-line) as causes of thrombocytopenia.
11. *Don't forget GI and DVT prophylaxis.*
    - Risk factors for stress-related GI bleeding are coagulopathy and mechanical ventilation for greater than 48 hours. These are the only situations where prophylaxis is indicated.
    - DVT prophylaxis is indicated in basically everyone who is bedridden for > 24 to 48 hours.

PROCEDURES

How do you hide something from an internist? Put a dressing on it.— Anonymous

The only thing we have to fear is fear itself.— Franklin Delano Roosevelt

If you have the manual dexterity to successfully feed yourself, you can probably perform most procedures.— Dr. Tyler Smith

Nuts and bolts should be explained at the bedside by your resident and fellow. Be aggressive about lines, dressings, tubes, etc. Just a few general points here:

- Don't be afraid to try new procedures under supervision.
- Be patient, flexible, and cool (can't be emphasized enough).
- Focus on the procedure (not about bleeding, pain, etc, except to keep the patient comfortable).
- Try not to dirty the bed (put chucks underneath, lest the nurses hate you).
- X-rays for neck and subclavian lines to assess placement and rule out pneumothorax.
- Internal jugular veins: anterior — easy but scary; posterior — little risk but a fishing expedition.
- You sometimes need to shallow the angle or pull the needle back to pass the wire (almost always you're too far in or at too steep an angle). *Never lose the wire.*
- Learn to be nimble with your left hand (you can and must). Never do a procedure from the other side; you lose perception and perspective. (We know, we're going against the attending physicians on this one, but the rewards of a useful left hand are great; trust us.)
- Lines are replaced if and when they get infected, not the traditional every 8 days.
- Intubating: check the light and the balloon; don't go without seeing the cords (let the fellows explain the rest).
- Make sure to take the lines out before the patient leaves the ICU.
- Oral-gastric tubes are preferable to NG tubes because the latter cause sinusitis.

EVALUATING

No reason for admission, no reason for discharge. — Anonymous

The philosophy of the ICU is that the doctors are the same, but it's the nursing care that's different (two patients per nurse, better nurses, etc). Core indications for ICU are as follows:

1. Ventilator
2. Invasive monitoring (A-line, Swan)
3. Titratable drips (hemodynamic drips, insulin, etc)
4. Risk of needing 1 to 3

15

Notes on Evaluating

1. The fellow will do what you say in general; when presenting, you should have a recommendation for accepting or rejecting with a cogent rationale.

2. If you don't know what to do, just present the facts; see if any core needs are present.

3. Don't be afraid to ask the fellow to look at the patient too (except at 3 AM).

4. Evaluations should be responded to within 15 minutes.

5. When getting an ER evaluation or any evaluation from any service that is not a reliable medicine team, don't take any information over the phone (what they say doesn't make sense and it's not true). Just take the name and bed number because you have to see the patient anyway; talking on the phone is just a waste of time.

6. When rejecting, remember to write a decent note (why you were called, pertinent history, physical, labs, x-ray, and recommendations on management and when they should call you back) (don't just write "not a candidate...").

7. If you accept, be sure to have the ER or whomever get stuff done that needs getting done (don't dump on your co-team) as the ER can get scans and tests quicker than anybody (your job is not just to evaluate but to ensure proper patient care).

8. Similarly, if there is a delay in transfer to the MICU, make sure the floor team has a plan of action to keep the patient alive until they arive. *If the patient possibly has sepsis, insist that the ED/floor gives antibiotics immediately (don't wait for a transfer).*

9. *Always write "discussed with fellow"* and local house staff.

ELECTROLYTES, ENDOCRINE ISSUES, AND MISCELLANEOUS

1. Hyponatremia: Try fluid restriction first; demeclocycline or fluids + furosemide (Lasix) are other options; hypertonic saline if seizures/lethargy; increase Na 1 mEq/1–2 h lest you get central pontine myelinolysis.

2. Hypernatremia. Replace half of the free water deficit over the first 24 hours.

3. Hyperkalemia. You know what to do (if you don't, you shouldn't be in the ICU). Caution: In digoxin patients with high potassium, *avoid* calcium (increased risk of arrhythmia).

4. Hypokalemia. This is important in cardiac disease and digoxin patients, and potassium is important to muscle strength.

5. Hypercalcemia. You know what to do (symptoms: stones, bones, groans, and psychic overtones).

6. Hypocalcemia. This can cause cardiac problems and refractory hypotension.

7. Hypomagnesemia. This can cause cardiac problems, refractory hypocalcemia, hypokalemia.

8. Phosphorus is important to muscle strength for weaning, etc.

9. Ratios of blood products to be given:
   - 10 U PRBC: 5 U platelets
   - 5 U PRBC: 2 U fresh frozen plasma
   - 3 U fresh frozen plasma: 10 U cryoprecipitate
   - Watch ionized Ca^{2+}

10. "It's better to bleed from a full tank than from a half tank." (Dr. Paul Mayo)

11. "All bleeding stops." Surgery's famous last words.

12. Octreotide drip is in vogue for all kinds of GI bleeding (reduces splanchnic blood flow).

13. Intracranial hypertension:
    - Dexamethasone (Decadron) to reduce edema and improve cerebral compliance (doesn't work for hemorrhagic or stroke edema)
    - Mannitol (controversy about use pre- or postherniation; use this to briefly bridge the patient to definitive treatment as its effect lasts 24 hours or less)
    - Phenytoin (Dilantin) for seizure prophylaxis
    - Hyperventilation

14. Be aware of the need for stress-dose steroids and presentation of addisonian crisis.

15. Malignant hyperthermia. This can occur with anesthetics, phenothiazines, and haloperidol; cool with ice, water, cooling blanket, fan, and fluids, consider dantrolene and bromocriptine (use the latter if neuroleptics are involved). Watch carefully for rhabdomyolysis, renal failure, and metabolic acidosis and treat accordingly.

15

16. For thyroid storm, give propylthiouracil and beta-blockers; consider potassium iodide.

17. For myxedema coma, give thyroxine + steroids (hydrocortisone 100 mg IV q.8h), as the body's reserve of steroids may be used quickly.

BIBLIOGRAPHY

References are included in Chapters 6 and 7.

PRIMARY CARE

16

Ambulatory Medicine

I desire no epitaph than the statement that I taught medical students in the wards, as I regard this by far the most useful and important work I do.
—Sir William Osler

The availability of good medical care is inversely related to its need in the population. —Terry Hart

WELCOME TO CLINIC

A. Clinic is a unique experience, loved by some and loathed by others. Make no mistake, you will *work* in clinic. Clinic affords a more long-term understanding of patients and their care and also lets you work on the nonemergent problems that make up 99% of medicine.

B. Time is your greatest enemy in clinic. As an intern, you will only be booked 1 to 4 patients a session, and you will initially develop a very ornate and detailed H&P for your patients. Alas, this does not last, and by second and third year, you'll be seeing up to 10 or so people in a 3-hour period. Don't take it too hard; after all, in outpatient practice, the average speed is 1 patient every 15 minutes (if that). Here are some tips on time management:

1. *Focus.* If the patient is in for a specific complaint, do *not* do a full physical; just check the affected area and look for other problems you may expect. Likewise, such a visit is *not* the time to explore psychosocial issues or to get into a discussion on smoking cessation or weight loss. The above are important parts of the primary care spectrum but are best done either at sessions specifically geared for such topics or at the initial intake interview, when you will have more time. Properly focused, you will get done in 10 to 15 minutes, and the patient will be happy that you addressed the problem so succinctly.

2. *Presenting.* Some attending physicians love to teach, and although this may be good for your learning process, it plays havoc with the day's schedule. It is worse if the attending physician is long-winded as there may be a two- to three-person line waiting. This can get very nerve-wracking when your patients in the waiting area begin to stalk you and throw you dirty looks. The only way around this is to (a) have a very focused presentation to the attending physican, (b) find fast attending physicians when possible, and (c) see "overlap" patients in other examination rooms (usually not feasible). *Do not* tell the attending physician to hurry up, but *do* let him or her know you have a serious backlog problem; remember, they want to leave by 5 PM too.

3. *Talkers.* Not all will come with a specific complaint. The weird, the disorganized, the intoxicated, the insane, and the very nervous will most likely defy all normal attempts at a focused H&P. To move things along is key here, and the best way to do that is to organize them yourself. Picking the major complaint to work on for the session is extremely helpful, and assurances that other, lesser problems will be worked out in future are usually enough for most "difficult" patients. Often, these people only want attention, and the simple fact of you helping with even one problem is enough for them.

4. *Somatizers.* These people are a specific subgroup of talkers and are very hard to manage. They present with vague, nonspecific stuff that defies work-up because nothing organic is there. You must never dismiss a somatizer's complaints as being "psychological" as this will simply cause an escalation in symptomatology. Rather, it is best to simply offer support and try remedies that may have a chance at working, even if homeopathic. Knowing the patient is your best defense.

5. *Organization.* You will find that your initial H&P visit can be much more regimented than the 20-minute follow-ups or walk-ins. Because of this, it helps to get down an H&P "speech" that covers all of the primary care bases. If you can stick to this and use it as a guide, it takes very little time in the long run. Below is an example:
   a. Introduction: "Are you here for a physical or is there a specific problem I can help you with?"

b. Discuss past history, medications, and allergies.

c. Discuss social history with an eye to (1) smoking, (2) ethanol abuse, (3) physical and/or sexual abuse (includes elder abuse), (4) family status and household situation, (5) environmental dangers (ie, pets in asthma), (6) sexual orientation and use of protection, and (7) seatbelt and firearm issues.

d. Discuss primary care history: (1) last PPD/TB status, (2) vaccinations, (3) need for Pap/pelvic examination and/or mammogram in females, (4) estrogen replacement therapy use in females, (5) need for flexible sigmoidoscopy in everybody for cancer screening, and (6) the patient's cholesterol level.

e. Discuss family medical history.

f. Do your examination.

g. Explain the plan in detail to the patient, repeating the most important parts again at the end.

h. Be sure to ask the patient for questions and if he or she needs any prescriptions (every visit).

6. *Non-English speakers.* Although you will invariably pick up a few medical and examination terms in other languages, it is not only impossible to do a real H&P with non-English speakers but also downright dangerous. Although irritating in the extreme to wait for translators, it is well worth it because it saves time in the end.

7. *How to keep things moving.* Here are some handy phrases to keep in mind for later use.

a. "Seems like you have a lot of medical problems; let's talk about the one that is bothering you most first."

b. "Uno momento señor, I will get a translator."

c. "What other problems do you have?" Believe it or not, this saves time because it prevents oddball stuff, like chest pain, from popping up at the end.

d. "Do you need any prescriptions?"

e. "Have you been to this clinic before?"

f. "Who is your regular doctor here?"

g. "Gosh, your back pain sounds terrible, but tell me a little about the…" (ie, change the subject).

h. "I'm sorry about the wait, but they keep overbooking me; I hate it as much as you do." You will use that a lot.

16

i. "How is the…" This is a good way to start an interview as it shows the patient you know his or her problems and gives you information on how he or she is doing.

COMMON DISORDERS

See Table 16–1 for screening guidelines.

Gastroesophageal Reflux Disease

1. GERD is a common complaint of many patients and may manifest as acid regurgitation, chest burning, swallowing pain, dysphagia, and even (with atypical symptoms) increased wheezing, hoarseness, and sore throat. People will describe a "little ball" in the lower chest, their teeth swimming in acid, and severe indigestion with certain foods (ie, chili dogs, pepperoni pizza, chocolate Armageddon cake, etc; you know, the stuff house staff eat). Helpful Spanish is "Tiene dolor con drage? Tiene acida? Acida con comeda?" to elicit symptoms.

2. This disease is caused by transient LES relaxation; there is no known treatment to control the basic pathophysiology (cisapride and other prokinetics only lower basal tone). As such, control is aimed at neutralizing stomach acid to correct symptoms.

3. Diagnosis is made mostly by a history of symptoms, but objective tests such as 24-hour pH monitoring and more frequently EGD are used for confirmation, especially in treatment failures.

4. Seven percent of the U.S. population have GERD and 2% have its major complication, erosive esophagitis, a precursor to Barrett's esophagus, which is an intestinal metaplasia of the squamous cell base of the esophagus. This has a high rate of change to esophageal cancer.

5. Management:

   a. First instruct the patient to avoid foods often responsible for lowering LES tone: onions, tomatoes, peppermint, chocolate, red wine/ethanol, fats, coffee, and garlic. The patient should also sleep with the head of the bed elevated. Look for medications (calcium blockers reduce LES tone).

   b. Failing this, the patient should be placed on an H_2-blocker such as ranitidine and, failing that, on a proton-pump inhibitor. It takes at least 4 to 6 weeks for esophageal healing to complete for erosive

Table 16–1. Screening in Primary Care

Screening Test	Indicated Population	Frequency of Testing
Breast cancer (mammogram + examination) (self-examination needed monthly)	Women aged 40–49 Women 50–75	Every 2 yr Annually
Chlamydia	Women at onset of sexual activity	Every 1–3 yr
Cholesterol	Men: age 35+ Women: age 45+	Every 5 yr
Colorectal cancer (rectal examination, guaiac + flexible sigmoidoscopy)	Average risk: age 50+ Moderate risk: age 40+ High risk (family history): age of earliest diagnosis in family	Every 3–5 yr Every 3–5 yr Every 2 yr (colonoscopy)
Diabetes	Family history, suggestive symptoms (polyuria, polydipsia, weight loss/gain)	As needed
Hepatitis B	High-risk groups (drug abuse, promiscuity)	Once
Hypertension	All adults	Every 2 yr
Influenza vaccine	Adults aged 65+, with comorbidities,* or health care workers	Annually
Mumps, measles, rubella vaccine	Those born from 1958–1980	Once

Table 16–1 continued on next page.

16

Table 16–1. Continued

Screening Test	Indicated Population	Frequency of Testing
Pneumococcal vaccine	Adults aged 65+ or with comorbidities†	Once
Influenza vaccine*		Annually
Prostate cancer (rectal examination; prostate-specific antigen still controversial)	Men over 50	
Testicular cancer	Men aged 20–39	Every 1–3 yr
Tetanus-diptheria booster	All adults	Every 10 yr

*Influenza vaccine should be given annually for all over 65, those with cardiac or pulmonary disease, and health care workers (including you).

†Pneumococcal vaccine is indicated for those with cardiac or pulmonary disease, diabetes, functional or anatomic asplenia, and those over 65 years.

esophagitis, and because the condition is chronic, this may recur if antacids are stopped.

c. Barrett's esophagus never goes away, and, depending on the degree of atypia, yearly EGD versus surgery may be needed.

d. Note that *H. pylori* is not associated with GERD and that its eradication may actually worsen the disease.

6. Pitfalls:

a. Beware of confusing GERD for anginal chest pain and vice versa. Unfortunately, GERD pain is often relieved by sublingual nitroglycerin as it works on the LES tone as well.

b. Uncontrolled asthma may be exacerbated by severe GERD; consider treatment with H_2-blockers. In these cases, *H. pylori* should not be treated in GERD or gastritis, only in PUD; therapies differ between treatment of PUD and GERD.

c. Try to avoid NSAIDs in GERD as for any other high acid condition.

d. Hiatal hernia is not always associated with GERD; only hernia types in which the LES is lowered below the diaphragm become symptomatic.

e. Finally, some drugs will increase GERD symptoms, such as calcium blockers and etidronate. Patients with more than 5 years of untreated GERD should probably be scoped to rule out Barrett's esophagus.

Hypertension

1. HTN, with the exception of diabetes, will be the most common problem for you to face in the general clinic setting. Like diabetes, this is an insidious disease that, to the patient, is usually without symptoms. This makes it hard to control as your treatments will offer no immediate gratification.

2. HTN can be grouped into two major categories: essential and secondary HTN:

a. Essential HTN is far and away the most common type; in the primary care setting, about 94% of your HTN is essential, which is to say that it has no definable medical etiology and its origins are lost in the dim jungles of speculative physiology.

b. Secondary HTN is, in some ways, good news for the patient, in that it is possibly curable. The bad news is that it's quite rare, comprising only about 5 to 10% of cases. The other bad news is that there are so many forms of secondary HTN that it is hard to know where to start your work-up.

3. Smoking does not cause HTN; alcohol does elevate BP.

4. Evaluation of HTN:

   a. All patients should be screened for HTN with the simple and quick BP cuff test.

   b. It is important to check BP over time to confirm HTN before consigning someone to a medicine or activity program. Usually, two elevated BPs over 1 month are enough, but at our clinic we like three.

   c. BP is categorized into four stages:
   - Stage 1 (140/90–159/99) is mild.
   - Stage 2 (150/100–179/109) is moderate.
   - Stage 3 (180/110–209/119) is severe.
   - Stage 4 (210/120 and up) is very severe.

   d. The risk of cardiovascular events goes up in a continuous and graded manner with HTN.

   e. Any BP that is very high (stages 3–4) and associated with symptoms such as vision change, chest pain, or headache will be classified as either hypertensive urgencies or emergencies.

   f. Urgency refers to high BP different in severity from the patient's baseline, with symptoms but without evidence of end-organ damage (see below).

   g. Emergency is when end organs, especially the kidney and retina, suffer from HTN, as evidenced by urinary protein on dipstick/urinalysis, hemorrhage in the retina on fundoscopy (yes, you must do fundoscopy on these people). Chest pain should prompt rapid MI work-up and BP control in this setting, and neurologic deterioration and signs of stroke are likewise medical emergencies.

   h. Hypertensive emergency necessarily requires transfer to the ER for admission, as the medicines used to treat it are often only available there or in a unit setting.

   i. Hypertensive urgency can be controlled in the office in the following ways:
   - First, administer the patient's own medications if he or she forgot to take them that day.
   - Second, try to maximize a present medication if not already done.

- Third, use either labetalol (200 mg PO) or clonidine (0.1–0.2 mg PO) for rapid control.
- *Do not* use nifedipine or sublingual nifedepine as this can drop BP inordinately fast, causing reflex tachycardia and ischemic stroke.
- Sometimes, judicious use of a benzodiazepine can help as well, especially if the patient is the overanxious type.

5. Treatment of HTN
   a. BP control is an art and not a science, especially considering that 94% of the time we don't know its actual cause.
   b. The biggest problem is that in most cases, patients will have no symptoms whatsoever from their increased BP, and you find yourself asking them to take bad-tasting, expensive, side-effect-producing pills essentially on faith. Patient education is your best hope in all of this, as is projecting your earnest care for the patient's long-term health. Don't use scare tactics; they don't work well (see Smoking).
   c. *Beta-blockers.* Probably the best all-around medicine, these work by beta-adrenergic blockade in the heart muscle and sinoatrial and atrioventricular nodes, reducing inotropy and rate, which leads to BP control. They are a "must-use" in those with prior MI and CAD for they have been shown to be cardioprotective. In long-term studies on antihypertensive use, patients on beta-blockers had the largest improvement in quality of life (same for diuretics). Potential pitfalls include the following: (1) depression and loss of mental arousal in the elderly, (2) they cannot be used in asthmatics, (3) type I diabetics may have their hypoglycemic warning signs masked by beta-blockade, and (4) impotence.
   d. *Diuretics.* Hydrochlorothiazide is another useful drug, especially in the African-American population, who tend to respond to this drug better than to others. In addition, they have little to no effect on cognition in the elderly and have been shown to also produce long-term cardioprotective effects. Low potassium states may occur.
   e. *ACE inhibitors.* A must-use in the diabetic patient, as they retard development of diabetic renal disease and can reverse microalbuminuria in those treated. These are nice drugs also as side effects (other than the infamous dry cough) are few and mentation is preserved. Increases in potassium may occur.

f. *Calcium channel blockers.* Although these drugs do appear to work well in the African-American population and in those with salt-sensitive HTN, so do thiazides. Calcium channel blockers have not been shown to improve long-term survival in hypertensives and are dangerous in those in the post-MI period. Their major problem is that the short-acting ones lower blood pressure too fast, resulting in reflex tachycardia. Note that nifedipine and amlodipine have mostly vasodilatory effects with little rate or inotropic alteration, whereas diltiazem and verapamil work more at the sinoatrial and atrioventricular nodes. These agents should basically be second line or ancillary and should never be used in their short-acting form.

g. *A word about nifedipine*: the *only* reasons to use this drug are the following:
  1. In patients with Raynaud's phenomenon
  2. In patients with esophageal spasm
  3. In patients on a β-blocker who are bradycardic but still hypertensive (adjunctive)
  4. When nothing else works

h. *Central agents.* Clonidine (alpha-2 agonist) is a very powerful vasodilator and antihypertensive with a few drawbacks. Its major problem is that there is a serious rebound effect after it is stopped. This leads to serious problems when compliance is poor, for if the patient forgets the dose, the consequences can be dire. The fact that the drug comes in a patch form is helpful, but clear and careful patient instruction is necessary when using it. For all that, it can often be the *only* drug that so much as dents a patient's pressure.

i. *Angiotensin antagonists* (eg, losartan [Cozaar]). These are pretty much the same as ACE inhibitors but not quite as well studied or proven to be cardioprotective. Most likely, they are just as good and lack the bradykinin effects purported to cause the "captopril cough." This is an ideal agent for the diabetic who cannot hack (ooooh...pun!!) ACE inhibitors.

j. *Nitroglycerin.* A reasonable agent for BP control in those with known angina or CAD, this is nonetheless only adjunctive and should never be used as a lone agent.

    k. *HTN in pregnancy*. Consider preeclampsia (look for proteinuria). Avoid ACE inhibitors and beta-blockers. You can use methyldopa and hydralazine.

6. *Causes of secondary HTN*:

    a. Renal (suspect when other tests reveal signs of dysfunction, ie, elevated BUN/Cr, proteinuria, polyuria/oliguria, history). Of course, many renal conditions may actually be due to untreated essential HTN, so this is tricky:

        1. Chronic pyelonephritis (should be evident from history)

        2. Acute and chronic glomerulonephritis (bad prognostic indicator).

        3. Polycystic renal disease (ultrasonography will confirm)

        4. Renovascular stenosis or infarction (work-up with nuclear medicine renography and treat with angioplasty; avoid ACE inhibitors in these patients). *Consider renovascular disease if HTN is abrupt in patients under 30 or over 50; if HTN is refractory, rapidly progressive, or very severe; if there is epigastric bruit; or if there is new or unexplained azotemia.*

        5. Diabetic nephropathy (note Rivan's syndrome)

        6. Reninomas (vanishingly rare)

    b. Endocrine

        1. Oral contraceptives (increase in intravascular fluid)

        2. Adrenocortical hyperfunction (Cushing's primary hyperaldosteronism; check morning cortisol levels especially if the patient has electrolyte abnormalities)

        3. Pheochromocytomas (everybody always checks for these; however, they are quite rare)

        4. Myxedema (all patients should have screening TSH)

        5. Acromegaly (you should be able to tell from examination)

    c. Psychological

        1. Don't scoff. We have had patients maxed out on nifedipine, clonidine, labetalol, nitroglycerin, verapamil, and furosemide with BPs of 210/100 who were immediately brought down to 140/90 by lorazepam. So there!

    d. Miscellaneous

        1. Coarctation of the aorta (check pulses on both arms)

        2. Polyarteritis nodosa

   3. Hypercalcemia
   4. Medications (glucocorticoids are notorious)
   5. But when do you do all of this work-up for secondary causes?
      a. When the HTN is in a young patient (ie, in their 20s)
      b. When the HTN is brand new in a previous normotensive
      c. When you suspect a secondary cause (see above)
      d. When your treatments are maxed out and have failed to pro-
         duce any good result
   e. Where to start:
      1. This largely depends on what you suspect. Lots of people rou-
         tinely send out urine metanephrines, vanillylmandelic acid, and
         the like when the chance of catching the elusive pheochromo-
         cytoma is very rare. If you do get a bonafide case of an adrenal
         tumor, you will see other abnormalites on the SMA-7 (low
         potassium and high sodium), you may note a visible tumor on a
         CT of the adrenals, and you may ask the nephrologist to do a
         renal vein sampling study, but, in all fairness, this is beyond the
         scope of your outpatient clinic.
      2. In any case, the best place to start is the H&P, which will yield
         most of the above secondary causes.
         a. Chronic pyelonephrits, acromegaly, and psychological prob-
            lems will all come out here, as will many cases of thyroid
            dysfunction and even Cushing's in most cases.
         b. Routine lab tests such as an SMA-7, urinalysis for protein,
            fingersticks, and TSH will help you determine many
            endocrine and renal causes.

Cholesterol

1. Hyperlipidemia is a common problem to be managed by the primary
   care physician, and high LDL and low HDL are both independent risk
   factors for CAD and cardiac events. Unfortunately, there is a bewildering array of medications for this disorder and an equally bewildering number of treatment recommendations based on cholesterol level.
2. A bit about lipids:
   a. LDL is the major bad guy, especially lipoprotein A (apoprotein
      B-linked LDL), the most atherogenic.
   b. HDL$_{(2)}$ is antiatherogenic.

    c. Triglycerides are probably atherogenic and can cause pancreatitis if levels > 1,000 mg/dL.

3. Screening management and use of fasting profile results (see Tables 16–2 and 16–3):

    a. Test adults over age 20 for nonfasting cholesterol/HDL. Risk factors are the CAD risk factors.

4. Goals of therapy:

    a. History of CAD, prior MI: < 100 LDL

    b. Two or more risk factors or diabetes alone: < 130 LDL

    c. Less than two risk factors: < 160 LDL

5. Diet therapy:

    a. Step 1 diet: total calories < 30% fat with less than 10% saturated fat and the remaining fat calories divided between omega-3 (fish

Table 16–2. Management Algorithm for Cholesterol Screening

Total Cholesterol	HDL > 35 mg/dL	HDL < 35 mg/dL
< 200	Repeat in 5 yr	Obtain fasting profile
200–239		
0 or 1 risk factor	Risk education; repeat in 1–2 yr	Obtain fasting profile
2 or more risk factors	Obtain fasting profile	Obtain fasting profile
> 239	Obtain fasting profile	Obtain fasting profile

Table 16–3. Use of Fasting Profile Results

LDL	0 or 1 Risk Factor	2 or More Risk Factors
< 130	Repeat in 5 yr	Repeat in 5 yr
130–159	Step 1 diet; repeat in 1 yr	Step 2 diet; work-up for hyperlipidemias
160–189	As above therapy	As above + drug
> 190	Step 2 diet; work-up for hyperlipidemias; drug therapy	Step 2 diet; work-up for hyperlipidemias; drug therapy

16

and flax oil) and polyunsaturated fat (vegetable oils, olive oil); < 300-mg cholesterol per day.

b. Step 2 diet: < 7% saturated fat and < 200-mg of cholesterol per day.

c. Check levels in 3 to 6 months or so to see if there has been an improvement.

6. Medications: HMG-CoA reductase inhibitors (lovastatin [Mevacor], simvastatin [Zocor], pravastatin [Pravachol], fluvastatin [Lescol], atorvastatin [Lipitor], N$statin) are the best overall medications (see Chapter 6).

Diabetes

See also Chapters 14 and 15.

1. Diabetes is a disease that we would not wish on our worst enemy. It causes damage to most bodily systems, which is often irreversible, and it is so insidious that most succumb to it through sheer inertia. Of what use is it to follow complex, irritating, and painful regimens if the disease doesn't even hurt? Compliance is always the greatest problem; and it increases geometrically with complexity. Only the most obsessive-compulsive of patients will be able to follow the regimens for tight control, and you must be, overall, realistic in your expectations.

2. *Screening.* All patients should be screened for diabetes. Type I diabetics will come to you with a known diagnosis, whereas type II not always will. As always, the H&P will be your best guide, and you must look for symptoms of polyuria, polydipsia, vision blurring, increased hunger, and neuropathic changes. Everyone should have initial lab work or at least a fingerstick to screen, especially those with positive family histories of type II diabetes.

3. *Lab tests.* Diabetes is defined as three fasting blood glucose levels above 126 g per deciliter or two measurements of random glucose above 200 with symptoms. A normal person should have a preprandial glucose level of < 115 and a bedtime level of < 120. Three fasting glucose levels of > 126 (consecutive) are indicative of diabetes. Other useful tests include checking a urine dipstick for glucose and checking a glycosylated hemoglobin in those with suspicion of disease. Normal people without DM will have glycohemoglobins below 6 (see below). In addition, lipid profiles must also be checked in those with suspicion of disease.

4. *Type I diabetes* is the result of the destruction of islet cells, usually at a relatively young age, from a presumed autoimmune reaction to a

viral pathogen (possibly coxsackievirus). Patients with DM type I suffer from an absolute lack of insulin and are very prone to DKA, as they have absolutely no insulin reserve. For DM type II patients, methods effective for control (see below) are worthless in this setting; insulin alone is effective. This is not a genetically inherited or common condition.

5. *Diabetes type II* is presumed to be the result of a decrease in receptor density at insulin target cells, possibly due to a combination of down-regulation from overproduction of insulin at the pancreas and to an increase of surface area (and thence a drop in receptor density) at fat-laden target cells in the liver, adipocytes, and skeletal muscle. The problem is a healthy pancreas in the face of an unhealthy periphery (the opposite of DM type I). The patient makes insulin, but the effect of the hormone is blunted or even lost in severe cases.

6. Pancreatic shock. Like the heart, the pancreas has a "starling curve" for insulin output. Simply put, the more sugar there is in the blood, the higher the output—to a point. Once the peak pancreatic output is reached, if the sugar level gets even higher, it begins to drop off. This accounts for the failure of sulfonylureas (see below) in very poorly controlled DM type II patients; the drug simply can't stimulate any more insulin output in the tired pancreas.

7. The hope for DM type II. If your patient has DM type II, he or she has some good news. The condition can be cured without resorting to shots or even drugs. The bad news is the patient will have to lose weight and exercise. Even a loss of 5 to 10% of body weight and a simple exercise regimen of 20 minutes of aerobic activity a day will markedly improve sugars and glucose tolerance. The downside, of course, is that motivation is—well—elusive to most people. DM type II doesn't hurt and rarely causes any discomfort, whereas dieting and exercise do. It is also, admittedly, not foolproof, as there are thin diabetes type II patients.

8. Medicinal treatment. There are a number of treatments for hyperglycemia, and these depend on the type of diabetes and other patient characteristics.

   A. Type I DM. Unfortunately, these people suffer from an absolute lack of insulin, so insulin is the only viable treatment. Overall, they should be followed by a diabetes specialist as their disease is extremely brittle and they are prone to both hypoglycemia (from treatment) and ketoacidosis (from failure of treatment), both of which are not within the scope of outpatient medicine. Nevertheless, tight control of blood glucose levels has been shown to significantly reduce morbidity in these patients (DCCT study), and that morbidity correlated well with HbA_{1C} levels. The goal of the trial was to keep the glycohemoglobin below 8.0 (they got down to 7.2%), and very tight control was needed, including fingersticks four to five times a day and very low glucose targets. Suffice it to say that, as in DM type II patients, the goal is to keep fasting glucose between 80 and 120, with changes in regimen if it is < 80 or > 140. Treat with insulin replacement; islet cell transplants are becoming a reality over the next few years.

B. Insulin
  a. Insulin comes in three major forms and is now almost all recombinant human insulin.
  b. Neutral protein hagedorn (NPH) is the long-acting form, its activity peaking 6 to 8 hours after administration.
  c. Regular insulin is intermediate, peaking at around 1 to 2 hours.
  d. Lispro is fast acting and peaks in about a half hour or less.

C. Regimens. Basically there are two major ways to go with this, standing and sliding scale regimens:
  a. Sliding scale up side: (1) tight control, (2) allows more dietary freedom, (3) closer to "natural physiology," (4) less chance of hypoglycemia, (5) more reactive in cases of infection
  b. Sliding scale down side: (1) diabetes becomes the patient's major hobby, (2) more painful, (3) hard to follow for patients with limited compliance ability
  c. Standing regimen up side: (1) only around two sticks a day, (2) easy to follow and administer
  d. Standing regimen down side: (1) needs more frequent physician adjustments

D. Type II DM. This is a bit easier to treat in that we have more varied medications.
  1. Sulfonylureas. These medicines are used frequently and act by increasing insulin production by the pancreas. They are capable of causing hypoglycemic reactions and can induce kidney dam-

age in the sensitive, so use with some caution. The up side is that they can be taken once a day.

2. Metformin (Glucophage). This is an excellent drug that literally attacks the lesion of DM type II by increasing receptor density and thus decreasing insulin resistance. Unlike the above class, it is effective even in states of pancreatic shock and can be combined with insulin or sulfonylureas. The down side is that in those with poor renal function (which unfortunately includes many with DM type II), a fatal lactic acidosis can occur, especially if the patient becomes dehydrated. This should not be used in elderly patients with poor GFR and propensity to dryness

3. Troglitazone (Rezulin). This is another drug that attacks the lesion and without that pesky kidney clearance problem. Unfortunately, this medicine has a nasty habit of burning the liver, so it has become less popular.

4. Acarbose (Precose). This unabsorbable sugar competes with glucose uptake in the gut, decreasing sugar levels. It is sort of a "diet in a pill." The down side is a pesky osmotic diarrhea that many dislike. It is, however, otherwise quite harmless.

5. Never forget that diet and exercise are the best first steps in the treatment of this disease.

E. The fingerstick

   a. Fingerstick checks are the bane of all diabetics, but they do help immensely in the control and management of this disease.

   b. For tight regimens of sliding scale control, fingersticks will need to be done at least four times a day.

   c. For those on standing regimens, you can usually use a twice-daily or even once-a-day regimen after good control is established; prior to this, a three-times-a-day regimen is usually needed for your assessment of how well the regimen is working.

   d. It should be noted that, overall, the HbA$_{1C}$ (glycohemoglobin) is actually more accurate in that it represents a sum of control over 3 months or more and does not suffer from the vagaries of poor documentation and diet cheating.

F. Diabetic complications:

   a. *Retinopathy*. This needs to be followed by a 6-month retinal examination to look for cotton-wool spots and other changes

16

indicative of poor glycemic control. Note that optical changes in diabetics may not represent actual retinopathy or retinal hemorrhage but may be due to clouding of the lens from high levels of blood glucose. Retinal detachment and cataracts need to be treated by an ophthalmologist and require referral.

b. *Polyneuropathy.* This is nerve damage resulting in the loss of (usually) sensory power over various areas of the body. Most frequently, the extremities (feet) are involved, and this can potentially be serious as these patients are often unaware that they have injured themselves. Testing with a monofilament for fine tactile sensation is useful in assessing this. In addition, occasionally, odd clusters of nerves are affected, such as the oculomotor cranial nerves, resulting in optic palsy. Another common site of neuropathy is the penis, with loss of erectile function or gastroparesis resulting in nausea or severe constipation.

c. *Foot ulcer.* This problem is a common one as the neuropathy, combined with a sluggish immune system, results in an easily infected extremity. The feet have the poorest blood supply and the highest chance for loss of sensation and thus are most affected. Foot ulcers initially can be treated with oral antibiotics, but it must be remembered that these lesions are usually polymicrobial (in diabetics) and often have anaerobes. Clindamycin and ciprofloxacin are a good combination treatment. If the ulcer is deep or not healing, it may require long- or short-term surgical débridement, and if it progresses to osteomyelitis, long-term IV antibiotics.

d. *Infection.* WBCs function poorly in high glucose concentration states, affecting diapedesis and oxidative burst. As such, diabetics with poor control are more likely to become infected with cellulitis, pneumonia, tinea pedis and cruris (important entry sites for bacteria), folliculitis and boils, and influenza. Wherever possible, steps such as Pneumovax, flu shots, foot inspection with tinea eradication, and PPD skin testing with prophylaxis should be initiated.

e. *CAD.* Diabetics have a high incidence of CAD (DM is an independent risk factor), and this must be followed and controlled for. Diabetics are usually hypertensive, and this needs to be controlled, preferably with an ACE inhibitor (see below) or beta-blocker. ASA is also useful if the patient tolerates it. An EKG should be done yearly in all diabetics (this is also useful in assessing autonomic neuropathy as there will be a loss of sinus arrhythmia). In addition, cholesterol risk profiles need to be done to correct for dyslipidemia (see above).

f. *Microvascular disease.* The destruction of small vessels in diabetes is another crippling complication. In addition to the destruction of the small vessels of the feet and extremities leading to many of the problems above, the kidneys also suffer with resultant glomerulonephrosis and proteinuria, ultimately progressing to renal failure. HTN concomitant to DM needs to be controlled as well as it can further hasten renal deterioration, and the agent of choice for this is an ACE inhibitor (failing that an angiotensin antagonist). A useful screening test for diabetic nephropathy is urine microalbumin testing, which may be positive before gross proteinuria is noted on urinalysis.

g. *Hyperosmolar coma and ketoacidosis.* These are both described in Chapters 14 and 15.

Preoperative Evaluation

1. Surgeons will often send you patients for evaluation prior to a procedure. This usually happens when the patient is a bit ill or medically complex, and if there is one thing a surgeon does not want to have to deal with, it's medical complexity. Overall, they just want medicolegal assurance that the person isn't going to die of an MI on the table and cause a lot of yelling and screaming in the operating room. The question then comes down to just what, if anything, we can do to avoid this.

2. The basic preoperative evaluation depends on age, sex, and comorbidity. Although the whole process seems confusing at first, remember that you are only trying to figure out if you need (1) a CBC, (2) an EKG, and (3) a CXR. Overall, the need for these tests is pretty intuitive.

3. Tests:

a. CBC. This is needed in (1) women over 12, (2) those with a history of blood-losing conditions (ie, active PUD, diverticulosis, etc), and (3) anybody over 40. Remember that in those without a bleeding problem, a CBC is good for 1 year. You don't need to stick the person again.

b. EKG. This should be done in anybody over 40, but note that like the CBC, the EKG is good for 1 year.

c. CXR: This should be done in those 50 or over; you do not need one in an asthmatic. This is also good for 1 year.

4. What about other tests?

a. SMA-7. This should only be done prior to procedures involving contrast and is routinely done in cardiac patients to assess kidney function. Overall, it should only be done rarely and in cases in which you are seriously concerned about renal function deteriorating after the operation.

b. Echocardiograms, stress tests, and catheters. These need to be done in conjunction with a cardiologist's consult. In patients with serious heart trouble, a consult is a good idea.

c. Fingersticks. These need to be done prior to the procedure as the patients invariably are NPO on the day of the surgery and have not taken their diabetic medications. Insulin or D_{50} (50% dextrose solution) may be needed before or after the procedure.

5. Other considerations:

a. *Diabetics.* In addition to the fingerstick, a diabetic's oral medications should be held prior to the operation. If on metformin, they will need to stop it at least 2 days in advance, and if on a sulfonylurea, 1 day in advance. Diabetics should skip their morning insulin but not the evening dose before the day of surgery.

b. *Asthmatics.* This is usually not a big issue, and an albuterol (Proventil) nebulizer can be given before the operation. However, asthmatics currently on steroids or who are steroid dependent may require stress doses to cover a potentially fatal adrenal crisis. IV methylprednisolone prior to the operation and every 6 hours after for two more doses is usually sufficient (100 mg).

c. *CAD.* BP needs to be checked before the procedure and is often in need of correcting as the patient may have skipped his or her medicine that morning. Usually, a good plan is to give some or all of the antihypertensive in a short-acting form (ie, no diltiazem [Cardizem] CD) prior to the operation. This is usually going to be the call of the anesthesiologist.

d. *Endocarditis prophylaxis.* This is a pain because no one can remember what to give. So here goes:

1. Prophylaxis is recommended in (1) dental procedures, (2) periodontal surgery, (3) root canals, (4) bloody cleanings, and (5) major nondental procedures (such as oral, respiratory, esophageal, GU, or GI work).
2. What you give depends on the surgery.
3. Dental. The standard is amoxicillin 2 g prior to the surgery and, if allergic to penicillin, clindamycin 600 mg, cephalexin 2 g, or clarithromycin 500 mg preoperatively. Note that the second dose is no longer needed and that 2 g is as good as 3 g.
4. Other, non-GU/GI surgeries (including esophageal) require the same prophylaxis as above.
5. GI/GU. This depends on how high a risk you are. The high-risk patients need ampicillin and gentamicin (2 g IV + 1.5 mg/kg IV), whereas the moderate ones need only ampicillin (2 g IM/IV) or amoxicillin (2 g). In the penicillin resistant, you can use vancomycin (1 g IV) plus the above gentamicin dose.
6. Remember that all of this needs to be done in those with (1) mitral regurgitation, (2) documented valve disease (ie, positive echocardiogram), (3) emergencies, and (4) those with prosthetic valves.

Back Pain

Quick Points

- H&P should look for sciatica and serious conditions (eg, fracture, tumor, cord compression). Look for anesthesia, sphincter dysfunction, and major motor weakness. See Table 16–4 for worrisome findings.
- Eighty-five percent of back pain is due to mechanical causes, 7% to sciatica, 4% to compression fracture, and 0.7% to cancer.
- Spinal stenosis causes bilateral buttock, back, and leg pain. It is increased by extension (downstairs) and decreased by going upstairs. It is increased by standing (vs. claudication) and relieved by sitting.
- Sciatica (nerve root compression) is suggested by pain on ankle dorsiflexion that is relieved by plantar flexion and pain on straight-leg raising or leaning forward. Pain shoots down the leg to below the knee. Nerve compression is suggested by absent reflexes.
- Disc herniation (usually affects L5 or S1 nerve roots) is relieved by lying down; 95% of clinically significant disc herniations have sciatica.

16

Table 16–4. Worrisome Findings in Back Pain

Findings	Worry About
Fever Percussion tenderness Urinary tract infection Intravenous drug abuse	Infection
Abnormal pulses Pulsatile mass in abdomen	Abdominal aortic aneurysm
Age > 50 Prior cancer Weight loss Failure to improve in 1 month Pain not relieved by rest Pain at night	Cancer
Age > 70 Trauma Prior steroid use	Compression facture
Urinary/fecal incontinence/retention Saddle anesthesia	Cauda equina syndrome

- Neurologic findings are listed in Table 16–5.
- A straight leg test is positive for radiculopathy if pain occurs below the knee at < 70 degrees.
- A crossed-leg test and rectal examination for tone, sensation, and voluntary control can also be helpful. Without worrisome history or examination, 90% of patients with back pain will improve within a month.

Initial Management
- For patients with low back pain < 4 weeks without neurologic deficit, treat conservatively:
  - Rest < 2 to 3 days
  - NSAIDs
  - Heat/ice (whichever is helpful)
  - Gentle exercise and gradual return to normal activities
- If symptoms persist more than 4 weeks or there are neurologic deficits, consider neurologic evaluation and/or MRI.

- Talk to patients about workplace ergonomics and good posture. Bedrest is inferior to maintenance of activity in terms of recovery; physical restriction should be used only for severe back pain.
- *Malignancy is not relieved by lying down. Rule out cancer if there are back pain changes in the elderly.*

Smoking and Quitting

- If you don't ask, the patient won't tell you how much he or she smokes.
- Tell the patient that after quitting, the risk for heart disease decreases 50% in the first year and returns to that of nonsmokers in 10 to 15 years. The risk of cancer also approaches that of nonsmokers over 15 years. The rate of pneumonia declines rapidly.
- For those interested in quitting, have the patient keep a diary, identifying triggers and cues. Enlist family and friends. Frame relapses as learning experiences, not failures.
- Adjuncts to behavioral therapy should be used once and not before a quit date is set. Contraindications to nicotine replacement are recent MI, CVA, or pregnancy. Methods include nicotine patch, gum, and spray. Antidepressants including bupropion (Wellbutrin; Zyban) are effective as well. Tapering should be done over 8 weeks.

Table 16–5. Key Neurologic Examination Findings in Back Pain Evaluation

Tested Level	Motor Tests	Involved Sensory Area
L4	Knee jerk	Medial heel
L4-5	Walking on heels	
	Foot dorsiflexion	
L5	Great toe extension	Medial foot
S1	Walking on toes	Lateral foot
	Ankle jerk	

16

GERIATRICS

The goal of geriatric medicine is to improve overall function, maintain independence, and impact on quality of life. The "i's" of geriatrics are as follows: intellectual decline, immobility, incontinence, instability, impoverished, isolation, insomnia, impotence, iatrogenesis, irritable colon, immune deficiency, and impaired eyes and ears.

Remember that it is often difficult for the geriatric patient to report symptoms. Often, they are limited by visual, auditory, or cognitive impairments. An important aspect of the physical examination is to assess overall appearance with respect to grooming, hygiene, and nutritional status. It is also important to take notice of the patient's attention level. The physical examination should be detailed and should include a Mini-Mental State Examination (MMSE) and gait assessment.

Some General Principles

- In terms of dosing, start at the lowest dose and titrate up slowly.
- Don't forget to calculate creatinine clearance and adjust antibiotics.
- Ambulation is always preferable to bed rest; call Rehabilitation as soon as possible.
- Use haloperidol (Haldol) sparingly, as some may become parkinsonian.
- Discharge planning starts the day of admission, especially if you think the patient may need skilled nursing facility care.

Dementia Work-up

- Delirium versus dementia. The diagnosis of dementia cannot be made until delirium is excluded.
- It is important to rule out any reversible causes of dementia, so check
  - MMSE (Table 16–6)
  - TSH, reactive plasma antigen (RPR), B_{12}, folate
  - CT scan or MRI of the brain

Alzheimer's Disease

Alzheimer's disease affects many of our elderly. It has an insidious onset and progresses gradually. The characteristics of the disease include progressive memory deficit along with one other cognitive function. There is no specific biologic marker for the disease, and Alzheimer's must be considered a clinical syndrome with several etiologies. Drugs such as

Table 16–6. Mini-Mental State Examination

Orientation
  What is the (year) (season) (date) (day) (month)?
  One point for each correct response (maximum 5 points)
  Where are we: (state) (county) (town or city) (hospital) (floor)?
  One point for each correct response (maximum 5 points)

Registration
  Name three common objects (eg, "apple, table, penny").
  One point for each correct response (maximum 3 points)

Attention and Calculation
  Serial 7s, backwards. Stop after five answers.
  Alternatively, spell "WORLD" backwards.
  One point for each correct response (maximum 5 points)

Recall
  Ask for the three objects above to be repeated.
  One point for each correct response (maximum 3 points)

Language
  Name a pencil and a watch. (*2 points*)
  Repeat the following: "No ifs, ands, or buts." *(1 point)*
  Follow a three-stage command: "Take a paper in your right hand, fold it in half,
    and put it on the floor." *(one point for each part correctly executed)*
  Read and obey the following: CLOSE YOUR EYES. *(1 point)*
  Write a sentence. *(1 point)*
  Copy a design (two intersecting pentagons). *(1 point)*
  Severity of cognitive impairment:
  Mild: MMSE ≥ 21; *Moderate:* MMSE 10–20; *Severe:* MMSE ≤ 9

tetrahydroaminoacridine (Tacrine) and donepezil (Aricept) seem to slow loss of memory and cognition.

Disability Assessment for Dementia

This is a functional scale developed to assess the disability in the performance of Activities of Daily Living (ADLs) for patients with Alzheimer's. It is part of the interview with the caregiver and measures actual performance in ADLs of the individual as observed over a 2-week period prior to the interview. Functional categories include

- Basic ADLs: hygiene, dressing, continence, eating
- Instrumental Activities of Daily Living: meal preparation, telephoning,

16

going out, finance and correspondence, medications, housework, ability to stay safely at home, leisure activities

Skin Care

Pressure ulcers are a serious complication in the elderly, as a result of immobility. There is a four-fold increased risk of death in the elderly with pressure ulcers. (See Table 16–7 for risk factors.)

Table 16–7. Risk Factors for Decubitus Ulcers

Prolonged immobility

Malnutrition

Urinary/fecal incontinence

Steroid use

Comorbidities (ie, diabetes, peripheral vascular disease)

Staging

Stage I—nonblanchable erythema, painful, clears in 24 hours without pressure

Stage II—partial-thickness skin loss involving epidermis ± dermis. Ulcer is superficial. May heal in 2 to 4 weeks.

Stage III—full-thickness skin loss, damage of subcutaneous tissue; may extend to fascia.

Stage IV—full-thickness skin loss with extensive destruction of muscle, supporting tissues, may extend to bone.

Treatment

- Remove pressure—air mattress, gel flotation pads
- Disinfection/cleansing—Dakin's solution; use only with a foul-smelling, not a clean, ulcer (impedes healing)
- Débridement (if necessary)
- Wound care—DuoDerm; adhesive wafers containing colloids and elastomers. Useful in high-friction areas. Used in deeper wounds. Change every 3 to 5 days.

Falls

- Major health problem in the elderly. Sixth leading cause of death among the elderly.

- Simple mnemonic for history of a fall (SPLAT):

  *S*ymptoms prior to fall

  *P*revious falls

  *L*ocation of fall

  *A*ctivity at time of fall

  *T*ime of day or night

A screening test used to identify these patients is the Performance Oriented Mobility Screen (POMS). Ask the patient to perform the following tasks:

1. Sit down in a chair.
2. Rise up from the chair (no cheating by using the side arms).
3. Stand without any assistance for 30 seconds with his or her eyes open.
4. Stand up, unassisted, with his or her eyes closed for 15 seconds.
5. Romberg's test.
6. Reach up and try to remove an object from a shelf.
7. Bend down and pick up something off the floor.

Incontinence

See Table 16–8 for classification.

Incontinence is often undertreated in the elderly. The prevalence is higher in the acutely hospitalized and nursing home residents. It is important to take a good history (acute or chronic, frequency, urgency). The following is a mnemonic for the reversible causes of incontinence (DRIP):

  *D*elirium

  *R*estricted mobility, retention

  *I*nfection, inflammation, impaction

  *P*olyuria, polypharmacy

Assessment should include a complete physical examination (don't forget the pelvic and rectal areas) and labs (urinalysis, culture and sensitivity, electrolytes, BUN/Cr); consider checking postvoid residual.

Depression in the Elderly

A high index of suspicion is necessary to detect depression. Depression may mask as dementia in the elderly. The questions in Table 16–9 are used to screen for depression.

Treat with selective serotonin reuptake inhibitors (first-line agent).

Table 16–8. Types of Persistent Incontinence

Type	Mechanism	Treatment
Stress	Loss of angle of bladder neck (eg, after multiple pregnancies)	Kegel exercises, estrogen cream (for atrophic vaginitis), pessary, surgery for vaginal prolapse
Urge	Detrusor instability or hyperreflexia	Oxybutynin (Ditropan) 5 mg PO bid, bladder training
Overflow	Anatomic obstruction (prostate), acontractile bladder (diabetes mellitus), detrusor-sphincter dyssynergia (spinal cord injury).	Treat cause; indwelling catheter
Functional	Barriers to toilet (cognitive deficit, environmental deficiency)	Adjust environment

Table 16–9. Geriatric Depression Scale—Short Form

Are you basically satisfied with your life? Yes/**NO**

Have you dropped many of your activities and interests? **YES**/No

Do you feel that your life is empty? **YES**/No

Do you often get bored? **YES**/No

Are you in good spirits most of the time? Yes/**NO**

Are you afraid that something bad is going to happen to you? **YES**/No

Do you feel happy most of the time? Yes/**NO**

Do you often feel helpless? **YES**/No

Do you prefer to stay at home, rather than going out and doing new things? **YES**/No

Do you feel that you have more problems with your memory than most? **YES**/No

Do you think it is wonderful to be alive now? Yes/**NO**

Do you feel pretty worthless the way you are now? **YES**/No

Do you feel full of energy? Yes/**NO**

Do you feel that your situation is hopeless? **YES**/No

Do you think that most people are better off than you are? **YES**/No

The answers indicating depression are in bold letters. Each of the bold answers receives 1 point (more than 10 points implies a strong risk for depression).

MISCELLANEOUS

- *BPH*. Symptoms include difficulty urinating and dribbling. Treat with avoidance of liquids prior to sleep, terazosin (Hytrin; beware of orthostatic hypotension), finasteride (inhibitor of 5-alpha reductase), and surgery.
- *Chronic fatigue* work-up includes H&P, psychiatric evaluation, CBC, SMA-20, thyroid function tests (TFTs), ESR, urinalysis, and consideration of Monospot and Lyme titer.
- *Depression*. Criteria include depressed mood, anhedonia, impaired function for > 2 weeks, weight loss, weight gain, insomnia (especially in the late portion of sleep), psychomotor retardation or agitation, feelings of worthlessness, and difficulty concentrating. No obvious external loss should be present. Older tricyclics are being replaced by serotonin reuptake inhibitors (fluoxetine [Prozac] and sertraline [Zoloft] are the most common). Doses should be gradually increased. Therapy should be continued for at least 6 months. *Always ask about suicidal ideation and do not hesitate to involve psychiatrists if there is any question.*
- *Eating disorders*. These should probably be referred promptly to specialists and psychiatrists if need be.
  - Features of anorexia include severe weight loss, female sex, amenorrhea, exercise, bradycardia, hypotension, hypokalemia, and preparation of elaborate meals for others.
  - Bulimia. Findings are binge eating, vomiting (with loss of posterior enamel and cracking of fingers due to induced vomiting), normal weight, and cardiac and endocrine status.
  - Obesity is extremely common and often intractable. Assess comorbidities, medication use, exercise ability, BP, and body mass index (BMI). Check fasting lipid profile, TSH, glucose, and sleep pattern. Consider pharmacotherapy for patients with BMI > 30 or BMI > 27 with comorbidities (HTN, DM, hyperlipidemia). To start therapy, the patient should have failed diet/exercise and be highly motivated. Options are orlistat (Xenical), which blocks pancreatic lipase and reduces fat absorption, and sibutramine (Meridia), a serotenergic and adrenergic agonist. Be aware that many of the oral treatments for obesity (including the latest, sibutramine [Meredia], and the pulled-

off-the-market phentirmine + phenylpropanolamine) cause pulmonary HTN and/or heart valve disease. Refer the patient to a nutrition specialist.

- *Hematuria.* Except in menstruating women, hematuria should prompt work-up for cancer and kidney stones. IVP urine cytology, cystoscopy, and probably ultrasonography are indicated. Look also for bleeding disorders, renal failure, and vasculitis if there is no clear cause.
- *Impotence.* Look for organic causes (vasculopathies, DM, medication, heart disease) or psychosocial problems. Assess nocturnal tumescence (if normal, then the etiology is likely psychosocial). Older therapies (implants, intracavernosal papaverine injections) have basically been rendered obsolete by oral sildenafil (Viagra). Sildenafil can cause bluish vision due to retinopathy.
- *Pruritus.* Look for skin problems, relation to weather or bathing, or contacts. Hodgkin's disease and polycythemia vera commonly present with pruritus (in polycythemia vera, itching occurs after hot showers), although cancer as a whole is a rare cause of itching. Treat with emollient cream, hydroxyzine (Atarax), antihistamines, and avoidance of triggers and drying soaps; treat localized tinea or psoriasis. Be aware that liver failure (with cholestasis) can present initially as pruritus, especially in primary biliary cirrhosis (in which ursodeoxycholic acid may be of use).
- *Sore throat.* The main issue is whether the etiology is viral or streptococcal. Streptococcal disease is characterized by tender anterior cervical nodes, tonsillar and pharyngeal exudates, and headache. Viral pharyngitis is often accompanied by cough and rhinorrhea. Mononucleosis is characterized by palatal petechiae, splenomegaly, and jaundice and hepatomegaly (the last two in those over 40). Do a culture or strep antigen; hold antibiotics for 24 hours while waiting for a result. Be aware that penicillin use in mononucleosis patients causes Jarisch-Herxheimer reaction (rash and myalgias) but is not a true allergy.

BIBLIOGRAPHY

Reviews

Alward WLM. Medical management of open-angle glaucoma. N Engl J Med 1998;339:1298–307.
Anand SS, et al. Does this patient have a DVT? JAMA 1998;279:1094–9.

Asher ML. Asking about domestic violence. JAMA 1993;269:237.

Chow J. The diagnosis and management of sinusitis. Compr Ther 1998;21:74–9.

Cook DJ, Simel DL. Does this patient have abnormal central venous pressure? JAMA 1996;275:630–4.

Cullen MR, et al. Occupational medicine. Part I. N Engl J Med 1990;322:94–601.

Cullen MR, et al. Occupational medicine. Part II. N Engl J Med 1990;322:675–83.

Cyr MG, Wartman SA. Routine screening questions in the detection of alcoholism. JAMA 1988;259:51–4.

Eatell R. Treatment of postmenopausal osteoporosis. N Engl J Med 1998;338:736–46.

Gillin JC, Byerley WF. The diagnosis and management of insomnia. N Engl J Med 1990;322:239–48.

Grover SA, et al. Does this patient have splenomegaly? JAMA 1993;270:2218–21.

Kapoor WN. Diagnostic evaluation of syncope. Am J Med 1991;90:91–106.

Koren G, et al. Drugs in pregnancy. N Engl J Med 1998;338:1128–37.

Leibowitz HM. The red eye. N Engl J Med 2000;343:345–51.

Marion MS, et al. Tinnitus. Mayo Clin Proc 1991;66:614–20.

McGee SR. Dizzy patients. West J Med 1995;162:37–42.

McKenzie R, Straus SE. Chronic fatigue syndrome. Adv Intern Med 1995;40:119–53.

Merli GJ, Spandorfer J. The outpatient with unilateral leg swelling. Med Clin North Am 1995;79:435–47.

National Institutes of Health. Methods for voluntary weight loss and control. Ann Intern Med 1993;119:764–70.

Naylor CD. Physical examination of the liver. JAMA 1994;271:1859–65.

Panju AA. Is this patient having an MI? JAMA 1998;280:1256–63.

Pratter MR, et al. An algorithmic approach to chronic cough. Ann Intern Med 1993;119:977–83.

Rife CM. Involuntary weight loss. Med Clin North Am 1995;79:299–313.

Rosenbaum M. Obesity. N Engl J Med 1997;337:396–407.

Sobel JD. Vaginitis. N Engl J Med 1997;337:1896–903.

Sumpio BE. Foot ulcers. N Engl J Med 2000;343:787–93.

Weinman E, Salzman E. Deep vein thrombosis. N Engl J Med 1994;331:1630–41.

Guidelines

American Psychiatric Association. Practice guidelines for eating disorders. Am J Psychiatry 1993;150:12–28.

Coley CM, et al. Screening for prostate cancer. Ann Intern Med 1997;126:480–4.

Donegan WL. Evaluation of a palpable breast mass. N Engl J Med 1992;327:937–42.

Drossman DA, et al. Physical/sexual abuse and GI illness. Ann Intern Med 1995;123:782–94.

16

Fiore MC, et al. Tobacco dependence and the nicotine patch. JAMA 1992;268: 2687–94.

Gardner P, et al. Adult immunization. Ann Intern Med 1996;40:1–94.

Guidelines for flexible sigmoidoscopy. Gastrointest Endosc 1988;34:S16–75.

Ito S. Drug treatments for breast-feeding women. N Engl J Med 2000;343: 118–26.

Mulrow CD, et al. Discriminating causes of dyspnea through clinical examination. J Gen Intern Med 1993;8:383–92.

National Cholesterol Education Program. Detection, evaluation, and treatment of high blood cholesterol. Circulation 1994;89:1333–445.

Zimethaum P, Josephson ME. Evaluation of palpitations. N Engl J Med 1998;338:1438–47.

Studies and Trials

Geriatrics

Fleischer AB. Pruritus in the elderly. Adv Dermatol 1995;10:41–59.

Inouye SK, Charpentier PA. Precipitating factors for delirium in hospitalized elderly persons. JAMA 1996;275:852–7.

King MB, Tinetti ME. Falls in community-dwelling older persons. J Am Geriatr Soc 1995;43:1146–54.

Mayeux R, Sano M. Treatment of Alzheimer's disease. N Engl J Med 1999; 341:1670–9.

Romero Y, et al. Constipation and fecal incontinence in the elderly population. Mayo Clin Proc 1996;71:81–92.

Scheitel SM, et al. Geriatric health maintenance. Mayo Clin Proc 1996; 71:289–302.

Hypertension

Johnson AG, et al. Do NSAIDS affect BP? Ann Intern Med 1994;121:289–300. (*A meta-analysis showing that NSAIDs elevated mean BP by 5 mm Hg and blocked the effects of beta-blockers. Piroxicam was the worst offender, aspirin the least.*)

Psaty BM, et al. Risk of MI in different antihypertensive therapies. JAMA 1995;274:620–5. (*Calcium blockers had a 60% greater mortality risk than beta-blockers.*)

Osteoporosis

Delmas PD, et al. Effects of raloxifene on bone mineral density, serum cholesterol, and uterine endometrium in postmenopausal women. N Engl J Med 1997;337:1641–7. (*Raloxifene increased bone density, lowered LDL and total cholesterol, and did not stimulate endometrial hyperplasia.*)

Hosking D, et al. Prevention of bone loss with alendronate in postmenopausal women under 60 years of age. N Engl J Med 1998;338:485–92. (*Alendronate prevents bone loss in this group almost as much as estrogen-progestin.*)

Kanf DB, et al. Preventing nonvertebral fractures by alendronate. JAMA 1997;278:1159–64. (*Using alendronate decreases the 3-year risk of nonvertebral fractures by 29%.*)

Orwoll E, et al. Alendronate for osteoporosis in men. N Engl J Med 2000;343:604–10. (*Alendronate lowers vertebral fractures 90%, reduces height loss, and increases bone density.*)

Walsh BW, et al. Effects of raloxifene on serum lipids and coagulation factors in healthy postmenopausal women. JAMA 1998;279:1445–51. (*Raloxifene, a selective estrogen agonist, lowered LDL, raised HDL, and did not affect triglycerides or coagulation factors.*)

Other

Cambridge Heart Antioxidant Study (CHAOS). A randomized clinical trail of vitamin E in patients with coronary disease. Lancet 1996;347:781–6. (*Vitamin E [400–800 mg/d] reduced the risk of nonfatal MI.*)

Campbell SS, et al. Alleviation of sleep maintenance insomnia with timed exposure to bright light. J Am Geriatr Soc 1993;41:829–36. (*Exposure to a bright white light [4,000 lux] increased sleep efficiency from 78 to 90%.*)

Colditz GA. Oral contraceptives and mortality. Ann Intern Med 1994;120:821–6. (*In a Nurses' Health Study, oral contraceptives did not affect mortality [12-year follow-up; 166,755 patients].*)

Fahs MC, et al. Cost effectiveness of cervical cancer screening for the elderly. Ann Intern Med 1992;117:520–7. (*Pap screening is effective for those over 65 who have not been screened routinely; for those who have undergone routine screening, Pap smears are not cost effective.*)

Goldstein I, et al. Oral sildenafil in the treatment of impotence. N Engl J Med 1998;338:1397–404. (*Sildenafil is safe and effective for impotence.*)

Gross PA, et al. The efficacy of influenza vaccine in elderly persons. Ann Intern Med 1995;123:518–27. (*Flu shots reduce pneumonia, hospitalization, and death. So give them.*)

Gullette MB, et al. Effects of mental stress on myocardial ischemia. JAMA 1997;278:1521–6. (*Stress can double the risk of myocardial ischemia in the next hour.*)

Hardcastle JD, et al. A randomized clinical trial of guaiac for colorectal cancer. Lancet 1996;348:1472–7. (*Stool guaiac screening reduces mortality from colorectal cancer.*)

Hart RD. A comparison of sustained-release bupropion and placebo for smoking cessation. N Engl J Med 1997;337:1195–202. (*Bupropion [Wellbutrin, Zyban] was effective in a dose-dependent manner for quitting and reducing weight gain.*)

La Croix AZ, et al. Does walking decrease the risk of CAD and death in older adults? J Am Geriatr Soc 1996;44:113–20. (*Walking more than 4 hours a week in healthy adults reduced the risk of CAD hospitalization over 4 to 5 years of follow-up.*)

McConnell JD. The effect of finasteride on the risk of acute urinary retention and the need for surgical treatment among men with BPH. N Engl J Med 1998;338:557–63. (*Finasteride [Proscar] for 4 years decreased urinary retention in BPH patients by 57% and the need for surgery by 55%.*)

Morin CM, et al. Nonpharmacologic interventions for insomnia. Am J Psychiatry 1994;151:1172–80. (*Sleep hygiene [stimulus control, sleep restriction, and relaxation] is effective.*)

Owens DM, et al. The irritable bowel syndrome. Ann Intern Med 1995;122:107–12. (*Positive physician-patient interactions were associated with fewer visits for irritable bowel syndrome.*)

Physicians' Health Study. Lack of effect of long-term supplementation with beta-carotene on the incidence of malignant neoplasms and cardiovascular disease. N Engl J Med 1996;334:1145–9. (*A large RCT showing that beta-carotene did not protect against cancer or CAD.*)

Redelmeier DA, Tibshirali RJ. Association between cellular phone calls and motor vehicle collisions. N Engl J Med 1997;336:453–8. (*Using cell phones while driving quadruples the risk of motor vehicle accidents.*)

Ross KS, et al. PSA screening strategy. JAMA 2000;284:1399–405. (*PSA testing at age 40 and 45, with biennial testing starting at age 50, was more effective and less costly than annual screening at 50. The threshold for biopsy should be 4.0 ng/mL.*)

Schapira MM, et al. Efficacy of ovarian cancer screening. Ann Intern Med 1993;18:838–43. (*Transvaginal ultrasonography and CA-125 are not effective for mass screening.*)

Sullivan M, et al. A randomized clinical trial of nortriptyline for severe chronic tinnitus. Arch Intern Med 1993;153:2251–9. (*An RCT showing that nortriptyline decreases depression, disability, and loudness of tinnitus.*)

17

Rheumatology, Allergy, Immunology, and Dermatology

Obviousness is the enemy to correctness. — Sir Bertrand Russell

Knowledge is power. — Attributed to Thomas Hobbes and Francis Bacon

RHEUMATOLOGY

General Points

History and Physical

1. Most rheumatic diseases occur in middle-aged women.
2. Ask how long morning stiffness lasts and how long until patients get exhausted.
3. African Americans have SLE more often and temporal arteritis less often.
4. Arthritis is usually worse on the dominant hand.
5. Occupations: jackhammers, Raynaud's phenomenon, carpal tunnel syndrome, secretaries.
6. Gout can cause explosive synovitis.
7. Spondyloarthropathy can cause heel pain, especially in young men.
8. Never forget HIV.
9. Assess mono- versus oligo- versus polyarticular, axial versus appendicular joints, tenderness, range of motion (ROM), swelling, deformity, and fever; examine skin (psoriasis), mouth (ulcers), retina, nodes, thyroid, chest (pulmonary fibrosis, cor pumonale, rubs), bruits, genitalia (ulcers), neurology (Bell's palsy, weakness, extraocular motions).
10. Steroids: dexamethasone (Decadron) 1 mg = methylprednisolone (Solu-Medrol) 4 mg = prednisone 5 mg = hydrocortisone 20 mg. Mnemonic: *Decadron is #1; St. Peter's House (SPH; 4 × 5 = 20).*

11. Celecoxib (Celebrex) is a Cox-2 inhibitor, which theoretically should not cause gastric mucosal toxicity, as the older NSAIDs did through inhibition of both Cox-1 and -2.

Labs (See Table 17–1.)

1. ESR is generally nonspecific; ESR > 90 is important for diagnosis of temporal arteritis and polymyalgia rheumatica.
2. Rheumatoid factor (anti-Fc portion of IgG) is 85% sensitive for rheumatoid arthritis (RA) but nonspecific; it correlates with systemic disease but not joint disease.
3. ANA has a 14% false-positive rate.

Synovial Fluid

1. Examine rapidly; normal fluid has < 95 WBCs/μL.
2. Fever plus monarthritis implies septic arthritis.
3. WBC > 3,000 implies inflammation; > 80,000 implies infection.
4. Septic arthritis risk is higher in RA and anyone with joint damage.
5. Gout has urate crystals (negative birefringence); calcium pyrophosphate deposition (CPPD) (pseudogout) has positive birefringence; hydroxyapatite crystals seen on alizarin red S stain.

Imaging

1. Use x-rays for fractures, erosions, and survey of axial skeleton for spondylitis and discogenic disease.
2. MRI is used for soft-tissue pathology, spinal canal, radiculopathy, disc problems, rotator cuff, bone avascular necrosis (AVN), cervical spine pannus, cord compression, and internal knee problem.
3. Bone scan is used for tumor, osteomyelitis, and nondisplaced fractures.
4. CT is not very useful.
5. EMG distinguishes myositis from noninflammatory disease.
6. Nerve conduction velocity distinguishes entrapment (do in carpal tunnel syndrome only if surgery is considered).

Treatment Modalities

1. When using steroids, watch for PUD, diabetes, infections, and osteoporosis and treat accordingly with H_2-blockers, vitamin D/calcium/estrogen, and insulin.
2. When using NSAIDs, watch for PUD and renal failure; Cox-2 inhibitors are a new class that hopefully won't have these side effects

Table 17–1. Rheumatologic Lab Findings

Lab Finding	Associated Disease
P-ANCA (antimyeloperoxidase)	Polyarteritis nodosa, ulcerative colitis, and many others
C-ANCA (antiprotease 3)	Wegener's disease
Antihistone	Drug-induced systemic lupus erythematosus (SLE)
Anti-Smith (Sm)	SLE
Anti U1RNP	Mixed connective tissue disease
Anti-Ro (SSA), anti-La (SSB)	Sjögren's disease, neonatal lupus (latter especially Ro, which also correlates with photosensitivity)
Anticentromere	CREST syndrome
Antitopoisomerase (Scl-70)	Scleroderma
Anti-Mi-2	Dermatomyositis
Anti-Jo-1	Polymyositis
P-ANCA	Ulcerative colitis, rheumatoid arthritis, nonspecific
HLA-B27	Ankylosing spondylitis
HLA-DR1, DR6, DR10, and DR4 (Dw4/14/15)	Rhematoid arthritis
Nucleolar ANA	Sjögren's disease, scleroderma
Diffuse or speckled ANA	Nonspecific
Anti–double-stranded DNA	SLE specific; correlates with renal disease

because Cox-1, which produces prostaglandins protective for PUD or kidneys, is not inhibited. Examples of Cox-2 inhibitors are celecoxib (Celebrex) and rofecoxib (Vioxx).

3. Surgery is indicated for incapacitating pain and disability due to joint damage or tendon rupture, refractory nerve entrapment syndromes, and refractory septic arthritis.
4. Physical therapy is good to improve ROM, decrease spasm and splinting, reduce pain and inflammation, and improve posture and for general rehabilitation.

17

Rheumatoid Arthritis

Quick Points
- RA affects 1% of adults; early diagnosis and treatment are important; the onset and course are insidious.
- Metacarpophalangeal, proximal interphalangeal, wrist, and ankle joints are most often involved first; 20% of patients have C-spine disease (C1–C2) (be careful when intubating) (in RA patients, occipital headache can mean cervical subluxation).
- To diagnose RA, four of the seven criteria in Table 17–2 are needed.
- Work-up includes ESR, CBC, SMA-7, LFTs, urinalysis, guaiac, CXR, and rheumatoid factor.
- Predictors of aggressive disease include number of criteria, number of joints involved, sustained disease active, positive rheumatoid factor, heterozygosity for HLA-Dw4 with Dw14, and extra-articular activity.
- Extra-articular manifestations include rheumatoid nodules (usually at bony prominences, sometimes in pleura), bursitis, nerve compression, anemia, lung (20% of patients have symptomatic disease; 60% have anatomic findings [pleural effusion with very low glucose, nodules, cavities, interstitial fibrosis]), vasculitis (ungual thrombi, leg ulcers, digital gangrene), pericardial effusions or constrictive pericarditis, Sjögren's disease, Felty's syndrome (RA, leukopenia, splenomegaly; 1% of RA patients have this triad and respond to splenectomy), large granular lymphocyte syndrome (clonal proliferation of CD8 cells, severe neutropenia with lymphocytosis, recurrent bacterial infections, which respond to cytotoxic drugs but not splenectomy), AA amyloidosis (think of this if the patient has RA, CHF, and nephrosis).
- Childhood onset: ½ seronegative; oligoarthritis; the only typical common systemic feature is uveitis (especially if ANA positive). Still's disease is 10% of juvenile RA; symptoms include rash, nodes, hepatosplenomegaly, and daily fevers. Adult Still's disease (evanescent, macular rash, with high fever) has a good functional prognosis.

Management
- Counsel the patient about diet, weight loss, joint protection, and energy conservation.

Table 17–2. Criteria for Diagnosis of Rheumatoid Arthritis

Morning stiffness > 1 hr

Simultaneous synovitis in > 2 joints

Synovitis in wrist or metacarpophalangeal or proximal
  interphalangeal joints

Symmetric arthritis

Rheumatoid nodules

Positive rheumatoid factor

Consistent radiographic changes

- Disease-modifying antirheumatic drugs (DMARDs) are safer than NSAIDs/steroids.
- Methotrexate is a mainstay of DMARDs and should be used early to reduce inflammation (it has not been proven to slow joint erosions).
  - Watch LFTs, check hepatitis B/C status; do liver biopsy if AST rises or albumin falls; pneumonitis is idiosyncratic (not dose related).
  - Other DMARDs include hydroxychloroquine (watch for GI and retinal toxicity), gold (proteinuria, bone marrow suppression, diarrhea, stomatitis), azathioprine (marrow and liver toxicity), and sulfasalazine (GI toxicity).

Osteoarthritis

Osteoarthritis (OA) often occurs in weight-bearing joints.

Quick Points

1. It is generally not inflammatory (vs. RA), except for erosive hand OA. Thus, warmth, redness, high synovial WBC, and fever should prompt a work-up for RA, gout, pseudogout, infection, etc. Diagnose by H&P. Assess ROM carefully. Table 17–3 lists distinguishing features of RA and OA.

2. Idiopathic OA is very common. It affects the distal interphalangeal (Heberden's nodes) and proximal interphalangeal joints (Bouchard's nodes) and the hip, knee, and spine. Secondary OA occurs after trauma, collagen disorders, neuropathy, abnormal joint alignment, and inflammation. If the patient is under 40, look for congenital or meta-

17

bolic diseases (Wilson's, hemachromatosis, DM, acromegaly, and hyperparathyroidism). Obesity is a correctable risk factor.
3. Rule out bursitis, which can mimic hip/knee OA. Knee OA is exacerbated more by going downstairs than upstairs.
4. Spinal stenosis and consequent radiculopathy due to OA in the elderly cause pseudoclaudication (different from vascular claudication because in the latter, leg pain is relieved by standing).

Management
- Treatment: avoid excessive finger use, warm soaks, splinting for finger OA. Topical capsaicin is good for knee OA, as well as physical therapy. Acetaminophen should be maximized first before starting NSAIDs (for mild to moderate disease, acetaminophen to a max of 1 g qid is as effective and safer). Intra-articular steroids are used for inflammation. Systemic steroids have no role.
- Joint replacement is required for severe pain and disability. Contraindications to total replacement include youth, lack of motivation for physical therapy, active infection, neuropathy, and severe osteoporosis. Young patients may be able to do with osteotomy to postpone arthroplasty.
- After arthroplasty, endocarditis prophylaxis is needed with dental procedures.

Gout

Quick Points
1. Gout is due to uric acid crystals (negatively birefringent, intracellular, needle shaped). Pseudogout is due to calcium pyrophosphate (positively birefringent, rhomboid).
2. Saturnine gout is due to lead (also renal and CNS disease). Thiazides, niacin, pyrazinamide, and cyclosporine increase uric acid and should be avoided in those with gout.
3. Gout causes severe joint inflammation and pain. Middle-aged men are the main group. It can also occur in Heberden's nodes in the elderly. Fever, high WBC, and chills can occur.
4. Gout affects the first metacarpophalangeal joint (big toe), ankles, knees, wrists, shoulders, and fingers. It is usually acute and monar-

Table 17–3. Osteoarthritis versus Rheumatoid Arthritis

	Osteoarthritis	*Rheumatoid Arthritis*
Signs and symptoms	Pain after joint use, bony enlargement, crepitus, no soft-tissue swelling	Morning stiffness, synovitis
Involved joints	Distal and proximal interphalangeal joints, wrist, hip, knee, spine, base of thumb (first carpometacarpal joint) (asymmetric)	Proximal interphalangeal and metacarpophalangeal joints, wrist, ankle, feet, C-spine (symmetric)
X-ray findings	Osteophytes, unequal joint space narrowing, subchondral sclerosis (eburnation)	Marginal erosions, equal joint space narrowing, periarticular osteopenia

ticular (can be insidious or polyarticular). Twenty percent of patients have a normal uric acid level in an acute episode.

Management
- *Acute attacks*: use NSAIDs (especially indomethacin [Indocin]). Also may give colchicine PO (0.6 mg q1h up to 10 times) or IV (1–2 mg q12h × 2); it blocks microtubules, inhibiting neutrophils. There are many side effects: GI toxicity; if > 0.6 bid, you can get colchicine myopathy in elderly patients with creatinine > 1.5; IV causes marrow suppression. (Use with caution. Intra-articular steroids and IM ACTH are also options; systemic steroids are not.)
- *Asymptomatic hyperuricemia* patients should not be prophylaxed for gout unless they have cancer and are at risk for tumor lysis. In those with two or more episodes a year, add urate-lowering agents. Use uricosurics (probenecid) if the uric acid excretion is < 750 mg/d; if the urate excretion is > 700 mg/d, use allopurinol (blocks xanthine oxidase). Allopurinol should be avoided in renal failure; also note that it slows metabolism of azathioprine and 6-mercaptopurine. *Do not give allopurinol in an acute attack (can prolong it)*. Side effects

17

of allopurinol are GI upset, rash, and hypersensitivity. Vitamin C decreases urate.
- *Guidelines for IV colchicine* in acute gout:
  - Single doses < 3 mg; maximum dose for one attack < 5 mg.
  - After a full IV dose, do not use colchicine for 1 week.
  - Adjust for liver or renal failure.
  - The IV dose is one half of oral dose.
  - Contraindications include combined renal and hepatic disease, creatinine clearance < 10 mL/min (including dialysis), and extra-hepatic biliary obstruction.
  - The maximum dose for those on maintenance colchicine is 2 mg IV.

Other Crystalline Arthropathies

- Pseudogout (due to calcium pyrophosphate deposition) is associated with hyperparathyroidism, hypothyroidism, hemochromatosis, Wilson's disease, amyloidosis, and trauma. The knee is the most commonly affected joint; it is usually monarticular. Chondrocalcinosis is one radiologic sign. Acute attacks are managed like gout (no chronic therapy).
- Milwaukee shoulder-knee syndrome (see Chapter 16) is due to hydroxyapatite plus CPPD (in snowball shape), causing idiopathic destructive arthritis.

Septic Arthritis

In inflamed monarthritis, do a synovial biopsy if the tap is negative for bugs.

Quick Points
- Gonococcal arthritis is more common in women.
  - Disseminated gonococcal infection (DGI) is the most common infectious arthritis in those younger than 40.
  - Acute monarthritis is *Neisseria gonorrhoeae* until proven otherwise.
  - More frequent in menses.
  - Symptoms include migratory oligoarthritis, tenosynovitis, and vesicopustular skin lesions on an erythematous base (this can also occur with meningococcus).
- *S. aureus* is the next most common cause.

- Spreads hematogenously or contiguously from infected soft tissue, bone, etc.
  - Risk factors are comorbidities (DM, steroids, other joint problems, immunosuppression), IDU, trauma, prosthesis, and arthroscopy.
- TB, Lyme disease, fungi, and parvovirus B19 can cause infectious arthritis as well.
- Rheumatic fever in adults may occur without prior pharyngitis and may not be migratory.
- Exaggerated inflammation in one joint of an RA patient requires a tap. The knee is the most commonly affected joint. Bone scan and MRI are useful.

Management
- In cases of suspected gonococcal infection, diagnose by culture (joint, pustule, blood, and cervical swabs). Treat with ceftriaxone plus doxycycline (presume chlamydial infection as well). Rule out HIV and syphilis as well. Tap affected joints (especially the knee) daily until fluid reaccumulation ceases. If DGI recurs, rule out complement deficiency by checking CH50. *Staph.* treatment is cephalosporins or vancomycin.
- Drain fluid completely (may require arthroscopy or open drainage). Use antibiotics for 4 to 6 weeks.
- Persistent synovitis with effusion after cure of septic arthritis can be treated with intra-articular steroids. Prosthetic joint infection requires removal (gram positive is more likely in the first 6 months after insertion; gram negative is more common afterward).

Systemic Lupus Erythematosus

Quick Points
- Female-to-male ratio is 9:1; complement deficiencies (C1, 2, or 4) increase the risk, as do African-American race and HLA-DR2 and DR3. Antibodies cause inflammation and immune complex disease.
- Procainamide, isoniazid, hydralazine, quinidine, and methlydopa cause SLE-like disease (without renal disease, low complement, or anti–double-stranded [ds] DNA).
- Diagnosis is made by meeting 4 of the 11 criteria outlined in Table 17–4.

17

- Life-threatening complications are renal, neurologic, and hematologic, as well as infections due to steroids and pulmonary hemorrhage, vasculitis, and myocarditis (rarer). *Salmonella* and S. *Pneumoniae* are increased by SLE itself. Bone avascular necrosis is due to SLE and steroids. High PTT due to lupus anticoagulant is a lab artifact (really hypercoagulable).
- Renal disease (glomerulonephritis or acute interstitial nephritis) presents clinically in 50% of patients. Biopsy in lupus acute renal failure only if steroids don't work and in mild renal disease diagnoses to assess the inflammatory component (trying to figure out how much is steroid responsive).
- ANA is positive in 95% of patients; anti–dsDNA or anti-Sm is more specific; rising anti–dsDNA and complement levels (falling C4, rising CH50) can predict renal disease flares.

Table 17–4. Criteria for Systemic Lupus Erythematosus

Malar rash	Renal disease (cellular casts, > 0.5 g/d proteinuria)
Discoid rash	Neurologic disease (seizures or psychosis)
Photosensitivity	Hematology hemolytic anemia, WBC < 4, platelet
Oral ulcers	< 100, or lymphocytes < 1,500/mcL
Arthritis	Serositis (more common in older patients)
Positive ANA	Miscellaneous: positive LE cells, anti-Sm, false-positive reactive plasma reagin, anti-DNA

Management

- Mild disease: NSAIDs, avoid sun, hydroxychloroquine (Plaquenil), low-dose prednisone (10–20 mg/d).
- Hydroxychloroquine is good for joint and skin disease and adjunct for visceral disease; check for retinopathy; withdrawal leads to flares.
- For life-threatening disease, give prednisone 1 mg/kg qd.
- Cyclophosphamide (Cytoxan) plus prednisone is good to prevent renal failure; monthly IV cyclophosphamide is as effective as oral qd

cyclophosphamide and less likely to cause hemorrhagic cystitis; the toxicity of cyclophosphamide includes infertility and late malignancy.

- Lupus nephritis: prednisone, cyclophosphamide, renal biopsy (plasmapheresis is worthless).
- Pregnancy: more miscarriages, may increase SLE flares, neonatal lupus (rash, congenital heart block associated with anti-Ro and sometimes anti-La). You may need to stop anti-SLE drugs. May be able to reduce fetal loss with ASA.

Antiphospholipid Syndrome

- Thromboses, low platelets, false-positive RPR, miscarriages, livedo reticularis, and skin ulcers are symptoms. It can be anticardiolipin or lupus anticoagulant.
- Thromboses need heparin and coumadinization to an INR of > 3. Thrombocytopenia responds to prednisone. It is unclear how to treat recurrent abortions.

Scleroderma (Systemic Sclerosis) and Variants

- Vasculopathy plus collagen deposition leading to Raynaud's phenomenon (digital pallor, cyanosis, then hyperemia and pain; giant loops on nail capillaroscopy are prognostic), skin tightening (no wrinkling), telangiectasia, pruritus, digital ulcers, and skin calcification.
- *Visceral disease*: Smooth muscle atrophy causes dysphagia, diverticulosis, and bowel obstruction. Interstitial lung disease, pulmonary HTN, and cardiomyopathy occur. Renal failure is another symptom. HTN, renal failure, and microangiopathic hemolytic anemia can occur suddenly.
- Signs and symptoms include symmetric thickening of the dorsum of the hand, sclerodactyly, basilar pulmonary fibrosis, and pitting of fingertips.
- CREST variant: *c*alcinosis cutis, *R*aynaud's phenomenon, *e*sophageal dysfunction, *s*clerodactyly, and *t*elangiectasia. It is a limited form of the disease (less renal failure, better prognosis).
- Treatment is supportive: steroids for myositis. Use calcium blockers for Raynaud's, omeprazole (Prilosec) for esophageal erosions, cisapride/metoclopramide (Propulsid/Reglan) for gastroparesis, and an ACE inhibitor for HTN.

17

- Eosinophilic fasciitis: skin wrinkles plus eosinophilia; no Raynaud's, hand, or visceral disease; responds to 20 to 40 mg of prednisone a day. Eosinophilic myalgia: occurs after rapeseed oil ingestion and in the 1980s after artificial tryptophan supplements.

Sjögren's Syndrome

- Dry eyes and mouth. Occurs often with RA and other rheumatic diseases. Can cause interstitial nephritis, renal tabular acidosis, neuropathy, interstitial pneumonitis, and thyroid disease. Treatment is artificial tears, hard candies, and dental care. Increased risk of B-cell lymphoma.

Dermatomyositis/Polymyositis

- Dermatomyositis is often paraneoplastic (lung, breast, colon, ie, more common tumors more often produce it). Dermatomyositis is due to CD4 cells; polymyositis is due to CD8 cells.
- Dermatomyositis: heliotrope rash on the upper eyelid, Gottron's papules over the knuckles, high CPK/aldolase, and a photosensitive rash on the face and neck (V-sign and shawl sign).
- Polymyositis: proximal weakness (difficulty climbing stairs, placing objects on a bookshelf, and combing hair), muscle pain, dysphagia, high CPK/aldolase (don't confuse with polymyalgia rheumatica, which is in the elderly, associated with temporal arteritis, and does not have high CPK [but may have high ESR]. EMG shows decreased amplitude with an increased spike amplitude).
- Zidovudine (AZT), HMG-CoA reductase inhibitors, and colchicine can cause myositis.
- A muscle biopsy is needed. Treat with steroids; for dermatomyositis, IV gamma globulin may be of benefit.
- Mixed connective tissue disease has elements of SLE, CREST, and polymyositis.

Vasculitis

See Table 17–5 for classification.

Key Points

See Chapters 4 and 9 for cryoglobulinemia and Henoch-Schönlein purpura (HSP).

Table 17–5. Vasculitides

Disease	Vessels and Pathology	Organs	Associations	Therapy
Polyarteritis nodosa (PAN)	Medium arteries, immune complex	Kidney, GI tract, nerves (mononeuritis multiplex), spares lung and spleen	Hepatitis B/C (intravenous drug abusers)	Cyclophosphamide + prednisone; for hepatitis B-PAN, prednisone, plasmapheresis, and interferon
Wegener's	Small and medium veins, granuloma	Sinuses, lung, kidney, eye		Cyclophosphamide + prednisone
Temporal arteritis	Extracranial carotid (especially ophthalmic arteries), granulomas	Eye	Elderly, polymyalgia rheumatica, ESR > 90	High-dose steroids (start 60 mg of prednisone even before biopsy)
Takayasu's	Aorta and great vessels, granulomas	Heart, brain, pulseless extremities	Young women	Steroids
Churg-Strauss	Small and medium veins	Skin, lung, kidney	Asthma, hypereosinophilia, allergic rhinitis	Steroids
Buerger's (hypersensitivity)	Capillaries and venules	Skin, kidney, GI tract, nerve	Young smokers	Quitting smoking, possibly steroids

17

1. Palpable purpura imply small vessel, leukocytoclastic vasculitis (differential diagnosis = drugs, HSP, SLE, RA, Goodpasture's, and cryoglobulinemia).

2. Initial prednisone for serious disease is 1 mg/kg/d; cyclophosphamide is 2 mg/kg/d.

3. *Temporal arteritis*. Signs and symptoms include temporal headache, scalp tenderness, fever of unknown origin, anemia, jaw claudication, visual loss, and bruit; the ESR is very high (> 100); get a long section of artery (lesions skip areas; look for granulomatous inflammation; if the biopsy is negative, biopsy the other side); taper steroids over at least 9 months. Temporal arteritis increases the risk for aortic dissection. Polymyalgia rheumatica alone responds to prednisone 10 to 20 mg/d and does not need biopsy if there are no symptoms.

4. *Polyarteritis nodosa*. Mononeuritis multiplex causes pain and weakness in a distribution (eg, footdrop due to peroneal nerve infarction). Renal involvement causes HTN. Biopsies of affected nerves or muscles are 65% sensitive; mesenteric angiogram is 60% sensitive (microaneurysms, alternating stenosis, and dilation). Note that for patients with HBV-associated polyarteritis nodosa, drop cyclophosphamide and use plasmapheresis and IFN along with prednisone.

5. *Wegener's granulomatosis* causes pulmonary hemorrhage and cavities, sinusitis, glomerulonephritis, and retro-orbital pseudotumor (causing proptosis of the eye). Biopsy the affected sites. TMP-SMX (Bactrim) may reduce the relapse rate.

6. *Takayasu's arteritis* is pathologically identical to temporal arteritis. It occurs in young women and causes bruits and absent pulses, along with high ESR. Use steroids and surgery as needed.

7. *Goodpasture's syndrome*. The anti–basement membrane antibody also causes hemoptysis and hematuria (like Wegener's).

8. *Henoch-Schönlein purpura* affects the skin, kidney, and GI tract and causes buttock and leg purpura. There are IgA deposits with leukocytoclastic vasculitis on biopsy. It is usually self-limited. Treat with IV gamma globulin.

9. *Renal biopsy* shows necrotizing glomerulonephritis with crescents in polyarteritis nodosa, Wegener's, Goodpasture's, and rapidly progressive glomerulonephritis.

Spondyloarthropathies

1. Seronegative spondyloarthropathies: sacroiliitis, spondylitis, enthesopathy (inflamed tendon and ligament attachments to bone), arthritis, tenosynovitis, HLA-B27 (which is 80% sensitive but only 10% specific).
2. Sausage-shaped digits (dactylitis) occur in ankylosing spondylitis, Reiter's syndrome, and psoriatic arthritis.
3. In inflammatory bowel disease (subclinical inflammatory bowel disease is more common in these patients), arthritis and erythema nodosum herald flares, whereas uveitis and spondylitis do not correlate.

Ankylosing Spondylitis

The onset of ankylosing spondylitis is in the 20s; it is more common in Caucasians and men).

- Symmetric sacroiliitis (tenderness, low back stiffness, bamboo spine if untreated), iritis in 25% of patients, peripheral arthritis (knees, hips), aortic regurgitation.
- Back stiffness causes brittleness (increased risk for spine fracture with minor trauma, eg, rear-ending in motor vehicle accidents). Patients have prolonged buttock stiffness in the morning.
- Measure lumbar spine mobility with Schober test. Draw a line from the midpoint between the posterior iliac spine to 10 cm above it; on forward bending, the normal distraction of the line is to at least 16 cm; in aortic stenosis patients, it may lengthen only 1 or 2 cm.
- Treat with indomethacin (maximum at 75 mg bid), physical therapy, and sulfasalazine. Pain is decreased with exercise.

Reiter's Syndrome

- The triad in Reiter's syndrome is arthritis, urethritis, and conjunctivitis. Symptoms also include circinate balanitis, keratoderma blennorrhagicum (psoriasiform rash on the palms and soles), palatal ulcers, and uveitis. It occurs after *Chlamydia, Shigella, Salmonella, Yersinia, Klebsiella, Campylobacter*, and *Ureaplasma* infections of the GI or GU tract. The risk is increased by HLA-B27.
- Treat with NSAIDs, sulfasalazine, intra-articular steroids, and doxycycline therapy for 3 months if *Chlamydia* is proven. You must rule out HIV if *Chlamydia* is present.

Finer Points of Rheumatology

See also Orthopedics in Chapter 18.

- Amyloidosis
  - The AA type (due to chronic disease) causes nephrotic syndrome. Treat the underlying disease.
  - The AL type (Ig associated, eg, myeloma) causes CHF, CRF, liver failure, macroglossia, ecchymoses, and neuropathy. Chemotherapy may be needed.
- *Avascular necrosis* = osteonecrosis. Risk factors include steroid use and lupus. The most common site is the femoral head (also in the scaphoid of the wrist, navicular of the foot, and the humerus). Core decompression may be of value early.
- In patients with OA or RA of the knee with new calf swelling, think of a ruptured Baker's cyst (pseudophlebitis) causing venous compression.
- *Behçet's disease* causes painful aphthous ulcers (oral, anal, and genital), vasculitis, uveitis, synovitis, erythema nodosum, DVT, CNS changes, and fever. The skin is hyperreactive to needle sticks. Treat with steroids and cyclosporine.
- In bursitis, active motion is very painful, but passive motion is not.
  - Lateral epicondylitis = tennis elbow
  - Olecranon bursitis = student's elbow
  - Prepatellar bursitis = housemaid's knee
  - Anserine bursitis causes pain at the medial and below knee (occurs more in OA patients)
  - Treat with rest and occasional intrabursal steroids.
- *Carpal tunnel:* entrapment of the median nerve (occurs with repetitive stress, RA, and in dialysis patients due to β_2-microglobulin). Check nerve conduction velocity. Treat with splinting and surgery; yoga may be useful.
- De Quervain tenosynovitis: repetitive stress causing inflammation of the abductor longus pollicis of the thumb, causing pain over the distal radius.
- Diabetes can cause Dupuytren's contracture (thickening of the palm causing finger flexion; treat with surgery) and Charcot's disease (foot neuropathy causing bone damage).
- Ehlers-Danlos can be autosomal dominant and causes joint hypermobility.

- Familial Mediterranean fever = recurrent fever, pleuritis, and pericarditis. Treat with colchicine.
- Ganglion cyst = swelling of the wrist tendon. Treat with slamming a phone book (in the old days, the family Bible) on it.
- Marfan syndrome causes long limbs, aortic regurgitation, and lens dislocation. Beta-blockers slow the progression of aortic regurgitation.
- A neuropathic joint (Charcot's) can be due to DM, amyloidosis, intra-articular steroids, myelocele, syphilis, leprosy, and syringomyelia.
- Osteogenesis imperfecta can also be autosomal dominant and causes blue sclera.
- Paronychia = abscess in the distal finger; felon = infection of the nail pulp. It is caused by *S. aureus.* Treat with incision and drainage.
- Pigmented villonodular synovitis: idiopathic, unilateral hemarthrosis of the knee. Treat with synovectomy or radiation.
- Pseudoxanthoma elasticum (autosomal recessive) gives angioid streaks in the retina and UGIB.
- Psoriatic arthritis causes nail-pitting (onycholysis), arthritis mutilans, pencil-in-cup deformity of the distal interphalangeal joints, and sacroiliitis. Treat with indomethacin and methotrexate
- Reflex sympathetic dystrophy occurs after trauma, inflammation, or major medical events and causes symptoms in the affected limb. Diagnose with a three-phase bone scan. Treat with sympathetic blockade, physical therapy, and steroids.
- Relapsing polychondritis causes arthritis, iritis, aortic regurgitation, and recurrent inflammation of cartilage of the head and neck, leading to hoarseness, saddle-nose, and ear deformity.
- Rotator cuff tear: arm drop sign. Pain on active more than passive abduction mandates MRI.
- Trigger finger means the index finger is stuck in full flexion. Treat with surgery.
- Volkmann's contracture: supracondylar fracture (after elbow trauma) causing brachial artery ischemia leading to unwillingness to extend the fingers and wrist due to pain.
- Whipple's causes arthritis, abdominal pain, and CNS changes.

ALLERGY

Eosinophilia

Quick Points
- Increased levels of eosinophils can be seen in allergic diseases, parasitic infections, and cancer. Worldwide, the most common cause is helminthic infections.
- Sometimes, an accumulation of eosinophils may be seen in certain organs: Well's syndrome (eosinophilic cellulitis), eosinophilic pneumonia (Löffler's syndrome), and eosinophilic fasciitis (Shulman's syndrome). Churg-Strauss syndrome is the association of eosinophilia with vasculitis, neuropathy, and asthma.
- Eosinophilia is classified in the following ways:
  - Mild (351–1,500 cells/mm^2)
  - Moderate (> 1,500–5,000 cells/mm^2)
  - Severe (> 5,000 cells/mm^2)

Management
- Conduct careful review of a patient's history of atopy (eczema, wheezing, rhinitis), travel history (endemic helminthic areas), presence of pets, cancer symptoms, or drug use (hypersensitivity drug reaction).
- Initial laboratory studies should include a peripheral blood smear, urinalysis, and stool for ova and parasites (at least three times).
- It is important to diagnose *Strongyloides stercoralis* because it can be fatal in immunosuppressed patients.
- Patients with persistent, mild eosinophila do not need therapy. These patients should have periodic echocardiograms to detect eosinophil-mediated cardiac damage.
- It may be reasonable to attempt a trial of steroids (prednisone 1 mg/kg) to see if there is a clinical response. Other options include IFN-α and myelosuppressive drugs.

Allergic Rhinitis

Quick Points
- The symptoms of allergic rhinitis (hay fever) are similar to that of viral rhinitis (common cold), but they are seasonal. Pollens are the most common allergens.
- Patients often have nasal congestion and watery eyes. On examination, the mucosa may appear pale or violaceous (this is due to venous engorgement).
- Keep in mind that the mucosa is beefy red in viral rhinitis, whereas it is boggy in allergic rhinitis.

Management
- Treatment consists of environmental controls for the most part. Oral decongestants are usually enough to alleviate symptoms (pseudoephedrine), but antihistamines target the allergy itself.
- Commonly used antihistamines are loratadine (Claritin), cetirizine (Zyrtec), and fexofenadine (Allegra). Nasal steroid sprays are an integral part of treatment (beclomethasone [Beconase] or fluticasone [Flonase]). It may take 1 to 2 weeks to see an effect.

Urticaria and Angioedema

Quick Points
Urticaria is usually a hypersensitivity reaction mediated by IgE. The most common causes of urticaria are foods, viral and parasitic infections, and medications. Lesions are usually itchy red swellings ranging in size and forming "geographic" patterns. In familial angioedema, there is usually a family history of angioedema of the extremities and GI or respiratory symptoms. Hereditary angioedema is due to deficiency of the C1q esterase inhibitor; the treatment is danazol, which stimulates its production by the liver. Patients may also develop angioedema as an idiosyncratic response to ACE inhibitors. It is important to try to localize the cause of the acute urticaria. Nonallergic causes are usually drugs (ie, morphine). Physical factors (heat, cold, sunlight) may also be the culprit. Allergic causes may be from medications (penicillin), foods (shellfish), or external contacts (cosmetics).

17

Initial treatment is with H_1-blockers (hydroxyzine). The offending agent, if possible, should be avoided.

Drug Eruption (Dermatitis Medicamentosa)

Rashes are the most common adverse drug reactions and are seen in 2 to 3% of hospitalized patients. Common offenders are amoxicillin, TMP-SMX, ampicillin, and penicillin. These drugs commonly produce urticaria and maculopapular rashes. Sulfonamides and anticonvulsants can produce toxic epidermal necrolysis and Stevens-Johnson syndrome.

Only a few drug reactions are truly allergic. Patients with allergic drug reactions usually have been exposed to the drug in the past. There is a so-called "incubation" period, and reactions are usually at doses below the therapeutic range of the drug. These patients may have a severe reaction (anaphylaxis, urticaria, vasculitis). These reactions are usually reproducible. Treatment must be tailored to the individual drug reaction.

IMMUNOLOGY

Classification of immune reactions (often asked on tests):

I: Allergic reactions (IgE and histamine mediated): for example, hay fever (these are immediate, occurring within 1 hour after exposure)

II: Antibody-dependent cytotoxicity: humoral immunity

III: Immune complexes: antibodies complex with antigen (eg, Arthus reaction causing hemorrhagic induration following tetanus or insulin shots, serum sickness, etc)

IV: Delayed hypersensitivity (cellular immunity): T-cell–mediated response, for example, tuberculin sensitivity, granulomatous diseases, and contact dermatitis

Table 17–6 lists immune deficiency disorders.

DERMATOLOGY

Translation Guide for Dermatology

See Table 17–7.

Nonmelanoma Skin Cancer

(Melanoma is covered in Chapter 10.)

Table 17–6. Immune Deficiencies

Name	Deficiency	Comments
Hereditary angioedema	C1 esterase inhibitor absent	Recurrent edema; treat with danazol
Chédiak-Higashi syndrome	Microtubular defect compromising neutrophil chemotaxis	
Chronic granulomatous disease	Defective oxidative burst of neutrophils causing immune reliance on T cells (granulomas)	Nitroblue tetrazolium test for diagnosis
	C1, C2, C4 deficiency	Recurrent ear and respiratory infections
	C5–C9 deficiency	Infections with encapsulated bacteria (meningococcus, gonococcus)
Bruton's agammaglobulinemia	No antibodies or B cells	X-linked; Treat with IVIg for life
Common variable hypogammaglobulinemia	IgG deficiency	Bronchiectasis and giardiasis are common
	IgA deficiency	Most common Ig deficiency; increased autoimmunity, sprue, giardiasis, and sinusitis
Wiskott-Aldrich	Low IgM	Triad (eczema, thrombocytopenia, + infections); treat with bone marrow transplantation

Table 17–6 continued on next page.

17

Table 17–6. Continued

Name	Deficiency	Comments
Ataxia telangiectasia	Cellular and antibody deficiency	Bronchiectasis, telangiectasia, and ataxia
Severe combined immunodeficiency	Adenosine deaminase deficiency (no T or B cells)	X-linked or autosomal recessive; fatal unless early bone marrow transplant
DiGeorge syndrome	Absent thymus due to third and fourth pharyngeal arch defects	Loss of T cells and parathyroids (fungal infections, hypocalcemia)

Table 17–7. Common Dermatologic Terms and Meanings

Urticaria	Itchy rash
Erythema	Redness
Macule	Flat spot
Papule	Raised spot
Plaque	Area of mild elevation
Epidermis	Surface skin
Dermis	Deep skin (full of vasculature)
Wheals	Hives
Vesicle	Shiny, fluid-filled bleb

A. Basal cell cancer is the most common in the U.S., comprising 80% of all skin cancers; squamous cell comprises only 20%.
B. Both are caused by a multitude of factors, but the overall greatest cause is sun exposure. Other factors include
   1. Celtic descent (or anybody with very fair skin)
   2. Arsenic exposure
   3. Xeroderma pigmentosum
   4. Radiation exposure
   5. Thermal burns
C. *Basal cell cancer*
   1. Arises from epidermal basal cells.
   2. Is usually a noduloulcerative nodule with telangiectasia on the surface, occuring in sun-exposed areas; if large, it may have central ulceration.
   3. Other types include morpheaform (flat, indurated, yellow to white plaque), which is more aggressive and recurrent.
   4. Pigmented basal cell cancer behaves like noduloulcerative but may look like a melanoma.
   5. Treatment is usually electrodessication and curettage for low-risk tumors, whereas excision is indicated for the morpheaform type or if the patient is having the removal on an aesthetically important area.

17

Other modalities used in nonaggressive tumors are cryosurgery, topical chemotherapy and intralesional IFN.

6. This lesion does not really metastasize, and the major problems it causes are through local spread and invasion.

D. Sézary syndrome and mycosis fungoides are cutaneous T-cell lymphomas.

E. *Squamous cell cancer*

1. This is a far more serious neoplasm.
2. It usually appears as an ulcerated nodule or a superficial erosion of the skin or often the lower lip, but it can also be a verrucous plaque or papule. Telangiectases are rare. Margins are ill defined, and it may be attached to underlying structures.
3. Usually, it occurs in a sun-exposed area.
4. Actinic keratosis and cheilitis are premalignant forms of this, representing areas of hyperkeratotic plaques. The risk of getting full squamous cell cancer increases with the number of these premalignant lesions, even though the transformation potential of any given lesion is low.
5. *Treatment*: surgical excision or radiation; however, in very small lesions, cryosurgery may be adequate.
6. Prognosis depends on position.
   a. There is a higher metastasis rate if it arises on nonactinically damaged skin.
   b. Cutaneous cancers metastasize more than mucosal.
   c. Cancers arising in burn scars, chronic ulcers, and genitals also have a higher rate.
   d. The overall rate of metastasis is 3 to 3.7%.

Rashes and Sores

A. *Rashes* are a common problem on the floors and are usually due to one of two major etiologies. It is always important to notice the pattern and distribution of the rash as this may give some clue to its cause.

1. Viral exanthems occur in the setting of other viral symptoms such as myalgias, URI, and headache.
2. Drug rash can be caused by almost any drug, usually occurs within 2 weeks of starting it, and may take quite a while to go away even after removal of the offending medication. Key drug reactions include

a. Penicillin (immediate anaphylaxis or delayed morbilliform eruption)

b. Phenytoin (erythema multiforme)

c. Warfarin: necrotic patches of skin (purpura fulminans in patients with protein C/S deficiency)

d. Tetracycline (photosensitivity)

3. Dermatitis will often occur in a distribution, suggesting a particular piece of clothing or a wristband, or over an area exposed to cosmetics or soaps.

4. Treatment is always the removal of the offending agent first, followed by use of antihistamines for itch, topical creams (menthols), and, if severe, a steroid taper.

B. *Urticaria* (the English translation is hives) have similar causes as the above, but if they last more than 24 hours, they may be due to a vasculitis or erythema multiforme. This condition is usually not one with an identifiable source unless it is of recent onset. One interesting thing is that NSAIDs can induce a flare-up of the problem.

C. *Erythema multiforme*

1. This is characterized by cutaneous target lesions with central vesiculation, purpura, and a peripheral urticarious (itchy) erythematous area. Lesions often heal, leaving a hyperpigmented area.

2. Erythema multiforme minor has no mucosal involvement.

3. Erythema multiforme major blends in with Stevens-Johnson syndrome (see below).

4. Toxic epidermal necrosis, which is as bad as it sounds, has a 30% mortality rate.

5. This is caused by hypersensitivity to drugs (which is the cause of the severe cases), herpes simplex, pregnancy, malignancy, collagen vascular disease, or inflammatory bowel disease (which are probably the same thing anyway).

6. Treatment is, of course, the removal of offending agents and, in the full-blown Stephens-Johnson syndrome, treatment in a burn unit to avoid dehydration and infection.

D. *Tinea* (nails, head, body, or foot) and *Candida*

1. Tinea is a fungus that affects various body parts, usually the feet (tinea pedis) or scalp (tinea cruris). Patients will also often get *Candida* yeast infections on the skin, usually in folds under the breasts or stomach in the obese. The tinea lesions present with sharp bor-

17

ders with erythema clearing toward the center of the macule. The *Candida* rash is also well defined, but there isn't as much central clearing; this and position are your major clues.

2. On skin scraping with a potassium hydroxide (KOH) preparation, tinea organisms have branching hyphae that look like bamboo, whereas *Candida* have pseudohyphae and are less distinct. Treatment involves appropriate antifungal topical agents, *but be careful.* If you use topical corticosteroids, you can seriously hurt your patient as the fungi will have a field day. However, topical steroids are useful for tinea capitis to prevent hair loss.

E. *Bed sores* (also known as decubitus ulcers)

1. An unfortunate result of being very aged, infirm, paralyzed, or critically ill is lack of movement and the development of pressure sores. Such things are a common cause of severe pain and fevers of unknown origin that are labelled as such because nobody likes to look under the dressing. They have four stages:
   * Stage one is a painful erythema with essentially unbroken skin.
   * Stage two is broken skin, but no extension through the dermis.
   * Stage three has dermal involvement.
   * Stage four has involvement of subdermal tissues like muscle, fat, and bone.

2. Treatment involves a bewildering array of wraps, tapes, plastics, and salves, which will vary from hospital to hospital. Basically, stages 1 and 2 will usually not require débridement and can be treated with dressings and turning the patient and applying antipressure booties or pillows.

3. Treatment of the worst stages (3 and 4) involves surgical débridement if severe or the famous "wet-to-dry" dressing, which is a euphemism for débridement because when the dry dressing is peeled off, so is all of the dead tissue.

4. Never forget that this is a significant cause of morbidity and even mortality in the aged and be sure to write out of bed→chair in your orders if the patient is in any way able to tolerate it.

Dermatologic Conditions

A. *Acne.* Acne vulgaris happens in the young. Treatment, if needed, is with topical benzoyl peroxide or oral tetracycline. Retinoic acid derivatives

(Accutane, Retin-A) are effective but may be mutagenic. Acne rosacea is a disease of the middle-aged and can be treated with oral doxycycline or topical metronidazole.

B. *Psoriasis.* Characteristics include silvery scales in symmetric fashion. Nail pitting is common. It can be exacerbated by antimalarials, gold, beta-blockers, and lithium. Treat with topical steroids, methotrexate for severe disease, PUVA (oral psoralen + ultraviolet light), and calcipotriene (a vitamin D analogue).

C. *Erythema nodosum.* This consists of red, painful, warm nodules, usually on the shins. Causes include sarcoidosis, inflammatory bowel disease, TB, streptococcal disease, and fungi.

D. *Pyoderma gangrenosum.* This is an inflammatory ulcer on the legs associated with inflammatory bowel disease, leukemia, RA, and chronic active hepatitis.

E. *Erythrasma.* This is a reddish lesion with scaling in intertriginous areas (mimicking fungal infection) due to *Corynebacterium minutissimum.*

F. *Ecthyma gangrenosum.* This is a shallow skin ulcer due to *Pseudomonas* (which can also cause hot tub folliculitis).

G. *Migratory necrolytic erythema.* This is a skin lesion of glucagonoma (a favorite question tests).

H. *Cellulitis.* See Chapter 5. Be aware of *Strep.* causing impetigo (perioral crusting), furuncles, folliculitis, erysipelas (superficial cellulitis that can spread in streaks along the lymphatics), and scarlatina (sandpaper-like rash). Also know that *Staph.* causes toxic shock syndrome (classically with tampons, this is abrupt shock, rash, and desquamation of the palms and soles).

I. *Warts.* These are due to human papilloma virus (HPV) and can be treated with liguid nitrogen or surgery.

J. *Molluscum contagiosum.* This is due to a pox virus and consists of smooth, umbilicated, pearly papules. It is sexually transmitted.

K. *Pemphigus vulgaris.* An antibody against desmosomes, which causes acantholysis (separation of epidermal cells from each other), leading to bullae with Nikolsky's sign (sliding of the blister with pressure, found also in toxic epidermal necrolysis). Oral mucosa is commonly involved. Treat with steroids and immunosuppression.

L. *Bullous pemphigoid.* These are tense blisters with anti–basement membrane antibodies. They are often paraneoplastic. Treat with steroids.

M. *Pityriasis rosea.* This papulosquamous rash (unknown cause) starts off with a herald patch and then annular trunk lesions. It is self-limited. Treatment is symptomatic (topical steroids).

N. *Tinea versicolor.* This is caused by *Pityrosporum* (don't confuse with the previous) and causes scaly trunk patches. See bugs on KOH preparation. Treat with selenium or antifungal creams.

O. *Lichen planus.* These papulosquamous patches over the wrists, back, and genitals occur with thiazides, antimalarials, and hepatitis C.

P. *Sweet's syndrome.* Also known as febrile neutrophilic dermatosis, this is usually seen in those with neutropenic cancers (generally acute leukemias). It presents as red or purple papules that coalesce into plaques. Lesions are solid and usually on the face, neck, or arms. Fevers are present. Treat with steroids (60-mg prednisone qd, tapered over 2–3 weeks).

Treatments

In general, most internists aren't comfortable with treating rashes. For mild xerosis, aquaphor and moisture creams are effective. Eucerin is an emollient (retains moisture). Lac-Hydrin is indicated for itching with xerosis or ichthyosis vulgaris. Calomine lotion is effective for pruritus of poison ivy. Antifungals (eg, clotrimazole [Lotrimin]) are handy for tinea infections. For nailbed infections, systemic treatment with itraconazole (Sporanox) is required. Don't use steroids without experience and don't continue them for long without dermatologic consultation.

BIBLIOGRAPHY

Allergy and Immunology

Reviews

Chan-Yeung M, Malo JL. Occupational asthma. N Engl J Med 1995;333:917–34.

Charlesworth EN. Urticaria and angioedema. Ann Allergy Asthma Immunol 1996;76:484–50.

Corbrige TC, Hall JB. The assessment and management of adults with status asthmaticus. Am J Respir Crit Care Med 1995;151:1296–316.

Delves PJ, Roitt IM. The immune system. N Engl J Med 2000;343:37–49, 108–117.

Dwyer JM. Manipulating the immune system with immune globulin. N Engl J Med 1992;326:107–16.

Greaves MW. Chronic urticaria. N Engl J Med 1995;332:1767–72.

Nelson HS. Beta-adrenergic bronchodilators. N Engl J Med 1995;333:49–56.

Newman LS, et al. Sarcoidosis. N Engl J Med 1997;336:1224–34.

Primer on allergic and immunologic disease. JAMA 1997;278:1797–2034.

Sampson HA, Metcalfe DD. Food allergies. JAMA 1992;268:2840–4.

Shapiro G, Rachelefsky G. Introduction to sinusitis. J Allergy Clin Immunol 1992;90:417–81.

Guidelines

NAEP Expert Panel Report 2. Guidelines for the diagnosis and management of asthma. National Institutes of Health publication number 97-4051A, Washington, DC: National Institutes of Health, May 1997.

Ratko TA, et al. Recommendations for off-label use of intravenously administered immunoglobulin. JAMA 1995;273:1865–70.

Richerson HB, et al. Guidelines for the clinical evaluation of hypersensitivity pneumonitis. J Allergy Clin Immunol 1989;84:839–44.

Studies and Trials

Abramson MJ. Is allergen immunotherapy effective in asthma? Am J Respir Crit Care Med 1995;151:969–74. (*A meta-analysis of 20 RCTs showing that allergen immunotherapy provided symptomatic improvement [odds ratio of 3.2] and reduction in bronchial hyperreactivity [odds ratio of 6.8].*)

Dermatology

Reviews

Anhalt GJ. Paraneoplastic pemphigus. N Engl J Med 1990;323:1729–35.

Asherson RA, et al. Antiphospholipid syndrome. J Invest Dermatol 1993;100:2–7.

Fine JD. Management of acquired bullous skin diseases. N Engl J Med 1995;333:1475–84.

Frank W, Rogers GS. Second primary melanoma. J Dermatol Surg Oncol 1993;19:427–30.

Gallagher RP, McLean DI. The epidemiology of acquired melanocytic nevi. Dermatol Clin 1995;13:595–605.

Gould JW. Cutaneous photosensitivity diseases induced by exogenous agents. J Am Acad Dermatol 1995;33:551–73.

Hogan PA, et al. Viral exanthems. Curr Probl Dermatol 1992;4:37–95.

Laman SD, Provost TT. Cutaneous manifestations of lupus erythematosus. Rheum Dis Clin North Am 1994;20:195–212.

17

Levenson DE, et al. Cutaneous manifestations of adverse drug reactions. Immunol Allergy Clin North Am 1991;11:493–507.

National Institutes of Health. Diagnosis and treatment of early melanoma. NIH Consens Statement 1992;10:1–25.

Piette WW. The differential diagnosis of purpura from a morphologic perspective. Adv Dermatol 1994;9:3–24.

Studies and Trials

Augenbraun M, et al. Increased genital shedding of HSV-2 in HIV-seropositive women. Ann Intern Med 1995;123:845–7. (*Asymptomatic shedding of HSV is linked to HIV infection and rises with increasing immune deficiency.*)

Black HS, et al. Effect of a low-fat diet on the incidence of actinic keratosis. N Engl J Med 1994;330:1272–5. (*Low fat intake reduced the development of new actinic keratoses.*)

Chuang TY, Reizner GT. Bowen's disease and internal malignancy. J Am Acad Dermatol 1988;19:47–51. (*This case-control study showed no association between Bowen's disease and internal malignancy.*)

Cornell RC, et al. Intralesional interferon therapy for basal cell carcinoma. J Am Acad Dermatol 1990;23:694–700. (*Injection of IFN-α-2b improved cure rates for basal cell carcinoma four-fold in this RCT. The authors recommend its use for patients who cannot undergo surgery.*)

Hofmann H, et al. Treatment of toenail onychomycosis. Arch Dermatol 1995;131:919–22. (*An RCT showing that terbinafine had a higher cure rate [60%] than griseofulvin [39%] and that use of the former required a shorter course of therapy.*)

Karagas MR, et al. Risk of subsequent basal cell carcinoma and squamous cell carcinoma of the skin among patients with prior skin cancer. JAMA 1992;267:3305–10. (*There was a 50% risk of developing second cancer within 5 years of the original diagnosis.*)

Khamashta MA, et al. The management of thrombosis in the antiphospholipid syndrome. N Engl J Med 1995;332:993–7. (*High-dose warfarin [INR > 3] was better at preventing recurrence than low-intensity warfarin or aspirin.*)

Misiani R, et al. Interferon alfa-2a therapy in cryoglobulinemia associated with hepatitis C virus. N Engl J Med 1994;330:751–6. (*Interferon reduces HCV-associated vasculopathies.*)

Tatnall FM, et al. A double-blind, placebo-controlled trial of continuous acyclovir in recurrent erythema multiforme. Br J Dermatol 1995;132:267–70. (*Even patients without clear evidence of HSV improved with acyclovir; recurrent erythema multiforme may occur in patients with subclinical HSV infection.*)

Thompson SC, et al. Reduction of solar keratoses by regular sunscreen use. N Engl J Med 1993;329:1147–51. (*This RCT confirmed that regular sunscreen use reduced the number and development of new lesions, even after many years of sun exposure.*)

Tucker MA, et al. Clinically recognized dysplastic nevi. JAMA 1997;277: 1439–44. (*One dysplastic nevus doubles the melanoma risk; 10 such nevi multiply the risk by 12.*)

Rheumatology

Reviews

Boumpas DT, et al. Systemic lupus erythematosus. Part I. Ann Intern Med 1995;122:940–50.

Boumpas DT, et al. Systemic lupus erythematosus. Part II. Ann Intern Med 1996;123:42–53.

Brooks PM, Day RO. NSAIDS. N Engl J Med 1991;324:1716–25.

Caldwell JR, Furst DE. The efficacy and safety of low-dose corticosteroids for rheumatoid arthritis. Semin Arthritis Rheum 1991;21:1–11.

Conaghan PG, Brooks PM. Rheumatic manifestations of malignancy. Curr Opin Rheum 1994;6:105–10.

Esterhai JL, Gelb I. Adult septic arthritis. Orthop Clin North Am 1991;22:503–14.

Fries JF, et al. Reduction in long-term disability in patients with rheumatoid arthritis by DMARDs (disease-modifying anti-rheumatic drugs). Arthritis Rheum 1996;39:616–22.

Hoffman GS, et al. Wegener's granulomatosis. Ann Intern Med 1992;116:488–98.

Jennette JC, Falk RJ. Small vessel vasculitis. N Engl J Med 1997;337:1512–23.

Kaandorp CJ, et al. Risk factors for septic arthritis in patients with joint disease. Arthritis Rheum 1995;38:1819–25.

Kerr GS, et al. Takayasu's arteritis. Ann Intern Med 1994;120:919–29.

Larsson LG, Baum J. The syndromes of bursitis. Bull Rheum Dis 1986;36:1–8.

Mankin HJ. Nontraumatic necrosis of bone. N Engl J Med 1992;326:1473–9.

Miller PD, et al. Clinical utility of bone mass measurements in adults. Semin Arthritis Rheum 1996;25:361–72.

Munoz FS, et al. Rheumatic manifestations of HIV. Semin Arthritis Rheum 1991;21:30–9.

Nicholas NS, Panayl GS. Rheumatoid arthritis and pregnancy. Clin Exp Rheum 1988;6:179–82.

Olin JW. Thromboangiitis obliterans. N Engl J Med 2000;343:864–9.

Pam AG, et al. Desensitization to allopurinol in patients with gout and cutaneous reactions. Am J Med 1992;93:299–302.

Ruddy S. Rheumatic diseases and inherited complement deficiencies. Bull Rheum Dis 1996;45:6–8.

Sakene T, et al. Behcet's disease. N Engl J Med 1999;341:1284–91.

Shuman S, et al. Compression neuropathies. Semin Neurol 1987;7:76–87.

Smith DL, Campbell SM. Painful shoulder syndromes. J Gen Intern Med 1992;7:328–39.

Vianna JL, et al. Comparison of the primary and secondary antiphospholipid syndrome. Am J Med 1994;96:3–9.

Guidelines

American College of Rheumatology. Guidelines for medical management of osteoarthritis. Arthritis Rheum 1995;38:1535–46.

American College of Rheumatology. Guidelines for monitoring drug therapy in rheumatoid arthritis. Arthritis Rheum 1996;39:723–31.

American College of Rheumatology. Guidelines for the initial evaluation of the adult patients with acute musculoskeletal symptoms. Arthritis Rheum 1996;39:1–8.

American College of Rheumatology. Methotrexate for rheumatoid arthritis. Arthritis Rheum 1994;37:28–36.

Carias K, Panush RS. Acute arthritis. Bull Rheum Dis 1994;43:1–4.

Evans TI, et al. A comprehensive investigation of inpatient IV colchicine use. J Rheumatol 1996;23:143–8.

Kwoh CK, Simms RW. Guidelines for the management of rheumatoid arthritis. Arthritis Rheum 1996;39:713–22.

Studies and Trials

Arthritides.

Bradley JD, et al. Comparison of an anti-inflammatory dose of ibuprofen, an analgesic dose of ibuprofen, and acetaminophen in the treatment of patients with osteoarthritis of the knee. N Engl J Med 1991;325:87–91. (*Over 4 weeks, acetaminophen, 1,200 mg of ibuprofen/d, and 2,400 mg of ibuprofen/d were equivalent in efficacy for knee arthritis.*)

Cushnaghan J, et al. Taping the patella medially. BMJ 1994;308:753–5. (*Medial knee taping reduced pain by 25% in osteoarthritis [superior to lateral or neutral taping].*)

Ferraz MB, O'Brien B. A cost effectiveness analysis of urate-lowering drugs in nontophaceous recurrent gouty arthritis. J Rheumatol 1995;22:908–14. (*Urate-lowering drugs were cost effective in those with two or more episodes of gouty arthritis a year.*)

Garfinkel MS, et al. Yoga for carpal tunnel syndrome. JAMA 1998;280:1601–3. (*In this RCT, yoga was more effective than wrist splinting or no treatment in relieving the signs and symptoms of carpal tunnel syndrome.*)

Jawaheer D, et al. Homozygosity for the HLA-DR shared epitope contributes the highest risk for rheumatoid arthritis concordance in twins. Arthritis Rheum 1994;37:681–6. (*HLA-DRB1 homozygosity accounts for the increased risk of RA in twins.*)

O'Dell JR, et al. Treatment of early rheumatoid arthritis with minocycline or placebo. Arthritis Rheum 1997;40:842–8. (*An RCT showing that minocycline 100 mg bid was effective for early RA.*)

Simon LS, et al. Anti-inflammatory and upper GI effects of celecoxib in rheumatoid arthritis. JAMA 1999;282:1921–8. (*Celecoxib was as effective and had fewer endoscopic ulcers than naproxen in patients with RA.*)

Collagen-Vascular Disorders and Vasculitides.

Dalakas MC, et al. A controlled trial of high-dose intravenous immunoglobulin for dermatomyositis. N Engl J Med 1993;329:1993–2000. (*An RCT showing that IV gamma globulin was safe and effective for dermatomyositis.*)

Evans JM, et al. Increased incidence of aortic aneurysm and dissection in temporal arteritis. Ann Intern Med 1995;122:502–7. (*Patients with temporal arteritis were 17.3 times more likely to develop thoracic aortic aneurysms and 2.4 times as likely to get abdominal aortic aneurysms.*)

Guillevin L, et al. Prognostic factors in polyarteritis nodosa and Churg-Strauss syndrome. Medicine 1996;75:17–28. (*Patients with idiopathic polyarteritis nodosa and good prognosis should receive just prednisone those with a bad prognosis [cardiac, CNS, GI, or renal disease] should receive prednisone and cyclophosphamide. Those with HBV-associated polyarteritis nodosa should be given prednisone briefly, followed by plasmapheresis and antivirals [vidarabine or IFN-α-2b].*)

Spondyloarthropathies.

Kirwan J, et al. The course of established ankylosing spondylitis and the effects of sulfasalazine over 3 years. Br J Rheumol 1993;32:729–33. (*An RCT showing that sulfasalazine reduced peripheral arthritis but did not affect spinal mobility in these patients.*)

Leirisalo-Repo M, et al. High frequency of silent inflammatory bowel disease in spondyloarthropathy. Arthritis Rheum 1994;37:23–31. (*Forty-four percent of patients with chronic spondyloarthropathies had silent endoscopic lesions in the ileum and colon; 26% met criteria for Crohn's disease.*)

18

Office Specialties: Ophthalmology, Orthopedics, Otolaryngology, and Gynecology

In matters of conscience, first thoughts are best; in matters of prudence, last thoughts are best. —Robert Hall

The key to everything is patience. You get the chicken by hatching the egg, not by smashing it. —Ellen Glasgow

OPHTHALMOLOGY

General

1. Like all subspecialties, there are important conditions (which the specialist wants to be called about) and unimportant conditions (which the specialist does not want to hear about), and, of course, the consultant would like the general physician to make those distinctions.
2. One of the great things about ophthalmology is that just about everything can wait at least an hour to be taken care of, often even a day.
3. You should be able to do a basic H&P with respect to the eye: See Table 18–1 for a discussion of eyedrops.
   - Ask about change in vision, change in color vision, diplopia, pain, itch, foreign body sensation, flashing lights, floaters, gray spots, history of eye problems, and history of trauma.
   - *Check vision* (at least with a near card). Use a pinhole to correct for refractive error. In people over 40, make sure they are wearing their reading glasses for near cards.

Table 18–1. Common Eyedrops and Systemic Side Effects

Medication	Systemic Side Effects
Brimonidine (Alphagan)	Bradycardia
Timolol (Timoptic) and other beta-blockers	Bradycardia, asthma exacerbation, depression
Dorzolamide (Trusopt)	Metabolic acidosis
Prednisolone (Pred Mild, Pred Forte)	All of the side effects of steroids

- You should also be able to check extraocular motions, pupils (look for afferent pupillary deficit—discussed below), and basic anterior segment evaluation (see below).
- When the eye is red, look for ciliary flush (a rim of hot pink around the cornea distinct from diffuse redness). Ciliary flush indicates corneal pathology (eg, abrasion) or intraocular inflammation, thus helping you decide what is important versus what is not important.
- You can check for cataract by holding a direct ophthalmoscope at arm's length from the patient and setting power to +2 (green) (the optical distance of arm's length is about 2 diopters). A cataract will appear as dark patches in the red reflex. Diabetics will have a spoke-and-wheel configuration.
- When using a direct ophthalmoscope, leave your own glasses on.
- If you want to look at the retina and optic disc, you must dilate the patient. Use phenylephrine (Mydfrin, Neo-Synephrine) and tropi-camide (Mydriacyl) eyedrops. Don't worry about causing angle-closure glaucoma (the incidence with dilation is 1/40,000). Further, if it does happen, you have diagnosed the patient in a controlled setting where treatment is immediately available (ie, you have done the patient a favor). If it does happen, use pilocarpine eyedrops and call Ophthalmology. If you don't dilate, you will never see the retina, and your examination will be horrible.
- Check the cornea using a fluorescein strip (if there is an abrasion or infiltrate, it will light up as bright green under blue light).

- If the eye is swollen, don't be afraid to forcefully open the lids (looking at the eye is key).
- Screen optic nerve function with a pupil check and color vision.

4. Basic anatomy:
   - The anterior segment includes the cornea (the clear part on the front of the eye; we don't mean to be condescending, but a lot of people don't know), iris (the color part of the eye), angle of the eye (at the junction of the iris and cornea, this is where the drainage of the eye is), and lens (behind the eye). The sclera is the white part of the eye. Hyphema is blood in the anterior chamber (between cornea and iris), and hypopyon is pus in the anterior chamber.
   - The anterior chamber is the space between the iris and the cornea and is filled with aqueous humor (in patients with narrow angles, it is shallow); the posterior chamber is between the lens and the iris.
   - The posterior segment is everything behind the lens (includes the vitreous and retina).

5. Pupils:
   - Afferent pupillary defect is known as Marcus Gunn pupil (indicates optic nerve dysfunction). The affected pupil will not respond to direct light but retains consensual response. So, the affected pupil dilates when light is swung from the unaffected to the affected eye. Also, the unaffected eye's pupil significantly constricts with the converse.
   - Argyll Robertson pupil (prostitute's pupil) can accommodate but not react (indicates syphilis).
   - Adie's pupil is tonic dilation of pupil due to idiopathic loss of cholinergic fibers. It is usually benign and self-limited. The differential includes pharmacologic dilation (from plants, medicine cabinet, belladonna make-up, etc). Diagnose by its response to 1% pilocarpine. Don't let this scare you (if someone is talking to you, he or she probably doesn't have intracranial bleeding just because one pupil is dilated).
   - The playful pupil constricts and dilates while light is shone directly. This is a NORMAL variant.
   - In physiologic anisocoria, both pupils respond normally to light but are slighly asymmetric. This is a NORMAL variant.

Clinical Entities and Treatments

1. The focus will be on things that are common and things that are important to recognize and refer. Going against the grain, we have not grouped these by presentation because many things can present in many ways. You should have a working knowledge of the conditions below.

2. *Angle closure glaucoma.* Key signs and symptoms are pain, headache, nausea and vomiting, decrease in vision, redness with ciliary flush, and visual halos. The pupil is usually not reactive on the affected side, and the eye is hard due to elevated pressure. Give pilocarpine drops and get the ophthalmologist quickly.

3. *Bell's palsy.* Look for corneal exposure and assess the blink; have the patient tape the eyelids and use lots of lubrication. If there is corneal abrasion, use erythromycin ointment. Due to research showing viral involvement, start famciclovir (Famvir) 500 mg PO tid or valacyclovir (Valtrex) 1 g PO bid for 10 days, with prednisone 60 mg PO qd for 5 days and prednisone taper for an additional 5 days.

4. *Blepharitis:*
   • The bane of ophthalmology, this exceedingly common problem presents with chronic irritation, foreign body sensation, and dryness (it's the fibromyalgia of ophthalmology). On examination, swollen meibomian glands, inspissated secretions, and telangiectasia of the eyelids can be seen. It is correlated with poor facial hygiene, acne rosacea, dandruff, long-term eye problems, age, and high anxiety levels. Often, it is a garbage diagnosis (ophthalmologists diagnose it when they don't see anything wrong). Fortunately, it is not serious (it does not affect vision or damage the eye). Treat with warm compresses, artificial tears, and lid scrubs (with a Q-tip in baby shampoo and hot water). For severe cases, use Blephamide drops or oral doxycycline. You must explain to the patient that it is not serious but it is chronic (there is no cure).

5. *Conjunctivitis:*
   • Bacterial: usually occurs in children; easy to diagnose (very purulent). Treat with erythromycin or sulfacetamide ointment + cold compresses + artificial tears.
   • Viral: very common (especially after exposure to others with a red eye, URI). Presents with severe redness (often asymmetric), tear-

ing, foreign body sensation, pain, itch (pain is greater than itch), and preauricular nodes. Treat with cold compresses, artificial tears, and ketorolac (Acular) eyedrops for severe pain. If there is corneal involvement, give erythromycin and refer to an ophthalmologist.

- Allergic: presents with severe itch, some pain (itch is greater than pain), mild redness, and often a history of allergies or exposure to allergens. Treat with cold compresses, artificial tears, and olopatadine (Patanol, Claritin for the eye) eyedrops qid.
- Medicamentosa. Chronic inflamed conjunctiva can be due to patients' taking frequent use of Visine, a vasoconstrictor that induces tolerance and dependence of the conjunctiva. So, the patient should go cold turkey and take lots of cold compresses and artificial tears (notice a theme?). As for you, stay away from Visine.

6. *Contact lens problems.* If there is severe pain, redness, and ciliary flush, a corneal abrasion or ulcer is likely. Start Ocuflox (at least q4h) eyedrops and refer to an ophthalmologist. If there is an obvious infiltrate (white spot on cornea), start Ocuflox q1h (some would say the patient should do q1h through the night, but we usually do it just q1h while awake and twice at night). The patient must not wear contacts during treatment and for at least a week after and must get a new pair of contacts. Explain that it will hurt a lot. Do not patch. Standard contact lens hygiene includes never sleeping in them, daily cleaning, replacement of contacts at least every 6 months, and limiting use to 8 to 10 hours at a stretch. If the patient has severe itch and big papillae on the eyelids (flip upper lid), then it is probably giant papillary conjunctivitis; treat with olopatadine (Patanol) qid and change contacts. Refer to an ophthalmologist.

7. *Corneal abrasion.* Usually, there is a history of trauma, and patient will report that it hurts when he or she blinks. Symptoms include pain, redness, ciliary flush, and photophobia. Look under the lower eyelid and flip the upper eyelid to make sure there is no foreign body. Treat with erythromycin ointment qid for 5 to 7 days. You must tell the patient that this will hurt a lot (the cornea has more nerve density than even the fingertips). Patching is not generally useful, except for comfort. If there is an obvious foreign body or a history of organic matter or flying metal, refer to an ophthalmologist.

8. *Diabetes*. Make sure diabetics are seen at least annually by an ophthalmologist. Cotton-wool spots (areas of nerve fiber layer infarcts in the retina) and dot-and-blot hemorrhages per se are not serious (but they do indicate a need for better diabetic management). Neovascularization is a major serious complication of diabetes.

9. *Diplopia* indicates nerve palsy or damage to muscle. Assess extraocular eye motion. Nerve palsies (especially of the III nerve but also of the IV and VI) occur very commonly in diabetics. Diabetic III palsies are usually painless and spare the pupil; if they involve the pupil (efferent pupil defect) or have pain, you must rule out posterior communicating artery aneurysm. Myasthenia gravis can cause ptosis and consequent diplopia, whereas multiple sclerosis can affect medial longitudinal fasciculus, causing internuclear ophthalmoplegia (see Chapter 8).

10. *Eyelid swelling*. Periorbital cellulitis is very common in children and also occurs after trauma. Usually, the lid is swollen, warm, red, and tender. In patients with chronic blepharitis, you can obtain very similar findings (generally no warmth and little tenderness), which is called a hordeolum, which is a prelude to a chalazion (a technical term for sty). For periorbital cellulitis, make sure there is no orbital involvement (key findings for the latter are restriction in motility, diplopia, proptosis, and change in vision). For hordeolum/chalazion, treat like blepharitis (warm compresses are crucial).

11. *Focal injection of conjunctiva*. You must distinguish episcleritis versus scleritis. Episcleritis is benign, painless, and red, without intraocular inflammation. Scleritis is serious, often has intraocular inflammation, is painful, and has a purplish/bluish hue. Episcleritis is treated with cold compresses and artificial tears, whereas scleritis requires further work-up by an ophthalmologist.

12. *Herpes*. It is very important to realize that just because there is involvement of eyelids by herpes (simplex or zoster) does not mean there is eye involvement. If the vision is okay and the eye is white, in all likelihood, there is no involvement. Herpes zoster ophthalmicus refers to involvement of the ophthalmic branch (V1) of the trigeminal nerve, not ophthalmic involvement. The eye is likely involved if there is eye redness, change in vision, flashing lights, floaters, or vesicles on the tip of the nose (nasociliary branch of V1 supplies the cornea and the tip of the nose; called Hutchinson's sign). You can see a corneal

18

dendrites pattern with fluorescein in HSV and pseudodendrites with VZV. The treatment for corneal herpes simplex is acyclovir + Viroptic eyedrops every 2 hours (refer to an ophthalmogist). For zoster, you can use Famvir 500 mg PO bid. IV acyclovir is reserved for immuno-suppressed patients or those with intraocular involvement.

13. *HIV.* If CD4 is < 75, there is a risk of CMV retinitis, and the patient should be screened every 3 months. *Toxoplasma*, HSV, and VZV are other major opportunistic ocular pathogens. *Don't call for a routine ophthalmologic screen on the day of discharge (it's not cool, especially on the weekend).* Symptoms include a change in vision, flashing lights, and floaters. See Chapter 11 for more information.

14. *Hypertension.* Arteriovenous nicking (nicking of arteries as they cross veins), copper/silver wire appearance of retinal arteries, and cotton-wool spots are evidence of hypertensive retinopathy. Diffuse hemorrhages and disc edema indicate malignant HTN.

15. *Hyphema.* Usually after blunt trauma, in this condition, blood is visible in the anterior chamber. The main risk is rebleed withing the first 72 hours, so the patient must be bedbound for that time. Give the patient Pred Forte six times a day and scopolamine bid, and do an ophthalmologic evaluation every day.

16. *Iritis.* Key symptoms are redness, severe photophobia, and pain (to both direct light and light shone into the uninvolved eye, as pupillary constriction causes pain). It usually occurs in men in their 20s to 30s. The anterior chamber is often cloudy. If you have a slit-lamp, look for cells. Treat with Pred Forte six times a day plus scopolamine bid (anti-inflammatory plus dilation to prevent synechiae formation and relieve pain) eyedrops; refer to an ophthalmologist. Approximately 50% of patients have only one episode. If there is recurrence or if both eyes are involved, do a work-up (HLA-B27, ANA, RF, RPR, FTA-Abs, Lyme titer, PPD). Do a CXR to rule out TB and sarcoid. Do a sacroiliac x-ray to rule out ankylosing spondylitis.

17. *Optic neuritis* usually occurs in young women. Symptoms include a slight decrease in vision but a dramatic decrease in color vision (test by asking patients to compare objects with each eye, and with Ishihara color plates). The sine qua non is afferent pupillary defect. Do MRI to look for enhancing lesions in the brain. Refer to an ophthalmologist. Be aware of the optic neuritis treatment trial (bottom line:

IV methylprednisolone followed by oral prednisone was good, whereas oral prednisone alone was bad). There is a risk of subsequent multiple sclerosis.

18. *Proptosis*/orbital compartment syndrome. Motility restriction, decreased vision, and optic neuropathy (color vision decline, afferent pupillary defect) indicate urgent intervention. For chronic thyroid orbitopathy, watch out for corneal exposure (have the patient tape the lids at night and use lots of artificial tears and Lacri-Lube ointment). Pseudotumor cerebri (occurs in young, obese women) presents with papilledema, disc hemorrhages, headache, and often without loss of vision. Treat with weight loss and acetazolamide (Diamox) 500 mg PO bid.

19. *Retinal detachment.* Key symptoms are flashing lights, burst of floaters, gray spots in vision (eg, curtain/shade across vision), and change in vision. Risk factors are prior retinal detachment, myopia, age, trauma, and family history. Get an ophthalmologist quickly.

20. *Subconjunctival hemorrhage.* This common condition is benign but scary. It is just a broken vessel on the conjunctiva overlying the sclera (not the cornea), is self-limited, and does not affect vision. However, it gets bigger initially (due to the spread of the hemorrhage) and changes colors before finally disappearing in 2 to 3 weeks. The causes of subconjunctival hemorrhage are idiopathic (most common), HTN, trauma, and straining (eg, constipation).

21. *Temporal arteritis.* Cardinal symptoms are headache, jaw claudication, diffuse myalgias (polymyalgia rheumatica), change in vision, and change in temporal pulse or bruit. If you have an elderly patient with an acute change in vision without another explanation, you must rule this out. Check ESR (generally over 80). If positive, start high-dose steroids (methylprednisolone 250 IV q6; taper to prednisone 60 mg PO bid, which should be continued for months). Get a temporal artery biopsy, but don't wait to start steroids.

22. *TIA.* Amaurosis fugax is a sudden unilateral loss of vision. You must rule out carotid and heart disease (check echocardiogram, carotid Doppler). Give ASA. Consider CT. If the vision does not improve, consider central retinal arterial occlusion and get an ophthalmologist quickly. Consider IV TPA (interventional radiology) and consider starting carbogen (an inhaled mixture of high oxygen and carbon dioxide).

23. Thus, you should be able to handle conjunctivitis, blepharitis, corneal abrasion, and subconjunctival hemorrhage (ie, don't call Ophthalmology unless it's serious).

24. *Things to refer immediately:*
    - Possible retinal detachment
    - Angle-closure glaucoma
    - Ruptured globe (eg, iris is hanging on the cheek, knife is through the eye)
    - Central retinal arterial occlusion
    - Optic neuritis
    - Hyphema

25. *Next-day referrals* include
    - Iritis
    - Cellulitis
    - Herpes
    - Bell's palsy
    - Anything else of concern

26. Miscellaneous: Roth's spots (hemorrhages with white centers) occur in endocarditis and leukemia. Pancreatitis can cause Purtscher's retinopathy (aggregations of WBCs in retinal vessels), causing sudden visual loss.

ORTHOPEDICS

Shoulder

1. Patients often present with pain on abduction above 90 degrees or lying on one side. The trigger is often overhead activity, which suggests impingement on the subacromial space or rotator cuff injury. Treat with NSAIDs, rest, and depot injection of corticosteroid plus local anesthetic in the posterior shoulder between the infraspinatus and teres minor into the subacromial space.

2. Weight lifters or contact-sports athletes often develop acromioclavicular arthritis, which has shoulder pain triggered by horizontal adduction of the arm. Treat with NSAIDs and rest. If persistent, get an x-ray; osteolysis of the distal clavicle may need to be resected in severe cases.

3. In chronic shoulder pain, if subacromial injection of a local anesthetic improves function, a rotator cuff tear is unlikely, and management is conservative. If weakness persists, a rotator cuff tear is likely pre-

sent; the patient should be referred to an orthopedist, and a lateral shoulder x-ray (outlet view) or MRI should be done to rule out bony encroachment.

4. Frozen shoulder is manifested by a great limitation of abduction and external rotation. Treat with depot injection of a local anesthetic plus corticosteroid, physical therapy, and referral to an orthopedist.

5. Shoulder separations (acromioclavicular dislocation) is treated with a sling and local-anesthetic injections. X-rays are done to rule out fracture. Traumatic unstable shoulders should be referred quickly to an orthopedist as arthroscopic surgery is often necessary. An atraumatic unstable shoulder may occur in connective tissue disorders. Surgery is rarely effective. Management of these is conservative.

Elbow

Lateral elbow pain is the most common problem; known as tennis elbow, lateral epicondylitis is due to repetitive or intense activity. Pain is triggered by wrist motion or gripping. Treat with NSAIDs and ice; injections aren't used. Golfer's elbow is known as medial epicondylitis. Olecranon bursitis occurs with repetitive elbow extension or a single blow. Treat with aspiration and steroid injection with NSAIDs and an elbow sleeve.

Wrist

1. Falls on an outstretched hand can cause Colles' fracture (of the distal radius) and scaphoid fracture (very bad as it often results in avascular necrosis of the scaphoid). Scaphoid fractures are not well seen on x-ray. If pain in the anatomic snuff box persists after 2 weeks with a splint, do a bone scan. The lunate is the most commonly displaced bone.

2. Carpal tunnel syndrome results from median nerve compression. Pain can go into the hand and forearm; thenar muscle weakness and atrophy can occur. It is a repetitive stress injury. Treat with a splint, physical therapy, ergonomic keyboards, etc. Patients with persistent pain should have decompression surgery after EMG/nerve conduction velocity to rule out other causes.

Hip

1. Repetitive flexion and extension of the hip can cause trochanteric bursitis (over the proximal lateral femur). Sleeping on either side is hard

to do in this case (sleeping on the contralateral side stretches the iliotibial band, which can apply force to the bursa, and sleeping on the same side causes direct compression of the bursa). Treat with NSAIDs, rest, ice, and physical therapy. Ischial pain (worse on sitting) is usually due to a hamstring injury or sciatic nerve pathology.

2. Hip pain is usually referred to the groin, anterior thigh, or knee. Limp is also a common finding. Hip stress fractures are best detected with bone scan or MRI. Avascular necrosis of the femoral head (Bo Jackson injury; occurs with trauma, steroids, and lupus) may require total hip replacement. Slipped capital femoral epiphysis occurs in children prepuberty. Treat with NSAIDs, analgesia, and referral to an orthopedist.

Knee

1. Anterior knee pain is often due to prolonged sitting and going up and down stairs and can be due to many mechanical causes. Pain is triggered by resisted quadriceps contraction. Treat with NSAIDs, rest, and occasionally intra-articular injections. Physical therapy is usually necessary.

2. Sorry triad = medial meniscus, medial collateral ligament, and anterior cruciate ligament (structures most likely to be torn in knee trauma). MRI and orthopedic referral are needed in probably all knee trauma cases.

3. Knee arthritis often causes pain and noninflammatory effusion after weight-bearing activity. Treat with analgesics, physical therapy, weight loss, and knee braces. Refer to an orthopedist if chronic.

Anterior Compartment Syndrome

Increased pressure in the anterior compartment of the lower leg can cause peroneal nerve compression, causing foot drop and sensory changes. It may be unmasked after exercise. Treat with fasciotomy.

Ankle and Foot

1. Lateral ankle sprains should be splinted for 1 to 2 days and mobilized early. Treatment involves physical therapy. Medial heel pain radiates to the plantar surface and plantar fasciitis. It is worsened by weight bearing, sitting, and dorsiflexion of the ankle and toe. Treat with rest, NSAIDS, ice, and heel taping.

2. Morton's foot refers to the short, hypermobile first metatarsal, which is inadequate for pushoff. A foot orthosis is often needed. It can lead

to Morton's neuroma, which often needs local anesthetic injection or surgical management.

Spine

1. Spinal stenosis is very commonly seen in the ambulatory setting. It is often seen as pain going down stairs. One can distinguish this from claudication as the latter's pain occurs with walking but not standing, whereas spinal stenosis causes pain even with standing. Treatment is analgesia. The role of MRI is controversial, as abnormalities seen are often not clinically relevant. If there is obvious nerve root compression or a radicular component to pain, decompression may be needed.

2. Low back pain is often seen in young adults. Contrary to old teachings, the patient should be mobilized early. If there is a radicular component (you can often discern this by a straight-leg test, which means that pain is elicited by passive raising of the leg above 45 degrees), you should do MRI to rule out disc pathology and refer as appropriate.

3. In a setting of trauma, always remember to clear the C-spine (you need a lateral view to visualize down to body of T1, and view through the mouth to view the dens and C1–C2 joint). Patients with RA or Down syndrome often have an unstable C1–C2 joint, so these patients should have that evaluated prior to elective intubation.

4. Finally, remember that *new back pain in patients with a history of cancer indicates metastases until proven otherwise.*

OTOLARYNGOLOGY

1. *Otitis externa* is due to pustules, local furuncles, perforated otitis media, or chronic eczema. It causes pain with movement of the pinna or mastication, unlike otitis media. Recurrent furuncles suggest DM, whereas chronic inflammation of the ear canal may be due to skin cancers. Treat with analgesia, avoidance of water, and topical antibiotics. If there is involvement of the ear, use oral antibiotics to cover *S. aureus* and *Pseudomonas. Pseudomonas* causes malignant otitis externa in diabetics, manifested by severe pain, purulent discharge, temporomandibular joint (TMJ) pain, and facial nerve involvement.

2. *Otitis media* is due to *H. influenzae, S. Pneumoniae,* and *Moraxella.* Treat with amoxicillin or cefuroxime. TMP-SMX (Bactrim) is an alternative. Chronic otitis media causes diminished hearing and dis-

charge without pain. Peripheral perforation can cause cholesteatoma. Unilateral serous otitis media can represent an obstructing nasopharyngeal tumor.

3. *Tinnitus* that is audible to the examiner can be due to arteriovenous fistulas, TMJ disorders, and palatal myoclonus. Tinnitus that is audible only to the patient is due to aging, Meniere's disease, and otosclerosis. HTN, thyroid disease, and depression can also cause it. Unilateral tinnitus plus unilateral hearing loss or imbalance requires a work-up for acoustic neuroma.

4. *Sinusitis* pain is exacerbated by bending over or head movement. Palpation and percussion can localize sinus involvement. Etiologies are usually respiratory suspects (*S. Pneumoniae* and *H. influenzae*). A CT scan is the best diagnostic modality and should be done if the patient does not respond to 10 to 14 days of therapy. Sinus puncture is not useful for acute sinusitis. Decongestants shrink mucous membranes but lose efficacy after 72 hours and can cause rebound rhinitis. Steam inhalation is also useful to reduce congestion. Saline nasal spray is sometimes of benefit. Chronic sinusitis is often due to *S. aureus* and oral anaerobes. Treat with amoxicillin (Augmentin) or clindamycin.

5. *Nasal congestion* causing cough implies postnasal drip. Treat with antihistamines (Claritin).

GYNECOLOGY

Benign Breast Disease

1. Fibrocystic disease occurs with the menstrual cycle and does not elevate the risk for breast cancer. It can also be associated with caffeine. Symptoms are worst in the premenstrual phase. Treat with diuretics and NSAIDs.

2. Fibroadenoma is a benign tumor that usually develops in the patient's teens and twenties. These tumors are smooth, mobile, and nontender but continue to grow. Masses should be evaluated with ultrasonography or aspiration up to age 35; in older patients, use a mammogram.

Premenstrual Syndrome

1. Symptoms include bloating, mastodynia, irritability, mood swings, and bowel changes.

2. Treat with symptomatic (withdrawal of caffeine, spironolactone for bloating, NSAIDs for cramps, bromocriptine for mastodynia) oral contraceptives to suppress ovulation.

Menopause

1. The main health issues are hot flashes, cardiac disease, and osteoporosis.
2. Postmenopausal estrogen reduces the risk for CAD by 30 to 50% and also reduces osteoporosis. *Progestin does not offset these beneficial effects.* Combination estrogen-progesterone therapy is thus effective in reducing cardiac mortality and osteoporosis without causing menstrual bleeding or increasing breast or endometrial cancer.
3. Alendronate is an alternative to estrogen to reduce osteoporosis.
4. Intake of 1.5 g of calcium or 1 g daily plus estrogen is recommended.
5. Hot flashes can be treated with short-term estrogen, clonidine, or megestrol.

Vaginitis/Cervicitis

1. Differential includes bacterial vaginosis (due to *Gardnerella vaginalis*), candidiasis, and trichomoniasis.
2. *Gardnerella* is characterized by clue cells (exfoliated vaginal epithelium with organisms on their surface), a pH of 5.0 to 6.0, and a fishy odor. Treat with oral metronidazole 500 mg bid for 7 days. In the first trimester of pregnancy, metronidazole is contraindicated, and the alternative is intravaginal clindamycin cream.
3. Candidiasis is characterized by a pH of 3.5 to 4.5, curd-like discharge, and yeast on KOH preparation. Treat with clotrimazole or terconazole cream.
4. Trichomonas is characterized by a strawberry-red cervix, mobile trichomonads (flagellated) on wet mount, frothy discharge, and a pH of 6.0 to 7.0. Treat with oral metronidazole. *It is vital to treat the sexual partner as well; otherwise, infection will recur.*
5. Atrophic vaginitis usually occurs in menopause. It can be treated with topical or oral estrogen.

Pregnancy

1. Clearly, a primary caregiver should defer to an obstetrician in most matters.

2. Be aware of agents that are contraindicated in pregnancy (Table 18–2).
3. Monitor patients with preexisting glucose intolerance or elevated BP closely for development of gestational diabetes (which can cause rapid progression of diabetic retinopathy and fetal complications) and preeclampsia (HTN and proteinuria). Eclampsia is preeclampsia plus convulsions. Treatment of preeclampsia is delivery of the fetus as soon as possible (you can give dexamethasone to speed fetal lung maturation). Magnesium can help prevent or treat convulsions.
4. HELP syndrome consists of hemolysis, elevated liver enzymes, and proteinuria. This is a variant of preeclampsia.
5. Asymptomatic bacteriuria in pregnancy may be associated with a higher risk of miscarriage and thus should be treated (ampicillin is a safe agent).

Gynecologic Cancers

- As a primary care physician, your role in gynecologic malignancies is principally early detection.
- Endometrial, ovarian, and cervical cancers are the most common gynecologic malignancies; ovarian cancer is the most lethal.
- Cervical cancer:
  - Risk factors include early sexual activity, promiscuity, infection with HSV or HPV (especially serotypes 16 and 18), HIV, other STDs, and smoking.
  - A Pap test is recommended to screen all sexually active women between 18 and 65 with three consecutive annual Pap smears and then every 3 years assuming that the results are benign.
  - Test factoid: if cervical cancer causes hydronephrosis (through impingement on ureters), then it is stage IIIb.
  - Treatment is excision and radiation.
- Endometrial cancer:
  - Risk factors are age, family history, history of hereditary nonpolyposis colon cancer syndrome (ie, Lynch syndromes, which affect the endometrium, breast, and GI tract), and long exposure to estrogen (early menarche, late menopause, unopposed estrogen therapy, and tamoxifen). Endometriosis is not a risk factor.
- Presentation is usually bleeding.
- Endometrial cells found in a Pap smear of postmenopausal women not on estrogen or atypical endometrial cells of any age should be worked up.

Table 18–2. Partial List of Teratogenic Agents and Effects

Drug	Teratogenic Effect
NSAIDs	Closure of ductus arteriosus, bleeding
Beta-blockers	Fetal loss
Warfarin (Coumadin)	Crosses placenta (unlike heparin) causing bleeding, nasal hypoplasia, bone stippling, growth retardation
Chloramphenicol	Gray baby syndrome (apnea)
Aminoglycosides	Vestibulocochlear nerve damage (deafness)
Sulfonamides	Hyberbilirubinemia, hemolytic anemia
Tetracycline	Staining of deciduous teeth
Anticonvulsants (phenytoin, barbiturates, diazepam)	Cardiac abnormalities, mental retardation, facial malformations (similar to fetal alcohol syndrome)
Valproate	Neural tube defects (spina bifida)
Sulfonylureas	Neonatal hypoglycemia
ACE inhibitors	Aplasia cutis, miscarriage
Antithyroid agents (methimazole, propylthiouracil)	Goiter
Quinolones	Arthropathy, hemolysis
Lithium	Ebstein's anomaly (tricuspid valve malformation + septal defect)
Chemotherapy	Intrauterine growth retardation, abortion, mental retardation, facial anomalies
Isotretinoin (Accutane)	Miscarriage, cardiac defects, CNS malformations
Azathioprine	Adrenal hypoplasia

- Work-up includes endometrial biopsy (which should be done in anyone on estrogen plus progesterone with unexpected bleeding or in patients with irregular bleeding) and ultrasonography.

18

- Ovarian cancer:
  - Usually occult, this tumor is usually widely metastatic at diagnosis. Risk factors include family history and the *BRCA1* gene.
  - Screening is a bimanual pelvic examination.
  - Work-up includes transvaginal ultrasonography.
  - The CA-125 marker is used for trending after therapy.

References are included in Chapter 16.

APPENDIX A
Toxicology

Absence of evidence does not equal evidence of absence. — Robert Wong

To study disease without books is to sail an uncharted sea, while to study books without patients is not to go to sea at all. — Sir William Osler

GENERAL

Call the Poison Control Center (in New York City, 212-POISONS), give charcoal and cathartics, and find out if dialysis or urine alkalinization is beneficial. Do not give ipecac for hydrocarbon poisonings (risk of aspiration).

1. Acetaminophen. Follow LFTs and PT (may need liver transplant), *N*-acetylcysteine within 24 hours (best if within 8 hours).
2. Anticholinergics (drugs, jimson weed). Symptoms include dry as a bone, red as a beet, and mad as a hatter. Pupils are large. Treat with physostigmine.
3. Arsenic. Acute symptoms include GI bleeding, shock, garlic-like breath, acute tubular necrosis, hemolysis, and cardiac arrest. Chronic symptoms include hyperkeratosis, Mees' lines (transverse white striae of fingernails), glove-and-stocking neuropathy, quadriplegia, cancer, and gangrene of the extremities. Treat with dimercaprol and support.
4. Aspirin causes respiratory alkalosis, metabolic acidosis, and then respiratory acidosis, as well as CNS depression. Treat by alkalinizing urine.
5. Barbiturates cause respiratory depression; alkalinize urine.
6. Benzodiazepines cause respiratory depression. Treat with flumazenil (Romazicon) (can also be used to reverse sedation in those who aren't waking up), which is very short acting. There is an increased risk of seizures in epileptics.
7. Beta-blockers. Symptoms include bradycardia and CNS depression. Treat with glucagon (beta receptor is blocked; this bypasses to the cAMP pathway).

8. Cadmium. Source includes mining and batteries. Acute symptoms include respiratory distress, nausea, vomiting, and diarrhea. Chronic symptoms include anosmia, yellow teeth, and osteomalacia. There is no specific treatment. Provide supportive care (vitamin D if osteomalacia).

9. Calcium blockers. Symptoms include bradycardia and CNS depression. Treat with calcium.

10. Carbon monoxide. Symptoms are respiratory and CNS depression. Treat with hyperbaric oxygen.

11. Cyanide. Symptoms include an almond odor, respiratory depression, and coma. Treat with amyl nitrite (nitrites cause methemoglobinemia, which preferentially binds cyanide, saving cytochrome oxidase), sodium thiosulfate (destroys cyanide that is on methemoglobin), and high oxygen.

12. Digoxin. Symptoms include vomiting, delirium, xanthopsia (things look yellow), bradycardia, atrioventricular block, and supraventricular tachycardia. Treat with digoxin immune Fab (Digibind) and phenytoin (Dilantin) for arrhythmias.

13. Ethylene glycol comes from antifreeze and windshield cleaners. Symptoms include metabolic acidosis, oxalate renal stones, and renal failure. Treat with ethanol.

14. Hydrocarbons. Sources are petroleum products. Symptoms include CNS depression, liver/kidney failure, aspiration, and pneumonitis. Treatment is supportive.

15. Ingestion of household products (lye, etc). Use milk and water to dilute and steroids for alkali burns.

16. Lead. Acute symptoms include include abdominal pain, irritability, lethargy, slurred speech, and ataxia (can lead to coma, seizures, and death due to cerebral edema). Chronic symptoms include anemia (can be sideroblastic), mental retardation, subtle cognitive deficits, peripheral motor neuropathy, headache, lead line at the gingiva-tooth border, interstitial nephritis, gout (saturnine), and renal failure. Treat with calcium ethylenediaminetetraacetic acid (EDTA).

17. Lithium. Symptoms include seizures, arrhythmias, and nephrogenic DI. Dialyze if the level is > 3.5; look for ataxia and nystagmus; give fluids.

18. MAOI. Symptoms include agitation, shock, and tachycardia. Treat with support (dialysis is not effective).

19. Mercury. Acute symptoms include pneumonitis, respiratory distress (inhalation), nausea and vomiting, abdominal pain, hematemesis (ingestion), shock, and renal failure. Chronic symptoms include "Mad Hatter" syndrome (irritability, insomnia, delirium) (happened in Minamata, Japan). It can cause fetal mental retardation. In children, mercury causes acrodynia (pink disease), which has itching, flushing, salivation, irritability, high pulse, high BP, and desquamation of the palms and soles. Treat with gastric lavage for acute, dimercaprol, or penicillamine.

20. Methanol comes from wood alcohol. Symptoms include acidosis, blindness, retinal edema, and shock. Treat with ethanol.

21. Methemoglobinemia is caused by nitrites, aniline, dapsone, nitroprusside, and primaquine. Symptoms include cyanosis and hemolysis. It gives a falsely high pulse oximetry. Treat with support, oxygen, and methylene blue (contraindicated in G6PD deficiency).

22. Neuroleptic malignant syndrome consists of QT prolongation, seizures, and hyperthermia. Treat with support, dantrolene, and bromocriptine.

23. Opiates. Symptoms include respiratory and CNS depression and pinpoint pupils. Treat with naloxone (Narcan).

24. Organophosphates (cholinesterase inhibitors, roach killers, etc). Symptoms include tachycardia, sweating, and seizures. Give atropine and pralidoxime.

25. Tricyclics. Symptoms include anticholinergic, prolonged QT. Treat by alkalinizing urine; give diazepam (Valium) for seizures. Bicarbonate is useful for cardiac toxicity.

APPENDIX B
Reading the Literature

I think it proper to suggest a more extended line of investigation which will promise abundant opportunities for practice. — René Descartes

It is astonishing with how little reading a doctor can practice medicine, but it is not astonishing how badly he may do it. — Sir William Osler

We are all pressed for time. Here's how you can keep up with your academics.

BOOKS YOU NEED IN YOUR POCKET (BESIDES THIS ONE, OF COURSE)

1. Drug book (*Clinical Pharmacopeia* or *Handbook of Commonly Prescribed Drugs* are our recommendations) (usually from your friendly neighborhood drug representative)
2. *Sanford Guides to Antimicrobial Therapy* and to *HIV Management*
3. *Facts and Formulas*
4. *ACLS Coderunner* (often courtesy of the Committee on Interns and Residents)

REFERENCE

1. *Harrison's Principles of Internal Medicine* (the gold standard)
2. *Atlas of Clinical Medicine* (an excellent way of correlating image to subject)

TEST REVIEW/PREPARATION

1. For USMLE, the *National Medical Series* are the gold standard. *The Family Practice Review Books* are also excellent, given the primary care bent of these examinations (for steps 2 and 3).
2. For the Medicine Boards, the *Medical Knowledge Self-Assessment Program* (MKSAP) are essential, both for text and questions. Focus especially on the tables in the MKSAP. The questions are excellent.

3. *Medstudy* is a good crash review, one that can be read on the run, in the bathroom, etc. The questions are weak, but do highlight the factoids.
4. *Mayo* is mainly geared for recertification purposes. The questions are fair.
5. *Harrison's Pretest Questions* are excellent.

GENERAL READING

To keep up with the field, read the *New England Journal of Medicine* (*N Engl J Med*) reviews. Go to the library every few weeks and digest them. If you have an appetite for more, go through the case presentations in the *N Engl J Med*. If you still want more, read the abstracts of the articles in the *N Engl J Med* and the *Journal of the American Medical Association* (*JAMA*).

Analysis of a Paper

1. Type of trial:
   - Prospective, randomized, double-blind, placebo-controlled, and crossover (where the two groups switch interventions after some time) types are the best.
   - Case-control trials are the second best.
   - Don't discount retrospective trials (although inconclusive, they often do point directions).
   - Case reports are anecdotes; they are what they are.
2. Don't just read the abstract and discussion, which you will be tempted to do.
   - Look at the methods and results and see if the methods they use are acceptable and if the results they generate answer the question (hard to do but well worth it).

APPENDIX C
Basic Statistics

There are three kinds of lies—lies, damned lies, and statistics. —Benjamin Disraeli

Do not believe hastily—what harm quick belief can do. —Ovid

- Prevalence = proportion of a population with a condition
- Incidence = rate of increase (generally annual) of a condition in a population
- Sensitivity = ability of a test to pick up a true test (ie, [true positives]/[true positives + false negatives])
- Specificity = ability of a test to confirm a true negative (ie, [true negatives]/[true negatives + false positives])
- *Sensitivity and specificity are intrinsic to a test.*
- Positive predictive value = confidence in a positive being true (ie, [true positives]/[true positives + false positives])
- Negative predictive value = confidence in a negative being true (ie, [true negatives]/[true negatives + false negatives])
- *Thus, positive predictive value increases with increasing prevalence and depends more on specificity than sensitivity (the opposite is true for negative predictive value).*
- P value = chance that an observed effect is due to a patient (P < .05 is good, meaning that there is a 95% chance that the effect is good)
- Power = probability that a true effect will be picked up by the study and not missed (generally want a power of at least 80%)
- Odds ratio is similar to relative risk, both of which reflect the amount of risk generated by an intervention
- 95% confidence interval = range of values for odds ratio/relative risk that the observed effect will have a 95% chance of being in (if the confidence interval includes 1.0, then there is a good chance that the effect is due to chance)

- Relative risk reduction (RRR) (percentage reduction in risk by an intervention, eg, if a risk of a disease is reduced from 6 to 3%, that is a 50% RRR)
- Absolute risk reduction (ARR) (using the same example above, this is only a 3% ARR; essentially, ARR = RRR times prevalence of disease)
- Number needed to treat (NNT) is equal to the number of people needed to treat with an intervention to have one patient benefit, so NNT = 1/ARR

APPENDIX D

Playbook of
Formulas and Numbers

Winners do what losers usually don't want to do. —H. Jackson Brown

Even if you're on the right track, you'll get run over if you just sit there.
—Will Rogers

I. Alveolar-arterial gradient =
$(FIO_2 \times 713) - PaO_2 - (PaCO_2 \times 1.25)$
(normal is < 10)

Conceptually, this is inspired oxygen (at room air, that would be 147) minus oxygen in blood minus oxygen used in metabolism (reflected by CO_2 produced times respiratory quotient). Each liter of O_2 in nasal cannula is estimated to add 3%, so 3 L nasal cannula is about 30% O_2. Even with a 100% nonrebreather mask, actual O_2 fraction is probably no more than 80%. Alveolar-arterial gradient rises with age (3 points for every 10 years over 20) and with O_2 concentration.

II. Creatinine clearance:
([140 – age] × [wt in kg])/(72 × Serum Cr mg/dL)

Normal > 100; mild renal failure: 40–100; moderate: 10–40; severe < 10

III. FENa (fractional excretion of Na):
(Urine Na/Plasma Na) × (Plasma Cr/Urine Cr)

FENa < 1 implies prerenal azotemia (intra-arterial volume loss due to dehydration, CHF, hypoalbuminemia, etc). If FENa is > 1, then azotemia is due to renal or postrenal causes.

IV. Free water deficit =
0.6 × wt (kg) × ([Na/140] – 1).

(First part of the equation represents the fluid compartment of the body and the second part the relative lack of water). Remember that half of the deficit should be replaced in the first 24 hours and the rest over the next 48 hours, lest there be cerebral edema.

V. Urine Electrolytes

Urine Na: Useful for FENa calculation and in hypo- and hypernatremia assessment.

The key concept is that properly functioning kidneys hold on to Na well, especially if the volume is low.

If the patient is hyponatremic, check volume status. For hypovolemic hyponatremia, urine Na < 10 implies extrarenal losses (diarrhea, vomiting, pancreatitis, etc). Urine Na > 20 implies renal causes (diuretics, adrenal insufficiency, renal failure).

For euvolemic hyponatremia, urine Na < 10 mEq/L implies polydipsia. Urine Na > 20 implies SIADH. For hypervolemic hyponatremia, urine Na < 10 implies intra-arterial volume loss (cirrhosis, CHF, nephrotic syndrome). Urine Na > 20 implies renal failure.

For hypernatremic patients, assess volume state as well. For hypervolemic hypernatremia (urine Na is generally > 20), the cause is Cushing's, Conn's, or drugs (eg, NaCl tablets, glycirrhyzzic acid in Swiss licorice, etc). Euvolemic hypernatremia (variable urine Na) can be due to DI, sweating, etc. For hypovolemic hypernatremia, urine Na < 10 implies dehydration. Urine Na > 20 implies renal losses (diuretics, renal failure).

Urine K: useful in assessment of hypokalemia.

Urine K < 20 implies nonrenal causes (diarrhea, fistulas, etc). For urine K > 20, check BP. If BP is high, check renin. High renin implies renovascular disease or tumors. Normal renin is Liddle's syndrome. Low renin implies Conn's, Cushing's, or licorice.

If BP is normal, check serum bicarbonate. If bicarbonate is low, then renal tubular acidosis is present. If bicarbonate is high, there is metabolic alkalosis; check urine chloride.

Urine Cl: useful for assessment of metabolic alkalosis.

The key concept is that volume contraction causes properly functioning kidneys to hold on to $NaHCO_3$ and dump KCl.

Urine Cl < 10, indicates saline-responsive alkalosis (there is volume contraction from vomiting, NG suction, villous adenoma, or diuretics). If urine Cl is > 10, check BP. If BP is normal, then there is Bartter's syndrome. If BP is high, there is mineralocorticoid excess (Conn's, Cushing's, drugs, licorice, etc).

VI. Gaps

Anion Gap = Na – Cl – HCO$_3$. Normal = 8–12.

High anion gap implies metabolic acidosis, unless there is infusion of sodium salts (dialysis, ticarcillin-clavulanate [Timentin], etc). Low anion gap can be due to hypoalbuminemia or hyperparaproteinemia (myeloma). Thus, a normal anion gap in a hypoalbuminemic patient is actually high.

Osmolal gap = measured osmolality (osm) – calculated osm.

Measured must always be higher than calculated (if not, check your math, or the lab has screwed up). Calculated osm = $(2 \times Na)$ + (Glucose/18) + (BUN/2.8). Normal gap < 10, and normal osm = 280–290 mmol/L. High osmolal gap implies unmeasured osms (eg, ethanol, methanol, ethylene glycol, etc). If osm gap is high, check pH. If pH is normal, then ethanol or isopropyl alcohol are present. If the patient is acidotic, then methanol or ethylene glycol are present.

VII. Corrections on SMA

1. *Very high glucose* can artificially lower Na. So, real Na = measured Na + 1.6 ([Na – 100]/100) (ie, every 100 of glucose over a 100 knocks down Na by 1.6).
2. *Albumin* affects calcium. So real Ca = measured Ca + 0.8 (4 – albumin) (ie, every 1 point of decrease in albumin lowers calcium by 0.8).
3. If total protein on SMA is more than twice the albumin, there is probably paraproteinemia (myeloma, MGUS, etc), so check serum protein electrophoresis/immune protein electrophoresis in that case.

VII. Body Fluids

1. In general, WBC:RBC ratio is 1:500, so if it is a traumatic tap, reduce fluid WBC accordingly.
2. Blood from trauma generally will clot, whereas blood that is already in a body cavity generally does not.
3. Send plenty of fluid for cytology (generally use ethanol, not formalin, but check with the lab).

PLEURAL EFFUSIONS

Transudates are due to CHF, nephrotic syndrome, and cirrhosis. Exudates are due to malignancy, TB, empyema, and parapneumonic effusions (reactive fluid that is exudative but not infected).

Lab Criterion	Transudate	Exudate
Specific gravity	< 1.016	> 1.016
Total protein	< 3.0	> 3.0
Protein/serum protein	< 0.5	> 0.5*
LDH	< 200	> 200
LDH/serum LDH	< 0.6	> 0.6*
WBC	< 1,000	> 1,000
RBC	< 10,000	> 10,000 (malignancy, TB, pulmonary infarction, or traumatic tap, hemothorax)
Glucose		< 30 implies RA, < 60 implies TB, empyema, or cancer
pH	~7.4	>7.3 is consistent with cancer; < 7.3 suggests TB; < 7.2 suggests empyema needing chest tube
Amylase		> 2X serum amylase indicates pancreatitis, cancer, or Boerhaave's syndrome (esophageal rupture)
Triglycerides (Sudan positive)		Chylothorax (lymphatic obstruction)
Cholesterol (Sudan negative)		Pseudochylothorax (RA, nephrotic syndrome, CHF)

Notes

1. Meigs' syndrome: ovarian tumor causing ascites + pleural effusion
2. Lupus pleuritis causes ANA + pleural effusion.
3. Mesotheliomas cause bloody effusions.

SYNOVIAL EFFUSIONS

1. Viscosity is high in normal or noninflammatory conditions. Viscosity is low in inflammatory or purulent conditions.
2. WBC is < 3,000 in noninflammatory conditions, with PMNs ~ 20%. Inflammatory conditions have WBC of 3,000 to 50,000, with PMN ~ 70%. Purulent conditions have WBC >50,000 (sometimes up to 300,000), with PMNs ~ 90%.
3. Crystal examination and cultures are key (see Chapter 17).

ASCITES

Transudates are due to CHF, nephrotic syndrome, and cirrhosis. Exudates are due to malignancy, TB, peritonitis, and pancreatic ascites (pancreatitis, pseudocyst).

Lab Criterion	Transudate	Exudate
Total protein	< 25	> 25
Protein/serum protein	< 0.5	> 0.5 suggests malignancy
LDH		Elevated in cancer
CEA		> 10 suggests malignancy
CEA/serum CEA		> 2 suggests malignancy
LDH/serum LDH	< 0.6	> 0.6 suggests malignancy
WBC	< 300–500	> 500 (infection, cancer)
RBC	< 10,000	> 10,000 (malignancy, TB, pulmonary infarction, or traumatic tap, hemothorax)
Glucose		< 60 implies TB or cancer
Amylase		Elevated in pancreatic ascites
Triglycerides (Sudan positive)		Chylous effusion

Notes

1. Serum-ascitic albumin gradient (SAAG) is crucial. Serum – ascites albumin > 1.1 occurs in cirrhosis, CHF, and nephrotic syndrome. SAAG < 1.1 in cancer, TB, peritonitis, and pancreatic ascites.

2. Negative AFB stain does not exclude TB. Laparoscopic peritoneal biopsy is needed to rule it in or out definitively.

CEREBROSPINAL FLUID

1. Should do CT before LP if mass lesion is suspected (otherwise may theoretically induce herniation). Thus, if there is a focal neurologic deficit that may be due to focal mass, do CT.

2. Send fluid for glucose, protein, cultures, India ink, *Cryptococcus* antigen (India ink not sensitive enough), and cytology (last only if cancer is an issue). *Check opening pressure* (it's not that hard). If tap is bloody, send tube #2 or #3 for chemistry and tube #3 or #4 for cell count. Send #1 for culture. Always save #4 (labs more likely to lose body fluids that are scarce and hard to obtain).

3. Cytology requires three negative taps for 95% specificity (since each tap yields little fluid).

4. Protein is increased by any meningitis or encephalitis.

5. Normal CSF glucose is two-thirds that of serum. Less indicates bacterial or TB meningitis. Viral (aseptic) meningitis has normal glucose.

6. Normal CSF can have up to 5 WBC (mostly monocytes). Bacterial meningitis causes lots of PMNs. Fungal and TB meningitis give mostly lymphocytes. Carcinomatous meningitis causes mostly mononuclear cells.

7. Opening pressure can be elevated in hydrocephalus and any meningitis (especially fungal or carcinomatous meningitis).

8. Truly bloody CSF (where all tubes are equally bloody, indicating that trauma is not the cause of blood) occurs in acute subarachnoid hemorrhage and herpetic encephalitis.

9. Xanthochromia (yellow CSF) indicates prior subarachnoid bleed.

10. India ink stains *Cryptococcus*.

APPENDIX E

A Whirlwind Tour of Medical Spanish

This is a brief overview of common Spanish terms that will be helpful in a pinch (eg, late at night with no interpreter back-up.) It is not meant as a substitute for proper translation that should be available for elective problems. It is intended for the resident who does not have the time or available memory space to take up the language and therefore may border on the cursory. Spanish pronunciation without actual terms is listed for simplicity.

English Phrase	Spanish Pronunciation
Hello.	Oh-lah.
How are you?	Como esta?
Pain	Dolor
Does it hurt?	Duelle?
When?	Quando?
How?	Como?
How long?	Quanto tiempo?
Where?	Donde?
Breathe.	Respira.
Breathe deeply.	Respira profunda.
Come.	Benga.
Here.	Aki.
Open your eyes.	Abra la sohos.
Relax.	Relaho.
You have	Usted tiene

Continued on next page.

English Phrase	Spanish Pronunciation
One, two, three, four	Uno, dos, tres, quatro
Twice a day	Dos Behsehs al dia. (last 2 words = a day)
Water	Agua
Fever	Feebre
Today	Oy
A moment	Momentito
Month	Mehs
Do you speak English?	Habla inglis?
I don't speak Spanish	Non hablo español
Little	Pokito
Lot, great, much	Mucho; grande
Year	Annyo
What?	Qual?
Look	Mira
Up, down, to the right, to the left	Areba, abaho, del recha, elskiya
There	Aiyah
Do you have?	Tiene?
Going home	A la casa
Please	Por fabor
Thanks	Gracias
Tomorrow	Mañana
Blood	Sangre
You need	Usted necesita

For other common words, just put an "o" or an "a" at the end and make it sound Spanish (eg, problema, stomacho, vomito, nausea, etc) (no disrespect intended).

APPENDIX F
Signs and Syndromes

Our minds are finite, and yet even in these circumstances of finitude, we are surrounded by possibilities that are infinite, and the purpose of human life is to grasp as much as we can out of that infinitude. — Alfred North Whitehead

What we have to learn to do, we learn by doing. — Aristotle

SIGNS

Head

1. Babinski's: extension of the great toe and abduction of other toes in response to plantar stimuli (vs. normal flexion); indicates upper motor neuron disease
2. Bárány's: absence of nystagmus to irrigation of the ear canal, indicating labyrinthine disease (normally, cold water causes nystagmus to the opposite side and warm to the same side [mnemonic is COWS])
3. Battle's: mastoid/postauricular ecchymosis indicating basilar skull fracture
4. Brudzinski's: passive flexion of neck causes flexion of hips and knees; also can mean passive flexion of the leg causing flexion of the other leg; indicates meningitis
5. Chaddock's: stimulation of external malleolus causes extension of the great toe (indicates upper motor neuron disease)
6. Chvostek's: spasm of facial muscles after tapping of facial nerve (occurs in hypocalcemia)
7. Doll's eyes: eyes lower when the head is raised and reversed (indicates brainstem function)
8. Eyelash: stroking eyelashes produces movement of eyelids in hysterically unconscious patients but not in those with strokes or organic brain disease

9. Hoffmann's: nipping of middle finger causing flexion of terminal phalanx of thumb (when unilateral, indicates upper motor neuron disease in corticospinal tract)

10. Hutchinson's: vesicles on the tip of the nose indicate involvement with varicella-zoster virus (VZV) of the nasociliary nerve, which also supplies the cornea

11. Joffroy's: forehead does not wrinkle when eyes roll up (occurs in Graves' disease)

12. Kernig's: calf extension when the thigh is flexed gives severe back pain (meningismus)

13. Kestenbaum's: decreased number of arterioles crossing optic disc margin (indicates optic atrophy)

14. Lasègue's: ankle dorsiflexion causes posterior thigh pain when the hip is flexed (indicates sciatica)

15. Marcus Gunn pupil: afferent pupillary defect

16. Möbius': impaired ocular convergence (Graves' disease)

17. Romberg's: loss of steadiness on standing with feet together on closing of eyes (indicates loss of posterior columns of the spinal cord, eg, tabes dorsalis, subacute combined degeneration)

18. Shawl and V: photosensitivity of skin in the V of the neck and shoulders due to dermatomyositis

19. Stellwag's: infrequent and incomplete blink in Graves' disease

20. Trousseau's: carpal spasm when BP cuff squeezes the arm (hypocalcemia)

Chest

1. de Musset's: head bobbing indicating AR

2. Ewart's: dullness below angle of the left scapula indicating pericardial effusion

3. Hamman's: crunching sound in the chest coinciding with heartbeat (indicates pneumopericardium or mediastinal emphysema)

4. Hill's: femoral BP > 20 mm Hg more than brachial (indicates AR)

5. Kussmaul's: paradoxical rise in jugular venous distension with inspiration (characteristic of tamponade)

6. Scratch: by scratching precordium with stethoscope on chest, can measure heart size

Abdomen

1. Cullen's: periumbilical ecchymosis indicating retroperitoneal hemorrhage (pancreatitis, ectopic pregnancy, leaking AAA, etc)
2. Chadwick's: bluish discoloration of the cervix in pregnancy
3. Grey Turner's: flank ecchymosis indicating retroperitoneal hemorrhage (due to tracking of blood)
4. Groove: big, firm, fixed, tender inguinal nodes in the groove of the ligament (characteristic of lymphogranuloma venereum)
5. Kehr's: left shoulder pain due to referred pain from splenic rupture or pathology
6. Meniscus: on standing, ascitic fluid (if small amount) forms a meniscus over the bladder
7. Puddle: tapping out of abdominal fluid in a circular puddle when patient is on all fours (increased intensity of sound on percussion) as you move the stethoscope up the abdomen indicates level of fluid
8. Rovsing's: pain in the right lower quadrant at McBurney's point on pressure in the left lower quadrant

Extremities and Miscellaneous

1. Drawer: indicates laxity of anterior cruciate ligament or posterior cruciate ligament of the knee
2. Flag sign: bands of hypopigmented hair indicating a history of hypoalbuminemia
3. Homans': pain in the calf or popliteal area with dorsiflexion of foot when the knee is bent (indicates calf DVT)
4. Merke's sign: bands on fingernails indicate hypoalbuminemia
5. Nikolsky's sign: bullae slide over the skin when lateral pressure is applied (indicates separation of outer layers of skin from basal layer) (pemphigus vulgaris)
6. Osler's nodes: painful erythematous swellings on hands and feet (endocarditis)
7. Pastia's line: hemorrhagic transverse lines in skin creases (elbow, groin, wrist) (occurs in scarlet fever)
8. Romaña's: chagoma over the eye (trypanosomiasis)
9. Ruff's: petechiae on the arm after the BP cuff is pressurized, indicating meningococcemia

10. Winterbottom's: swelling of the posterior cervical nodes (sleeping sickness)

SYNDROMES

Neurologic

1. Adams-Stokes: heart block, slow pulse, and seizures
2. Brown-Séquard's: transsection of half of the spinal cord leading to ipsilateral paralysis and proprioception and contralateral loss of pain and temperature (remember, latereal spinothalamic tracts that carry pain fibers cross in cord)
3. Cervical: extra cervical rib compresses the brachial plexus, giving neck pain radiating to the shoulder, arm, and forearm
4. Dandy-Walker: obstructions of foramina of Magendie and Luschka in infants, causing hydrocephalus
5. Down: retardation, simian crease, prominent epicanthal folds, cardiac defects (due to trisomy 21)
6. Fetal alcohol: alcohol-abusing mothers give birth to growth-deficient babies with congenital anomalies
7. Froin's: xanthochromia + high protein in CSF due to blocked CSF outflow
8. Gerstmann's: acalculia, agraphia, right-left disorientation, and agnosia due to parietal lobe lesions
9. Guillain-Barré: viral/autoimmune polyneuritis causing ascending paralysis
10. Horner's: sympathetic cut (often with Pancoast tumor) leading to ptosis, miosis, anhidrosis, and enophthalmos
11. Kartagener's: ciliary dyskinesia (autosomal recessive) leading to sinusitis, bronchiectasis, and situs inversus
12. Klippel-Feil: fused cervical vertebra, short neck, low hairline, and brainstem anomalies
13. Korsakoff's: confabulation by alcoholics
14. Lambert-Eaton: small cell carcinoma mimicking myasthenia (but Lamberg-Eaton myasthenic syndrome is presynaptic defect vs. postsynaptic in myasthenia gravis)
15. Leriche's: distal aortic occlusion (leading to leg weakness and impotence)

16. Pancoast's: tumor in superior sulcus of lung (yields Horner's and muscle atrophy)
17. Ramsay Hunt: geniculate gangion of facial nerve infected by zoster, leading to facial palsy, ear vesicles, and hypogeusia
18. Riley-Day: familial dysautonomia
19. Sheehan's: postpartum pituitary necrosis (due to hemorrhage) leading to hypopituitarism
20. Wernicke's: thiamine deficiency in alcoholics causing ataxia, nystagmus, ophthalmoplegia, and amnesia

Heart

21. Barlow's: late systolic murmur or click at the apex due to a floppy mitral valve
22. Carcinoid: excess serotonin leading to flushing, diarrhea, tricuspid regurgitation, bronchial spasm (look for 5-hydroxyindoleacetic acid in urine)
23. Eisenmenger's: left-to-right shunt that after a long time causes pulmonary HTN causing right-to-left shunt (basically untreatable and terminal, except for heart-lung transplant)
24. Sick sinus: alternating bradycardia and tachycardia

Gastrointestinal

1. Acute radiation: 12 hours after exposure to radiation: vomiting, then prostration, fever, diarrhea, purpura, shock, death
2. Afferent loop: G-J loop obstruction proximal to a gastrojejunostomy.
3. Asherman's: adhesions inside uterus causing infertility (can be from endometriosis)
4. Banti's: splenomegaly + anemia due to cirrhosis/portal HTN or splenic vein thrombosis (latter can occur in pancreatitis)
5. Barrett's esophagus: premalignant columnar metaplasia of lower esophagus due to reflux
6. Budd-Chiari: hepatic vein thrombosis leading to hepatomegaly, ascites, and death (often occurs in paroxysmal nocturnal hemoglobinuria, polycythemia vera, and essential thrombocythemia)
7. Chinese food: monosodium glutamate leading to burning, chest pain, flushing
8. Cronkhite-Canada: GI polyps, diffuse alopecia, nail dystrophy, protein-losing enteropathy

9. Cruveilhier-Baumgarten: cirrhosis, caput medusae, and venous hum and thrill
10. Dubin-Johnson: mild jaundice due to a defect in excretion of conjugated bilirubin
11. Fitz-Hugh–Curtis: gonorrhea/*Chlamydia* causing perihepatitis post-pelvic inflammatory disease (violin-string peritoneal adhesions)
12. Gardner's: autosomal-dominant trait causing colon polyps, osteomas, epidermoid cysts, and fibromas
13. Meigs': ovarian fibroma with ascites and hydrothorax
14. Peutz-Jeghers: intestinal hamartomas (nonmalignant) with hyperpigmentation of mouth, lips, and buccal mucosal
15. Pickwickian: obesity, somnolence, erythrocytosis, and hypoventilation
16. Plummer-Vinson (or, in the U.K., Paterson-Kelly): upper esophageal web (premalignant) wih anemia
17. Reye's: fatty liver infiltration, seizures, unconsciousness when aspirin is given to kids with chickenpox
18. Yellow nail: nail thickening and growth cessation with yellowing due to lymphedema or bronchiectasis
19. Zollinger-Ellison: peptic ulcers (into jejunum), gastric hyperacidity due to gastrinoma of pancreas

MISCELLANEOUS

1. Bartter's: primary juxtaglomerular hyperplasias in kidney with hyperaldosteronism, alkalosis, hypokalemia, increased angiotension and renin but normal BP
2. Behçet's disease: aphthous orogenital ulcers, uveitis, optic atrophy, vasculitis
3. Conn's: primary hyperaldosteronism
4. Ehlers-Danlos: overelasticity and hyperextensibility of skin and joints (due to collagen defect)
5. Fanconi's: type 1, pancytopenia, marrow failure (congenital); type 2, aminoaciduria, glucosuria, phosphaturia, rickets, and cystine deposition (renal diseases or drugs)
6. Felty's: RA, splenomegaly, and neutropenia
7. Hamman-Rich: interstitial pulmonary fibrosis

8. Kimmelstiel-Wilson: intercapillary glomerulosclerosis (characteristic of diabetes)
9. Klinefelter's: XXY genotype leading to infertility, small testes
10. Lesch-Nyhan: deficient in HGPRTase (X-linked trait) causing gout, self-mutilation
11. Löffler's: eosinophilia with transient infiltrates in lungs
12. Marfan: connective tissue inherited disorder leading to arach nodactyly (long extremities and digits), lens subluxation, and aortic insufficiency
13. Mikulicz's: enlargement of lacrimal and salivary glands in leukemia, sarcoidosis, and TB
14. Munchausen: fabrication of organic pathology due to deep-seated psychopathology
15. Postrubella: congenital microphthalmos, cataracts, retardation, pulmonic stenosis, patent ductus arteriosus due to maternal rubella infection during pregnancy
16. Prader-Willi: congenital disease with short stature, obesity, and retardation
17. PMS: pain, irritability, edema, headache 2 to 3 days before menses
18. Reiter's: urethritis, iritis, arthritis (post-*Chlamydia*); also circinate balanitis and keratoderma blennorrhagicum can occur
19. Osler-Weber-Rendu: hemorrhagic hereditary telangiectasia (often causes severe nosebleeds)
20. Restless legs: leg restlessness causing insomnia
21. Stein-Leventhal: polycystic ovarian disease
22. Stevens-Johnson: erythema multiforme + bullae including mucosal membranes
23. Straight back: loss of kyphosis of thoracic spine leading to cardiomegaly, ejection murmur
24. Sudden infant death (SIDS): abrupt and unexplainable death of infant in the first few months of life
25. Superior vena cava: obstructed superior vena cava (from neoplasia) leading to SOB and edema of the head and arms
26. Testicular feminization: XY karyotype with feminine external features
27. Thorn's: salt-losing nephritis

28. Tietze's: costal chondritis
29. Toxic shock: tampon-related desquamation and shock in menses (due to *Staph.* toxins)
30. Turner's: XO karyotype with dwarfism, webbed neck, elbow valgus, sterility
31. Ulysses: iatrogenic sequelae of extensive work-ups due to one false-positive test
32. Waterhouse-Friderichsen: meningococcemia with adrenal hemorrhage and shock

APPENDIX G

Some Important
Drug Interactions

He who knows not, and knows not that he knows not, is a fool—shun him.
He who knows not, and knows that he knows not, is simple—teach him.
—Confucius

The battle against the use of drugs of the action of which we know little
(yet we put them into bodies of the action of which we know less), has not
been brought to a finish. —Sir William Osler

Drug	Increases Level of	Decreases Level of	Comment
Acetazolamide	Quinidine		Metabolic acidosis
Allopurinol	Azathioprine, cyclophosphamide, warfarin		
Aminoglycosides	Paralytics		Otologic and nephrologic toxicity
Amiodarone	Digoxin, quinidine, warfarin		
Antacids	Quinidine	Aspirin, iron, isoniazid, itraconazole, ketoconazole, tetracycline	
Barbiturates (affects P-450 system)	CNS depressants	Beta-blockers, chloramphenicol, quinidine, tetracycline, warfarin	
Beta-blockers	Chlorpromazine		
Carbamazepine	Isoniazid, lithium	Theophylline, warfarin	Hepatotoxicity
Chloramphenicol	Barbiturates, phenytoin, sulfonylureas, warfarin		
Chlorpromazine	Beta-blockers		

Continued on next page.

Drug	Increases Level of	Decreases Level of	Comment
Ciprofloxacin	Theophylline		
Cyclophosphamide	Allopurinol		
Digoxin	Amiodarone		Watch potassium closely
Disulfiram	Benzodiazepines, phenytoin, warfarin		
Erythromycin	Carbamazepine, theophylline, warfarin		Torsades de pointes when combined with terfenadine
Furosemide	Digoxin		
Ibuprofen	Lithium, methotrexate	Captopril, furosemide	
Indomethacin	Lithium, methotrexate	Captopril, furosemide	
Isoniazid	Carbamazepine, phenytoin		
Ketoconazole	Warfarin, cyclosporine		
Methotrexate	Sulfonamides		
Methyldopa	Lithium		
Metronidazole	Disulfiram, warfarin		
Sulfonylureas	Warfarin		
Phenytoin	Chloramphenicol	Quinidine, theophylline, warfarin	
Probenecid	Allopurinol, methotrexate, rifampin	Salicylates	
Quinidine	Digoxin, warfarin		

Continued on next page.

Drug	Increases Level of	Decreases Level of	Comment
Rifampin (affects P-450 system)		Beta-blockers, benzodiazepines, cyclosporine, digoxin, methadone, steroids, sulfonylureas, quinidine, theophylline, verapamil, warfarin	Protease inhibitors can increase rifampin
Salicylates	Methotrexate, sulfonylureas, warfarin		
Sulfonamides	Barbiturates, sulfonylureas, phenytoin, warfarin		
Theophylline		Lithium	
Thiazides	Digoxin, lithium		
Trazadone	Digoxin, phenytoin		
Triamterene	Potassium, indomethacin		
Tricyclic antidepressants		Clonidine	
Verapamil	Digoxin		

APPENDIX H

EKG and
Swan-Ganz Tracings

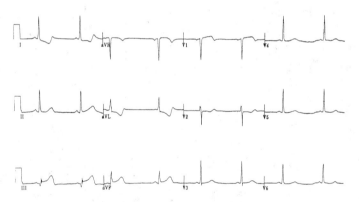

EKG 1: *Inferior myocardial infarction.* Q waves in III and F with ST elevation in the inferior leads indicate acute myocardial infarction. ST depressions in I and L denote "reciprocal changes," that is, they are an electrical reciprocal to the inferior ST elevation and not evidence of lateral ischemia. Note also the bradycardia, which ofter occurs in inferior wall myocardial infarction, possibly due to vagal responses (the vagus nerve runs near the inferior wall) and/or to underperfusion of the sinoatrial node (both the sinoatrial node and the inferior wall are generally supplied by the right coronary artery).

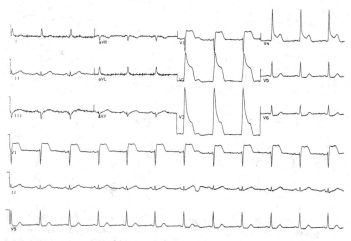

EKG 2: *Acute myocardial infarction.* Note the gross elevation of ST segments in VI-4 ("tombstones").

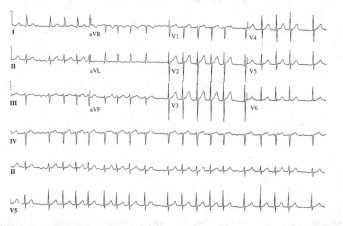

EKG 3: *Atrial fibrillation.* Note the absence of P waves, irregularly irregular rhythm, and narrow complexes signifying a supraventricular origin of the beats.

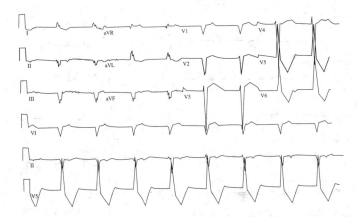

EKG 4: *Accelerated idioventricular rhythm.* This EKG has a rate of 50, with no atrial waves and wide complexes signifying a ventricular pacemaker. The pacemaker is most likely located in the right ventricle, as the EKG has a left bundle branch block pattern (indicating that the left ventricle is depolarizing later). The left bundle branch block characteristics include deep S waves with ST elevation in the inferior and right-sided leads (V1-3) and tall R waves with ST depression and inverted T waves in the lateral and left-sided leads (V4-6). If this rhythm was significantly faster, then it would be considered ventricular tachycardia.

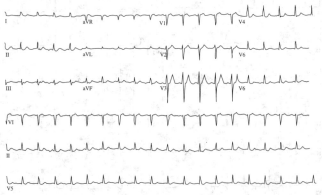

EKG 5: *Atrial flutter.* Note the sawtooth pattern on the rhythm strips. There is a 2:1 A-V block: for every two atrial beats, one gets through the atrioventricular node to stimulate a ventricular beat.

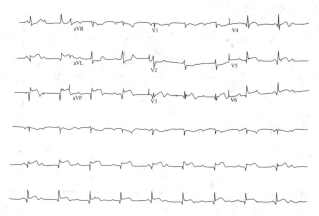

EKG 6: *Inferolateral myocardial infarction with complete heart block.* There are Q waves and ST elevation in the inferolateral leads. Note that the P waves "march right through" the ventricular beats (ie, there is no relationship between the atrial and ventricular beats, which defines complete heart block).

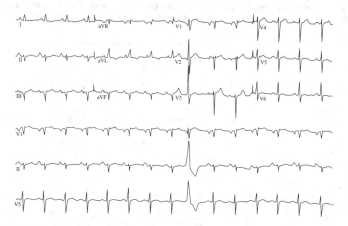

EKG 7: *Inferior infarct; left atrial enlargement.* Note the Q waves in III and aVF, which leads to left axis deviation. In V1, there is an inverted P wave, with the inverted portion having an area more than 1 mm², signifying left atrial enlargement.

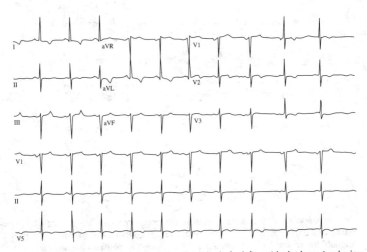

EKG 8: *Left ventricular hypertrophy.*   See the criteria for left ventricular hypertrophy in the text. ST depressions are common in the leads with upright QRS complexes in this condition; they denote "repolarization abnormality," not ischemia, much as in bundle blocks. Similarly, a diagnosis of left bundle block precludes a diagnosis of left ventricular hypertrophy, as the criteria go out the window when there is a left bundle branch block.

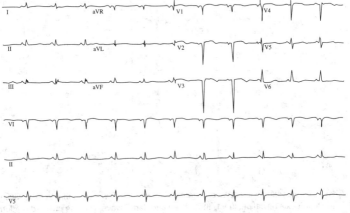

EKG 9: *Old septal myocardial infarction.*   Note Q waves in V1-4.

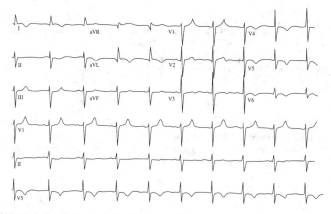

EKG 10: *Left anterior fascicular block, septal infarct, and lateral ischemia.* Note the small Qs in I and L, S waves in II, III, and aVF; and left axis deviation (upright complex in I with a mostly downright complex in aVF), all of which are criteria for left anterior fascicular block. There is a Q in V2, indicating a septal infarct (likely old), and Q in V2 is abnormal (in all other leads, a Q wave must be at least 1 mm in width to be considered significant for an old infarct). T wave inversions in I, L, and V4-6 indicate probable lateral ischemia.

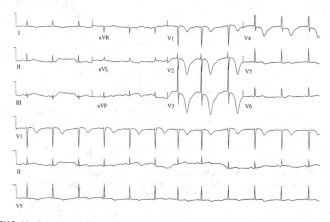

EKG 11: *Anterolateral ischemia.* Note the ST depression and T wave inversions of I, L, and the precordial leads (V1-6).

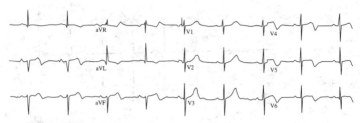

EKG 12: *Inferolateral ischemia.* Biphasic T waves are present in the inferior (II, III, aVF) and lateral (V4-5) leads. Biphasic T waves can indicate acute ischemia. There is also a left anterior fascicular block.

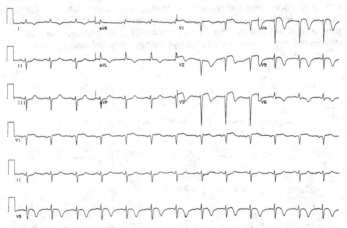

EKG 13: *Biphasic T waves.* Note the biphasic T waves across the precordium, indicative of acute anterolateral ischemia. Think of them as active progression of EKG findings: T wave inversions rising into ST elevation (the former, a sign of ischemia; the latter, one of infarction).

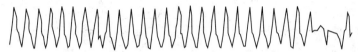

EKG 14: *Ventricular tachycardia.* See text for a full description. Note the extremely rapid and wide monomorphic complexes unrelated to P waves.

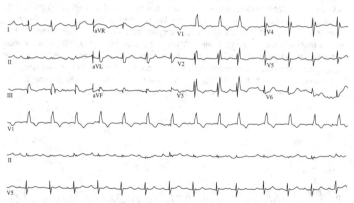

EKG 15: *Right bundle branch block.* There are RSR complexes in V2-4 and M-shaped complex in V1.

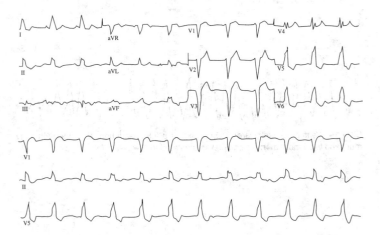

EKG 16: *Left bundle branch block.* The left bundle branch block characteristics include deep S waves with ST elevation in the inferior and right-sided leads (V1-3) and tall R waves with ST depression and inverted T waves in the lateral and left-sided leads (I, L, V5-6), also known as "M-shaped" complexes. With respect to the EKG, the RSR pattern (seen in V4) is equivalent to the M-shaped complex; commonly, the RSR is seen in right bundle blocks in the right-sided leads (V1-3). However, either the RSR or M-shaped complex can be seen in right or left bundle blocks; it is *where* they are located that makes the differentiation between right and left bundle. Further, in bundle blocks, ST depressions occur with upright QRS complexes and ST elevations with downright complexes; hence, detecting ischemia or infarction is complicated accordingly.

MONITOR
LEAD

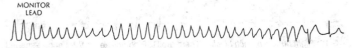

EKG 17: *Torsades de pointes.* Note the rotation of the complexes about the baseline, which also is rotating in a sinusoidal pattern.

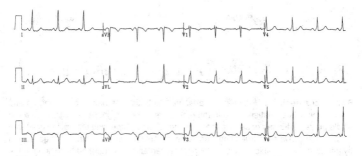

EKG 18: *Wolff-Parkinson-White.* There are delta waves (a slurred upstroke from the P wave to the QRS), signifying an accessory pathway that leads to early depolarization of the ventricles prior to the arrival of the atrial signal through the atrioventricular node.

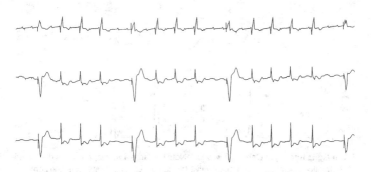

EKG 19: *Paced beats.* Note the paced beats that occur when there is a long interval after a normal beat. Note the pacing spike and the left bundle branch block pattern of the paced beats (as the pacemaker is in the right ventricle). This is a VVI pacemaker (see later in chapter).

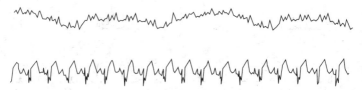

Swan-Ganz tracing 1: *Respiratory variation.* Note that the baseline is going up and down (in ventilated patients, the intrathoracic pressure is higher in inspiration, so the whole pressure tracing goes up a mountain, whereas in expiration the tracing goes into a valley; the converse is true in nonventilated patients, in whom inspiration is generated by negative intrathoracic pressure). Inspiration can also be confirmed by looking at the corresponding EKG tracing, in which the rate speeds up during inspiration. The a wave of the Swan follows the P wave on the EKG (so often it is at the same time as the QRS), while the v wave comes after the QRS; the c wave is the little wavelet in between that occurs due to closure of the AV valves. The true wedge is the nadir of the valley between the a and the c waves. (Pulmonary capillary wedge pressure tracing is over the EKG tracing.) See text for more.

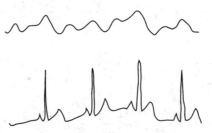

Swan-Ganz tracing 2: *Cannon a waves.* Note the large a waves, which are due to atrial contraction against a closed mitral valve (as can occur in mitral stenosis and complete heart block (a wave follows the P wave).

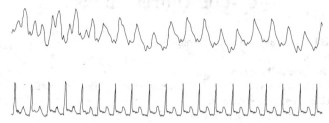

Swan-Ganz tracing 3: *Cannon v waves.* Note the large v waves, which can occur in mitral regurgitation (v wave follows the QRS complex).

List of Abbreviations

5-HT: 5-hydroxytryptamine serotonin
Ab: antibody
ABG: arterial blood gas
ABVD: Adriamycin (doxorubicin), bleomycin, vinblastine, dacarbazine
ACA: anterior cerebral artery
ACD: anemia of chronic disease
ACE(I): angiotensin converting enzyme (inhibitor)
ACLS: Advanced Cardiac Life
ACTH: adrenocorticotropic hormone
ADA: American Diabetic Association
ADH: antidiuretic hormone
ADLS: Activities of Daily Living
AFP: alpha-fetoprotein
AIDS: acquired immunodeficienncy syndrome
ALL: acute lymphocytic leukemia
ALS: amyotrophic lateral sclerosis
ALT: alanine aminotransferase
AMA: against medical advice
AML: acute myeloid leukemia
ANA: antinuclear antibody
ANC: absolute neutrophil count
ANCA: antineutrophil cytoplasmic antibody
ANP: atrial natriuretic peptide
Anti–dsDNA: anti–double-stranded DNA antibody
AP: anteroposterior
APD: afferent pupillary defect
AR: aortic regurgitation
ARDS: acute respiratory distress syndrome
ARF: acute renal failure
AS: aortic stenosis
ASA: aspirin
ASD: atrial septal defect
AST: aspartate aminotransferase
ATC: around the clock

ATP: adenosine triphosphate
ATRA: all-*trans* retinoic acid
AVM: arteriovenous malformation
AVN: avascular necrosis
AWMI: anterior wall myocardial infarction
AZT: zidovudine
BCG: bacille Calmette-Guérin
BEC: bleomycin, etoposide, cisplatin
BFB: bifascicular block
bid: twice daily
BMI: body mass index
BMT: bone marrow transplantation
BOOP: bronchiolitis obliterans with organizing pneumonia
BP: blood pressure
BPH: benign prostatic hyperplasia
BUN: blood urea nitrogen
C. difficile: Clostridium difficile
CI: cardiac index
Ca: calcium
CABG: coronary artery bypass graft
CAD: coronary artery disese
cAMP: cyclic adenosine monophosphate
CBC: complete blood count
CCU: critical care unit
CEA: carcinoembryonic antigen
CHF: congestive heart failure
CHOP: cyclophosphamide, Oncovin (vincristine), prednisone
Cl: chloride
CLL: chronic lymphocytic leukemia
CMF: cyclophosphamide, methotrexate, 5-fluorouracil
CML: chronic myelogenous leukemia
CMV: cytomegalovirus
CN: cranial nerve
CNS: central nervous system
COPD: chronic obstructive pulmonary disease
Cox-2: cyclooxygenase type 2
CPAP: continuous positive airway pressure

CPK: creatine phosphate kinase
CPK-MB: creatine phosphate kinase of cardiac type
CPPD: calcium pyrophosphate deposition
Cr: creatinine
CREST: calcinosis, Raynaud's phenomenon, esophageal dysfunction, sclerodactyly, telangiectasia
CRF: chronic renal failure
CSF: cerebrospinal fluid
C-spine: cervical spine
CT: computed tomography
CVA: cerebrovascular accident (stroke)
CVD: collagen vascular disease
CVP: central venous pressure
CXR: chest x-ray
D&C: dilation and curettage
DCT: distal convoluted tubule
DCCT: Diabetes Control and Complications Trial
DEC: diethylcarbamazine
DGI: disseminated gonococcal infection
DI: diabetes insipidus
DIC: disseminated intravascular coagulation
DKA: diabetic ketoacidosis
DLCO: diffusion capacity for carbon monoxide
DM: diabetes mellitus
DMARD: disease-modifying antirheumatic drug
DNA: deoxyribonucleic acid
DNR: do not resuscitate
DOE: dyspnea on exertion
DRE: digital rectal examination
DTR: deep tendon reflex
DVT: deep vein thrombosis
D$_5$W: 5% dextrose in water
E. coli: *Escherichia coli*
EBV: Epstein-Barr virus
EF: ejection fraction (generally of left ventricle)
EGD: esophagogastroduodenoscopy
EJ: external jugular

EKG: electrocardiogram
ELISA: enzyme-linked immunosorbent assay
EM: electron microscopy
EMG: electromyography
ER: emergency room
ERCP: endoscopic retrograde cholangiopancreaticography
ESR: erythrocyte sedimentation rate
ESRD: end-stage renal disease
ET: endotracheal tube
FAB: French-American-British (classification)
FAP: familial adenomatous polyposis
FDA: U.S. Food and Drug Administration
FENa: fractional excretion of sodium
FEV: forced expiratory volume (usually in first second)
FNA: fine-needle aspiration
FSH: follicle-stimulating hormone
FTA-(Abs): fluorescent-treponemal antigen (antibodies)
FU: fluorouracil
FVC: forced vital capacity
GABA: γ aminobutyric acid
GBM: glomerular basement membrane
G-CSF: granulocyte colony-stimulating factor
GERD: gastroesophageal reflux disease
GFR: glomerular filtration rate
GI: gastrointestinal
GM-CSF: granulocyte-macrophage colony-stimulating factor
Gn-RH: gonadotropin-releasing hormone
G6PD: glucose-6-phosphate dehydrogenase
GU: genitourinary
GVHD: graft-versus-host disease
H/H: hemoglobin and hematocrit
HACEK: *Haemophilus, Actinobacillus, Cardiobacterium, Eikenella,* and
  Kingella
HAV: hepatitis A virus
Hb: hemoglobin
HbA$_{1c}$: hemoglobin A$_{1c}$
HBcAg: hepatitis B core antigen

HBsAb: hepatitis B surface antibody
HBsAg: hepatitis B surface antigen
HBV: hepatitis B virus
hCG: human chorionic gonadotropin
HCL: hairy cell leukemia
HCV: hepatitis C virus
HDL: high-density lipoprotein
Hgb: hemoglobin
Hib: *Haemophilus influenzae* type b
H. influenzae: *Haemophilus influenzae*
HIV: human immunodeficiency virus
HLA: human leukocyte antigen
HOCM: hypertrophic obstructive cardiomyopathy
H&P: history and physical
HPV: human papilloma virus
H. pylori: *Helicobacter pylori*
HSP: Henoch-Schönlein purpura
HSV: herpes simplex virus
HTLV-1: human T-cell leukemia/lymphoma virus
HTN: hypertension
HUS: hemolytic-uremic syndrome
ICP: intracranial pressure
ICU: intensive care unit
IDA: iron deficiency anemia
IDL: intermediate-density lipoprotein
IDU: injection drug user
IFN: interferon
lg: immunoglobulin
IHSS: idiopathic hypertrophic subaortic stenosis
ILD: interstitial lung disease
IM: intramuscular
INR: international normalized ratio (for standardization of prothrombin time)
IPF: idiopathic pulmonary fibrosis
ITP: idiopathic thrombocytopenic purpura
IUD: intrauterine device
IV: intravenous
IVC: inferior vena cava

IVIg: intravenous gamma globulin
IVP: intravenous pyelogram
IWMI: inferior wall myocardial infarction
JAMA: *Journal of the American Medical Association*
JVD: jugular venous distension
K: potassium
LBBB: left bundle branch block
LA (H): left atrium (hypertrophy)
LAD: left anterior descending artery
LAE: left atrial enlargement
LAFB: left anterior fascicular block
LAP: leukocyte alkaline
Lcx: left circumflex
LDH: lactate dehydrogenase
LDL: low-density lipoprotein
LES: lower esophageal sphincter
LFTs: liver function tests
LH: luteinizing hormone
LH-RH: luteinizing hormone–releasing hormone
LLQ: left lower quadrant (abdomen)
LM: left main (artery)
LP: lumbar puncture
LPFB: left posterior fascicular block
LV(H): left ventricle (hypertrophy)
LVF: left ventricular function
LVMI: left ventricle myocardial infarction
MAC: *Mycobacterium avium-intracellulare* complex
MALT: mucosalassociated lymphoid tissue lymphoma
MAO(I): monoamine oxidase (inhibitor)
MAT: multifocal atrial tachycardia
MCA: middle cerebral artery
MCHC: mean corpuscule hemoglobin concnetration
MCP: metacarpophalangeal joint
MCV: mean corpuscular volume
MDI: metered-dose inhaler
MDS: myelodysplastic syndrome
MEN: multiple endocrine neoplasia

MGUS: monoclonal gammopathy of undetermined significance
MI: myocardial infarction
MM: multiple myeloma
MMSE: Mini-Mental State Examination
MMZ: methimazole
MOPP: mechlorethamine (nitrogen mustard), Oncovin (vincristine), procarbazine, prednisone
MR: mitral regurgitation
MRA: magnetic resonance angiography
MRI: magnetic resonance imaging
MRM: modified radical mastectomy
MRSA: methicillin-resistant *Staphylococcus aureus*
MS: mitral stenosis
MTHFR: methylene tetrahydrofolate reductase
MTX: methotrexate
MVAC: methotrexate, vinblastine, doxorubicin, cisplatin
MVP: mitral valve prolapse
Na: sodium
NASH: nonalcoholic steatohepatitis
NCV: nerve conduction velocity
N Engl J Med: *New England Journal of Medicine*
NG: nasogastric
NHL: non-Hodgkin's lymphoma
NIF: negative inspiratory force
NMTT: *N*-methylthiotetrazolium
NPO: nothing by mouth
NS: normal saline
NSAID: nonsteroidal anti-inflammatory drug
NSCLC: non–small cell lung cancer
OA: osteoarthritis
PA: posteroanterior
PADP: pulmonary artery diastolic pressure
PAN: polyarteritis nodosa
PAS: periodic acid–Schiff stain
PCA: posterior cerebral artery
PCO$_2$: carbon dioxide partial pressure
PCP: *Pneumocystis carinii* pneumonia

PCR: polymerase chain reaction
PCT: proximal collecting tubule
PCWP: pulmonary capillary wedge pressure
PD: peritoneal dialysis
PDA: posterior descending artery
PE: pulmonary embolus
PEEP: positive end-expiratory pressure
PEG: percutaneous endoscopic gastrostomy
PEJ: percutaneous endoscopic jejunostomy
PET: positron emission tomography
PFTs: pulmonary function tests
PI: protease inhibitor
PICC: peripherally introduced central vein catheter
PID: pelvic inflammatory disease
PML: progressive multifocal leukoencephalopathy
PMN: polymorphonuclear neutrophil leukocyte
PND: paroxysmal nocturnal dyspnea
PNH: paroxysmal nocturnal hemoglobinuria
PO: by mouth
PPD: skin test for tuberculosis
PR: per rectum
PRBC: packed red blood cells (transfusion)
PRN: as needed
PSA: prostate-specific antigen
PSGN: poststreptococcal glomerulonephritis
PSVT: paroxysmal supraventricular tachycardia
PT/PTT: prothrombin time and partial thromboplastin time (standard)
    coagulation profile
PTCA: percutaneous transcoronary angioplasty
PTH: parathyroid hormone
PTU: propylthiouracil
PUD: peptic ulcer disease
PVC: premature ventricular contraction
PWMI: posterior wall myocardial infarction
qhs: at bedtime
qid: four times a day
RA: rheumatoid arthritis

RAH: right atrium hypertrophy
RAIU: radioactive iodine uptake
RBBB: right bundle branch block
RBC: red blood cell
RCA: right coronary artery
RCT: randomized controlled trial
RDW: red cell distribution width
RF: rheumatoid factor
RIPA: ristocetin-induced platelet aggregation
RL: Ringer's lactate
ROM: range of motion
RML: right middle lobe (lung)
RPGN: rapidly progressive glomerulonephritis
RPR: reactive plasma reagin (for syphilis)
RSV: Respiratory Syncytial virus
RT: reverse transcriptase
RTA: renal tubular acidosis
RV (H): right ventricle (hypertrophy)
RVMI: right ventricle myocardial infarction
***S. aureus*:** *Staphylococcus aureus*
SAM: symmetric anterior motion
SBE: subacute bacterial endocarditis
SBP: systolic blood pressure
SCLC: small cell lung cancer
SIADH: syndrome of inappropriate antidiuretic hormone secretion
SIMV: synchronized intermittent mandatory volume
SLE: systemic lupus erythematosus
SMA-7: chemistry 7 (sodium, potassium, chloride, bicarbonate, blood urea nitrogen, creatinine, glucose)
SOB: shortness of breath
SQ: subcutaneous
***Staph.*:** *Staphylococcus*
STD: sexually transmitted disease
***Strep.*:** *Streptococcus*
SVT: supraventricular tachycardia
TB: tuberculosis
TEE: transesophageal echocardiography

TFTs: thyroid function tests
TGF: transforming growth factor
TIA: transient ischemic attack
tid: three times a day
TIPS: transjugular intrahepatic portosystemic shunting
TLC: triple-lumen catheter (aka "central line")
TMJ: temporomandibular joint
TMP/SMX: trimethoprim-sulfamethoxazole (Bactrim)
TNF: tumor necrosis factor
TNM: tumor size, nodes, metastases (staging concept)
TPA: tissue plasminogen activator
TPN: total parenteral nutrition
TR: tricuspid regurgitation
TRAP: tartrate-resistant acid phosphatase
TS: tricuspid stenosis
TSH: thyroid-stimulating hormone
TSS: toxic shock syndrome
TTP: thrombotic thrombocytopenic purpura
TURP: transurethral resection of prostate
U: unit
U/A: urinalysis
UC: ulcerative colitis
UGIB: upper gastrointestinal bleeding
URI: upper respiratory infection
UTI: urinary tract infection
V/Q: ventilation-perfusion scan
VDRL: venereal disease reactive laboratory (for syphilis)
VIP: vasoactive intestinal peptide
VLDL: very-low-density lipoprotein
VRE: vancomycin-resistant enterococcus
VT: ventricular tachycardia
VWF: von Willebrand's factor
VZV: varicella-zoster virus
WBC: white blood cell count
WHO: World Health Organization

Index